Treatment Companion

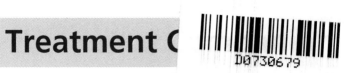

to the

DSM-IV-TR® Casebook

Treatment Companion

to the
DSM-IV-TR® Casebook

Edited by

Robert L. Spitzer, M.D.

Michael B. First, M.D.

Miriam Gibbon, M.S.W.

Janet B.W. Williams, D.S.W.

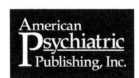

American Psychiatric Publishing, Inc.

Washington, DC
London, England

Note: The authors have worked to ensure that all information in this book is accurate at the time of publication and consistent with general psychiatric and medical standards, and that information concerning drug dosages, schedules, and routes of administration is accurate at the time of publication and consistent with standards set by the U.S. Food and Drug Administration and the general medical community. As medical research and practice continue to advance, however, therapeutic standards may change. Moreover, specific situations may require a specific therapeutic response not included in this book. For these reasons and because human and mechanical errors sometimes occur, we recommend that readers follow the advice of physicians directly involved in their care or the care of a member of their family.

Copyright © 2004 American Psychiatric Publishing, Inc.
ALL RIGHTS RESERVED
Manufactured in the United States of America on acid-free paper
08 07 06 05 04   5 4 3 2 1
First Edition

Typeset in Palatino and Frutiger

American Psychiatric Publishing, Inc.
1000 Wilson Boulevard
Arlington, VA 22209-3901
www.appi.org

Library of Congress Cataloging-in-Publication Data
Treatment companion to the DSM-IV-TR casebook / edited by Robert L. Spitzer ... [et al.].
    p. ; cm.
  Includes bibliographical references and index.
  ISBN 1-58562-194-3 (casebound : alk. paper)--ISBN 1-58562-139-0 (pbk. : alk. paper)
    1. Mental illness--Treatment--Case studies. 2. Mental illness--Diagnosis--Case studies. 3. Mental illness--Classification. I. Spitzer, Robert L. II. DSM-IV-TR casebook.
   [DNLM: 1. Mental Disorders therapy--Case Reports WM 40 T784 2004]
   RC465.T744 2004
   616.89'1--dc22

                                                      2003070870

British Library Cataloguing in Publication Data
A CIP record is available from the British Library.

Contents

Elephant Man

Diagnosis: Body Dysmorphic Disorder
Discussants: Katharine A. Phillips, M.D., and Rocco Crino, Ph.D.

Disco Di

Diagnosis: Borderline Personality Disorder
Discussants: John Gunderson, M.D.; Kathryn E. Korslund, Ph.D.,
   and Marsha M. Linehan, Ph.D.

Cocaine

Diagnosis: Cocaine Dependence
Discussant: Edward Nunes, M.D.

Unfaithful Wife

Diagnosis: Delusional Disorder, Jealous Type
Discussant: Lewis A. Opler, M.D., Ph.D.

Melancholy or Malarky?

Diagnosis: Depression
Discussant: Max Fink, M.D.

Junior Executive

Diagnosis: Dysthymic Disorder
Discussant: John C. Markowitz, M.D.

Dolls

Diagnosis: Gender Identity Disorder
Discussant: Kenneth J. Zucker, Ph.D.

Edgy Electrician

Diagnosis: Generalized Anxiety Disorder
Discussant: Laszlo A. Papp, M.D.

Cry Me a River

Diagnosis: Major Depressive Disorder
Discussant: Charles F. Reynolds III, M.D.

My Fan Club

Diagnosis: Narcissistic Personality Disorder
Discussant: Otto Kernberg, M.D.

Sitting by the Fire

Diagnosis: Schizotypal Personality Disorder
Discussants: Larry J. Siever, M.D.; Ming Tsuang, M.D., Ph.D.

Goody Two Shoes

Diagnosis: Self-Defeating Personality Disorder
Discussant: Arnold M. Cooper, M.D.

A Perfect Checklist

Diagnosis: Separation Anxiety Disorder
Discussant: Rachel Klein, Ph.D.

Frustrated Librarian

Diagnosis: Sexual Dysfunction
Discussant: Lawrence A. Labbate, M.D.

Mike DeBardeleben

Diagnosis: Sexual Sadism
Discussant: Michael Stone, M.D.

"The Jerk"

Diagnosis: Social Phobia
Discussant: Franklin R. Schneier, M.D.

Sickly

Diagnosis: Somatization Disorder
Discussant: C. Robert Cloninger, M.D.

About the Editors

Robert L. Spitzer, M.D.

Dr. Spitzer is Professor of Psychiatry at Columbia University and Chief of the Biometrics Research Department at the New York State Psychiatric Institute. He had his psychiatry residency training at the Institute and has worked there since 1961. He has achieved national and international recognition as an authority in psychiatric assessment and the classification of mental disorders. He is the author of more than 250 articles on psychiatric assessment and diagnosis.

In 1974, the American Psychiatric Association (APA) appointed Dr. Spitzer to chair its Task Force on Nomenclature and Statistics, and in this capacity he assumed the leadership role in the development of the *Diagnostic and Statistical Manual of Mental Disorders*, Third Edition (DSM-III), published in 1980, which became the authoritative classification of mental disorders for the mental health professions, not only in the United States, but internationally.

In 1983, Dr. Spitzer was appointed to chair the APA's Work Group to Revise DSM-III and coordinated that effort, which resulted in the publication of the *Diagnostic and Statistical Manual of Mental Disorders*, Third Edition, Revised (DSM-III-R), in the spring of 1987. He was active in the development of the *Diagnostic and Statistical Manual of Mental Disorders*, Fourth Edition (DSM-IV), as a Special Advisor to the APA's Task Force on DSM-IV.

In 1994, Dr. Spitzer received the APA's award for psychiatric research for his contributions to psychiatric assessment and diagnosis. In 2000, he was the Thomas William Salmon Medal recipient from the New York Academy of Medicine. He has pioneered the development of several widely used diagnostic assessment procedures, including the Research Diagnostic Criteria (RDC), the Schedule for Affective Disorders and Schizophrenia (SADS), the Structured Clinical Interview for DSM-IV (SCID), and the PRIME-MD Patient Health Questionnaire (PHQ).

Michael B. First, M.D.

Dr. First is a Research Psychiatrist in the Biometrics Department at the New York State Psychiatric Institute, is an Associate Professor of Clinical Psychiatry at the Columbia University College of Physicians and Surgeons, and maintains a schema-focused cognitive therapy and psychopharmacology practice in Manhattan. He is a nationally and internationally recognized expert on psychiatric diagnosis and assessment.

Dr. First is the editor and cochair of the *Diagnostic and Statistical Manual of Mental Disorders,* Fourth Edition, Text Revision (DSM-IV-TR); the Editor of Text and Criteria for DSM-IV; the editor of the DSM-IV Primary Care Version; editor of the APA's *Handbook of Psychiatric Measures;* and Medical Editor of the Quick Reference Guides to the APA's Practice Guidelines for the Treatment of Psychiatric Disorders. He has coauthored and coedited a number of books, including *A Research Agenda for DSM-V; Advancing DSM: Dilemmas in Psychiatric Diagnosis; Am I OK? The Layman's Guide to the Psychiatrist's Bible; DSM-IV-TR Guidebook; DSM-IV-TR Handbook of Differential Diagnosis;* the SCID; and *DSM-IV-TR Casebook,* and various software packages for psychiatric diagnosis. He has trained thousands of clinicians and researchers in diagnostic assessment and differential diagnosis.

Miriam Gibbon, M.S.W.

Ms. Gibbon is a Research Scientist in the Biometrics Department of the New York State Psychiatric Institute and is on the faculty of the Columbia University College of Physicians and Surgeons, Department of Psychiatry. She has been involved in the development of psychiatric evaluation and diagnostic instruments for 25 years and has served as a consultant to many research groups in the United States and internationally.

In the 1970s, Ms. Gibbon began working with the Biometrics group to develop the Schedule for Affective Disorders and Schizophrenia (SADS). She is a coauthor of the Global Assessment Scale (GAS), which was part of the SADS, and of the Global Assessment of Functioning (GAF), a revision of the GAS that became Axis V of DSM-III-R. She is a coauthor of the SCID and of the DSM *Casebooks,* and, with Dr. Michael First, produced the SCID 101 Videotape Training Program.

Ms. Gibbon has trained thousands of researchers and clinicians in the use of diagnostic and evaluation instruments, beginning with the

SADS and continuing with the GAS, the Hamilton Depression and Anxiety Scales, and the SCID.

Janet B.W. Williams, D.S.W.

Dr. Williams is Professor of Clinical Psychiatric Social Work in the Departments of Psychiatry and Neurology at Columbia University College of Physicians and Surgeons and Deputy Chief of the Biometrics Research Department at the New York State Psychiatric Institute. Her career has focused on the development of psychiatric classifications and instruments to measure psychopathology, and she is well known for her interview guides for the Hamilton Rating Scales. She was heavily involved in the development of DSM-III, DSM-III-R, and DSM-IV and was made an Honorary Fellow of the APA for her contributions. She collaborated on the development and testing of the PRIME-MD, an interview guide designed to help primary care physicians make mental disorder diagnoses, and its self-report version, the PHQ. Dr. Williams is the author of many rating instruments and interview guides and more than 230 scholarly publications. She serves on the editorial boards of several psychiatric journals and is an active consultant to clinical trials on depression and anxiety.

Dr. Williams holds a B.S. in biology from Tufts University, an M.S. in marine biology from the University of Massachusetts Dartmouth, and an M.S. and D.S.W. in social welfare from the Columbia University School of Social Work. In 1994, Dr. Williams founded the Society for Social Work and Research (SSWR, now with more than 1,300 members) and served as its President for 2 years. In 1999, she was inducted into the Columbia University School of Social Work Alumni Association Hall of Fame, and in 2000 she received the Lifetime Achievement Award from SSWR.

Preface

Next to the DSM manual itself, the most popular books published by the American Psychiatric Association and American Psychiatric Publishing have been the DSM Casebooks, beginning with the *DSM-III Casebook* in 1981. There are several reasons for this. First of all, the cases, based on actual patients, bring the DSM diagnostic criteria to life. In addition, the inclusion of cases covering virtually all of the diagnostic categories has enabled readers to become familiar with types of patients that they may not encounter in their work or studies. Finally, the discussions of each case are useful for teaching the principles of differential diagnosis.

One of the main purposes of the psychiatric diagnosis is to guide treatment selection. Although some of the cases in the *DSM-IV-TR Casebook* mentioned treatment that the patient received, the discussions were focused exclusively on diagnostic issues. In this book, we have taken the next step: For 34 cases (all but three from the *DSM-IV-TR Casebook*), we have invited experts—many world renowned—to discuss their approach to the treatment of a case in their specialized area. They were asked to discuss both how they would manage the specific case and the general principles of treatment for that disorder. We encouraged them to present their personal experience with such patients and their own approach to treatment with the understanding that other experts might have a very different approach. For three cases, we invited two experts, who we knew had very different approaches, to discuss the treatment.

We thank the contributors for providing informative and lively discussions that we enjoyed reading—as we trust the reader will as well. We also thank the contributors of the original cases; they are acknowledged in the *DSM-IV-TR Casebook* on pages vii–ix.

Robert L. Spitzer, M.D.
Michael B. First, M.D.
Miriam Gibbon, M.S.W.
Janet B. W. Williams, D.S.W.

Martini Man

George White was about 30 hours postoperative following a routine hernia repair when his doctor was called by the intensive care unit nurse. George appeared confused and agitated. His pulse rate was 150 beats/minute, he demonstrated a bilateral coarse tremor of the hands, and he was perspiring profusely. He had pulled the intravenous line out of his arm and was trying to find his clothes so he could leave the intensive care unit. He was persuaded to get back into bed and was calmer after being given 5 mg of haloperidol.

George is a 45-year-old tenured teacher of literature in a prestigious suburban high school. He has no history of treatment for any serious medical or mental health problems. The origin of his new symptoms is unknown. Orders are given for a neurological workup, and the hospital social worker is asked to obtain a more complete history from George's wife.

George grew up in a suburb of New York City. Along with many of his peers, he began drinking at age 15—mostly at weekend beer parties. His consumption of alcohol escalated through college, and by the time he graduated he was drinking almost every evening. He sometimes spent the night with friends because he could not remember where he had parked his car and several times had awakened the next morning unsure of what had happened the night before.

When he was age 25, he married his high school sweetheart and began working at his current job. By age 30, he routinely drank two martinis before dinner, shared a bottle of wine with his wife, and drank two or three beers while watching television. On weekends, he usually drank beer all day while doing chores or watching television, often consuming up to 12 bottles in a day.

When he was age 32, George had a minor automobile accident while returning home from an evening of heavy drinking but managed to talk his way out of a citation for driving under the influence. His wife was upset about his pattern of drinking, and the couple frequently argued, with George always pointing out that he was sober every morning and that he was able to hold a responsible job, thereby proving he was not an alcoholic. He insisted he could quit any time he wanted, and in fact, he often demonstrated abstinence for 2 or 3 months at a time in an effort to prove he could get along without alcohol. These periods of abstinence were always followed by several weeks or months of a return to drinking according to preset rules (e.g., "I'll only drink after 6:00 P.M."), but escalation of intake always followed.

When George was in his late 30s, his colleagues at school noticed that he was often short-tempered, and he began taking "sick Mondays" with increasing frequency. He had also begun to join friends at a local bar after school, where he would drink two or three beers before going home.

George had never mentioned his drinking problem to his primary care doctor nor had he been asked about it. The medical workup revealed symmetrical hyperactive deep tendon reflexes, no evidence of nuchal rigidity, a normal funduscopic examination, and absent Babinski signs. The blood workup revealed a slight macrocytosis (e.g., a mean corpuscular volume of 92.5 μm^3), no evidence of anemia, a very slightly elevated white blood cell count (with no shift in the differential), and a normal level of platelets. Although the usual liver function tests such as alanine transaminase and aspartate transaminase were high normal, his gamma glutamyltransferase values were 55 U/L, and his uric acid was a slightly elevated 7.1 mg/dL.

DSM-IV-TR Diagnosis of "Martini Man"

George presented with symptoms of delirium, including confusion and agitation, after his hernia operation. Postoperative delirium is not unusual and may be caused by a number of factors, including general medical conditions, reactions to medications, or withdrawal from substances. The possibility that George's delirium was a reaction to the anesthesia was ruled out by the time course—he had no evidence of psychiatric symptoms immediately following the anesthesia; in fact, an entire day elapsed without symptoms, indicating that the delirium was not likely to be related to the anesthetic used. The medical workup did not result in evidence pointing to a general medical condition as the cause of the delirium. In this case, the drinking history provided by his wife clinched the diagnosis. She reported that George had been a heavy drinker for years, with increasing tolerance for alcohol. Although he had been able to maintain his job, his drinking had caused problems in the marriage, and he appeared to have been drinking almost all the time that he was not actually teaching. Thus, it is pretty clear that George's postsurgery symptoms were those of Alcohol Withdrawal Delirium (DSM-IV-TR, p. 143). Surgery for hernia repair resulted in an abrupt cessation of his heavy drinking, and about 30 hours after surgery he suddenly became agitated and confused and demonstrated an elevated pulse rate, sweating, and a tremor. Most patients who develop severe alcohol withdrawal have a pattern of alcohol consumption that justifies a diagnosis of Alcohol Dependence, and this is certainly true in this case. George's combination of repetitive heavy drinking, spending a great deal of time using alcohol, continued use despite problems, and giving up time with his family in order to drink, along with consumption levels that imply tolerance and evidence of a withdrawal syndrome, all support a diagnosis of Alcohol Dependence (DSM-IV-TR, p. 213).

Discussion of "Martini Man" by Marc Schuckit, M.D.*

My interest in substance use disorders began more than 30 years ago as a medical student, and I've had the opportunity of directly treating or

---

*Dr. Schuckit is Director of the Alcohol and Drug Treatment Program at the Veterans Affairs San Diego Healthcare System. His major areas of research have focused on evaluating the importance of genetic influences in alcoholism and then searching for the biological factors that might interact with the environment to produce vulnerability toward severe alcohol problems. Other research efforts include a search for the optimal diagnostic criteria for substance abuse or dependence, which led to his appointment as a member of the Task Force and Chair of the Substance Use Disorders Committee for DSM-IV. His third focus has been on the relationship between alcoholism and drug use disorders and psychiatric syndromes, especially depression, states of anxiety, or psychoses. He is the Editor of the Journal of Studies on Alcohol and has served on the editorial boards of major journals covering alcohol and drug use issues in the United States and Europe. He has been fortunate to be recognized for a number of awards in the alcoholism field, including the Middleton Award for the best research within the Veterans Affairs system and the American Psychiatric Association's Hoffheimer Award for Research in Psychiatry.

supervising the care of thousands of alcohol-dependent individuals. I've also gained perspective as a member of the faculty at a medical school and through serving as director of alcohol and drug treatment programs in both the public and private sectors. These experiences convince me that George is fairly typical of the usual alcohol-dependent individual. Few alcoholics meet the stereotype most physicians have regarding how an alcohol-dependent man or woman is likely to present for treatment. It is probable that the lifetime risk for alcohol dependence is at least 15% for men and perhaps 8% or so for women regardless of level of education, and the usual alcohol-dependent individual has a job and family and functions moderately well in life despite his or her alcoholism. Therefore, a patient with George's background is fairly representative of the alcohol- (or drug-) dependent individual likely to be seen by most practitioners.

The fact that the physician did not consider a diagnosis of Alcohol Withdrawal Delirium is, unfortunately, more likely to be the rule than the exception. In this instance, the postoperative problems could have been avoided if the physician had recognized the importance of establishing a history of major life problems (e.g., in George's marriage and job) and then probed to see whether alcohol or drugs might have been involved. An additional important step would have been to pay special attention to a series of blood tests that are likely to be high normal or just above the normal range in the usual alcoholic individual. These state markers of heavy drinking include gamma glutamyltransferase values greater than 35 U/L (still well within the normal range but higher than that observed in the usual otherwise-healthy patient), a mean corpuscular volume value only slightly higher than normal (reflecting the direct effects of alcohol on red blood cell stem cells), and a slightly elevated uric acid level. Such results are likely to be observed during heavy alcohol intake (about six to eight or more standard drinks per day on a regular basis), with values returning toward (or to) normal within several weeks of abstinence.

The treatment of the usual alcohol-dependent individual often begins by considering the possibility of alcoholic withdrawal. Had George's alcohol dependence been recognized and appropriately treated early on with benzodiazepines (e.g., 25 mg of chlordiazepoxide approximately three times a day on day 1, with progressive decreases in dosages to zero over the subsequent 5 days), a withdrawal-related delirium could have been avoided. An unrecognized alcohol dependence and the physical stresses associated with surgical recovery probably combined to markedly enhance the risk of a withdrawal delirium.

Once alcohol withdrawal delirium (also called *delirium tremens* or *DTs*) begins, it is likely to run a course of 3–5 days. Many clinicians would prefer to treat the condition with whatever doses of benzodiazepines are required; others, fearing excessive sedation (but ignoring the possibility that antipsychotic drugs lower the seizure threshold), might favor antipsychotic medications such as haloperidol; and some would use the two categories of drugs in combination. I prefer benzodiazepines alone, but there are few data to demonstrate a clear superiority of any specific approach, and the key is recognizing the development of alcohol withdrawal, beginning appropriate treatment, and correcting any associated medical difficulties.

Once the acute emergency of preventing withdrawal delirium is addressed, the challenge (perhaps the most difficult aspect of treatment) is to work with the individual to enhance his or her motivation to stop using alcohol. Actually, such work is no different from approaches that help patients alter their habits because of any long-term disorder that requires lifestyle changes, such as diabetes or hypertension. An effective technique called *motivational interviewing* can be used to enhance motivation to change. Following the tenets of this approach, George is addressed in an empathic way, concerns regarding future problems are shared with both him and his spouse, and he is encouraged to voice any reservations regarding whether abstinence might cause him distress. It is important to emphasize that George, alone, controls the steps that need to be taken. In the usual outpatient setting, this process of enhancing motivation (also known as *intervention*) often takes several sessions and sometimes develops over a series of weeks or months as the patient considers his or her options. Inclusion of a spouse in the process can be important both to help the couple make plans and to enhance the probability that the patient will choose abstinence.

The next phase of care, "rehab," centers on cognitive-behavioral approaches (e.g., cognitive-behavioral therapy [CBT]) for modifying thoughts and behaviors regarding drinking. Not only are steps taken to continue to optimize motivation, but the person also is encouraged to alter his or her ways of handling stress, to acquire a sober peer group, and to optimize relationships with important individuals in his or her life. George would be advised to avoid his usual drinking buddies and, with counseling, to work through conflicts that are likely to have developed with his wife over the years. As is true of any life changes associated with a long-term condition, the possibility of a relapse into prior behaviors must be considered and planned for, and a script for how to address and remedy any return to drinking needs to be proposed.

Most of these rehabilitation steps can usually be carried out in an outpatient setting, either through a one-on-one relationship with a clinician, as part of a group, or by referral to a formal treatment regimen. Affiliation with other individuals going through a similar process (e.g., through a "12-step" program such as Alcoholics Anonymous) can be very helpful. The clinician should help the patient find the program with which he or she will be most comfortable. Important considerations in program selection include the patient's desire for a greater or lesser emphasis on religion, preference for a gender-specific versus a mixed-gender group, comfort with the socioeconomic stratum of the program members, and so on.

In addition to cognitive and behavioral approaches such as motivational interviewing and more formal CBT, several medications are worth considering in the rehabilitation phase of the treatment of alcohol dependence. These medications are probably not appropriate in the absence of a rehab program but sometimes can be a useful adjunct. Both ReVia (naltrexone) (50–100 mg/day) and (although not yet available in the United States) acamprosate (approximately 2 g/day) have been reported to improve the outcome (i.e., maintenance of abstinence) by between 10% and 20% for the average patient. Although no hard and fast guidelines exist, it makes sense to continue the medications for approximately 6 months, as this is the period during which relapse is most likely to occur. In this case it seems that George can afford the medications, so I would offer him the possibility of using naltrexone. There are few systematic data that would support the superiority of Antabuse (disulfiram) over placebo for the average alcohol-dependent individual, and this drug carries with it the risk for moderate to severe side effects, including neuropathies, depression, and impaired liver functioning. I rarely prescribe this drug.

Once a relatively high-functioning individual such as George recognizes a problem and participates in treatment, the probability is between 60% and 70% that he or she will remain fully abstinent for at least 1 year. One year of sobriety predicts a high probability of 5 years of abstinence; few studies have gone beyond the 5-year window. Thus, there is a high probability of an excellent outcome.

Suggested Reading

Conigrave KM, Degenhardt LJ, Whitfield JB, et al: CDT, GGT, and AST as markers of alcohol use: the WHO/ISBRA collaborative project. Alcohol Clin Exp Res 26:332–339, 2002

Connors GJ, Tonigan JS, Miller WR: A longitudinal model of intake symptomatology, AA participation and outcome: retrospective study of the Project MATCH outpatient and aftercare samples. J Stud Alcohol 62:817–825, 2001

Fleming MF, Mundt MP, French MT, et al: Brief physician advice for problem drinkers: long-term efficacy and benefit-cost analysis. Alcohol Clin Exp Res 26:36–43, 2002

Kaner EFS, Wutzke S, Saunders JB, et al: Impact of alcohol education and training on general practitioners' diagnostic and management skills: findings from a World Health Organization collaborative study. J Stud Alcohol 62:621–627, 2001

Kiefer F, Jahn H, Tarnaske T, et al: Comparing and combining naltrexone and acamprosate in relapse prevention of alcoholism. Arch Gen Psychiatry 60:92–99, 2003

Mason BJ: Treatment of alcohol-dependent outpatients with acamprosate: a clinical review. J Clin Psychiatry 62 (suppl 20):42–48, 2001

Morgenstern J, Longabaugh R: Cognitive-behavioral treatment for alcohol dependence: a review of evidence for its hypothesized mechanisms of action. Addiction 95:1475–1490, 2000

O'Brien CP, McLellan AT: Myths about the treatment of addiction. Lancet 347:237–240, 1996

Rice JP, Neuman J, Saccone NL, et al: Age and birth cohort effects on rates of alcohol dependence. Alcohol Clin Exp Res 27:93–99, 2003

Schuckit MA: Drug and Alcohol Abuse, 5th Edition. New York, Kluwer Academic Press, 2000

Schuckit MA, Tipp JE, Reich T, et al: The histories of withdrawal convulsions and delirium tremens in 1648 alcohol dependent subjects. Addiction 90:1335–1347, 1995

Schuckit MA, Smith TL, Danko GP, et al: Similarities in the clinical characteristics related to alcohol dependence in two populations. Am J Addic 11:1–9, 2002

The Hiker

A 61-year-old high school science department head who was an experienced and enthusiastic camper and hiker became extremely fearful while on a trek in the mountains. Gradually, over the next few months, he lost interest in his usual hobbies. Formerly a voracious reader, he stopped reading. He had difficulty doing computations and made gross errors in home financial management. On several occasions he became lost while driving in areas that were formerly familiar to him. He began to write notes to himself so that he would not forget to do errands. Very abruptly, and in uncharacteristic fashion, he decided to retire from work, without discussing his plans with his wife. Intellectual deterioration gradually progressed. He spent most of the day piling miscellaneous objects in one place and then transporting them to another spot in the house. He became stubborn and querulous. Eventually he required assistance in shaving and dressing.

When examined 6 years after the first symptoms had developed, the patient was alert and cooperative. He was disoriented with respect to place and time. He could not recall the names of four of five objects after a 5-minute interval of distraction. He could not remember the names of his college and graduate school or the subject in which he had majored. He could describe his job by title only. In 1978 he thought that Kennedy was president of the United States. He did not know Stalin's nationality. His speech was fluent and well articulated, but he had considerable difficulty finding words and used many long, essentially meaningless phrases. He called a cup a vase and identified the rims of glasses as "the holders." He performed simple calculations poorly. He could not copy a cube or draw a house. His interpretation of proverbs was concrete, and he had no insight into the nature of his disturbance.

An elementary neurological examination revealed nothing abnormal, and routine laboratory tests were also negative. A computed tomography (CT) scan, however, showed marked cortical atrophy.

DSM-IV-TR Casebook Diagnosis of "The Hiker"

This patient has memory impairment, impairment in abstract thinking (concrete interpretation of proverbs), and other disturbances in higher cortical functioning (aphasia). These signs of global cognitive impairment, severe enough to interfere significantly with work and social activities and not occurring exclusively during the course of Delirium, indicate a Dementia. There is an insidious onset, beginning before age 65, with a generally progressive, deteriorating course and no specific cause. Thus, the most likely diagnosis is Dementia of the Alzheimer's Type, With Early Onset (DSM-IV-TR, p. 157). Because of the absence of clinically significant behavioral problems (most of the patient's problems are related to the cognitive impairment), we note the subtype to be Without Behavioral Disturbance.

Given that some degree of supervision is necessary, the severity of the Dementia is noted as Moderate. We note the presence of the neurological disease, Alzheimer's disease, on Axis III.

Follow-Up

This man's condition progressed, and he required admission to the hospital within a year of his initial assessment. Over the next year, he became essentially mute, and mental status testing was virtually impossible. He had a tendency to pace back and forth constantly on the ward; on one occasion he managed to get out of the locked ward and was found some miles from the hospital. (Note that, at this point in the course, the subtype With Behavioral Disturbance would have been warranted.)

His retained physical appearance was in striking contrast to his devastated intellectual capacities for a long time, but eventually he began to lose weight, took to his bed, and developed contractures (permanent muscular contractions).

He died at age 72 of pneumonia. Autopsy revealed cerebral atrophy and, microscopically, the plaques and tangles diagnostic of Alzheimer's disease.

Discussion of "The Hiker" by Marshal Folstein, M.D.*

Clinical and Pathological Features of Alzheimer's Disease

In 1907, Alzheimer published a description of a case of early-onset Dementia—a disease that came to be called by his name. The patient was a "51-year-old woman who showed as one of her first disease symptoms a strong feeling of jealousy toward her husband. Very soon she showed rapidly increasing memory impairments; she was disoriented carrying objects to and fro in her flat and hid them. Sometimes she felt that someone wanted to kill her and began to scream loudly…. After 4 years of sickness she died. She had a striking cluster of symptoms that included reduced comprehension and memory, as well as aphasia, disorientation, unpredictable behavior, paranoia, auditory hallucinations, and pronounced psychosocial impairment" (Maurer et al. 1997; an abstract of the record of this patient can also be found at http://www.zarcrom.com/ users/alzheimers/w-09.html, accessed 17 December 2003).

The cognitive symptoms progress from memory loss to aphasia, apraxia, and agnosia and then to a final stage of gait disorder and incontinence (Folstein and Whitehouse 1983). On average, death occurs 10 years after onset. The symptoms correspond to the progression of

---

Dr. Folstein is Professor of Psychiatry at Tufts University School of Medicine. Marshal Folstein began his work in geriatric psychiatry in 1970 when, in collaboration with Susan Folstein and Paul McHugh, he developed the Mini-Mental State Examination (MMSE). With Jason Brandt, Marshal Folstein published the Telephone Interview of Cognitive Status and other tools for the assessment of disability and noncognitive symptoms. He was an author of the National Institute of Neurological and Communicative Diseases and Stroke/Alzheimer's Disease and Related Disorders Association (NINCDS-ADRDA) criteria for Alzheimer's disease prior to working on the DSM-IV criteria for Dementia and Delirium. He began to study the phenotype of Alzheimer's disease and published observations with John Breitner based on family studies that suggested that major genes caused Alzheimer's disease in both the early- and late-onset cases. His work with Barry Rovner, Cynthia Steele, Mary Jane Lucas, and others in 1986 indicated that nursing homes were becoming mental hospitals that needed psychiatrists and psychiatric nurses. Folstein, Rovner, Lucas, and Steele published the first randomized trial of treatment of behavior disorder in patients with Dementia in long-term care. Their work informed the 1987 Omnibus Budget Reconciliation Act (OBRA) regulations for the use of restraints and medications in nursing homes. From 1993 until 2003, Dr. Folstein was Chairman of the Department of Psychiatry at Tufts University. Currently, he is President of the Boston Society of Neurology and Psychiatry, principal investigator in a population study of nutrition and memory in the homebound elderly of Boston, and Medical Director of the psychiatric inpatient service of the Merrimack Valley Hospital.

the disease from the entorhinal cortex and amygdala to the parietal and the frontal cortex (Braak and Braak 1991). Cell loss also occurs in the nucleus basalis of Meynert, causing a depletion of acetylcholine, and in the locus coeruleus and central raphe, causing a depletion of norepinephrine and serotonin (Zweig et al. 1988). An inflammatory cascade leads to free radical formation and cell death. The loss of synapses correlates with the degree of cognitive impairment.

Early-onset disease is caused by several genetic mutations that interfere with the metabolism of a transmembrane protein, which leads to the deposition of extracellular amyloid and intracellular neurofibrillary tangles (Blacker et al. 2003).

Case Discussion

We are not told of the chief complaint or family history of The Hiker. Because the man's diagnosis is early onset, we would expect to see other family members affected and concern in family members about their own susceptibility.

"*A 61-year-old high school science department head who was an experienced and enthusiastic camper and hiker became extremely fearful while on a trek in the mountains.*" Although the defining features are cognitive, the noncognitive symptoms of depression, anxiety, delusions, hallucinations, sleep disturbance, and other behavior disorders are often of most concern to caregivers (Loreck et al. 1994). Anxiety or depression occurs frequently in Alzheimer's disease and sometimes occurs prior to onset of cognitive impairment, as in the patient Alzheimer described (Loreck and Folstein 1993). The mood changes sometimes occur out of the blue and may be related to changes in monoaminergic nuclei, which are affected early in the disease (Rovner et al. 1989; Zweig et al. 1988). An alternative explanation for the patient's fear while on a trek is that he had a catastrophic reaction because of his loss of capacity to orient himself in the woods (Goldstein 1963). Victims of cerebral diseases react emotionally to task difficulty or failure.

"*Gradually, over the next few months, he lost interest in his usual hobbies. Formerly a voracious reader, he stopped reading.*" Apathy and inertia are more often early symptoms of a frontal dementia, such as Pick's disease, as opposed to Alzheimer's disease. The patient with Alzheimer's disease usually wants to maintain customary activities until 4 or 5 years into the illness. Given the emotional reaction of The Hiker, his loss of interest could be a symptom of depression.

"*He had difficulty doing computations and made gross errors in home financial management.*" This is expected early in Alzheimer's disease.

"On several occasions he became lost while driving in areas that were formerly familiar to him. He began to write notes to himself so that he would not forget to do errands." Carrying notes may reflect loss of memory, feelings of anxiety, or obsessional checking. Some patients find notes to be useful memory aids, but others forget to use them. Orientation to place depends on hippocampal cells, which are affected early in the course of Alzheimer's disease.

"Very abruptly, and in uncharacteristic fashion, he decided to retire from work, without discussing his plans with his wife." When cognitive impairment reaches the severity demonstrated by The Hiker, retirement from work is necessary. However, many patients, especially men, want to continue to work and drive in the face of serious impairment of attention. Interpretation of The Hiker's failure to inform his wife of his retirement depends on his reasons and their relationship. The psychiatrist caring for the patient with Alzheimer's disease must understand the previous, current, and future roles of the family members.

"Intellectual deterioration gradually progressed." The rate of deterioration of function in Alzheimer's disease is variable, but, before the introduction of the cholinesterase inhibitors in the treatment of Alzheimer's disease patients, the duration of the disease from onset of memory disturbance to death was 8–10 years. In the first years of illness, memory and attention are primarily affected. Some 3–4 years later, the patient develops communication problems because of the onset of semantic aphasia. In the final stages, the patient becomes incontinent and develops a gait disorder. Delusions and hallucinations appear as the MMSE score falls (Loreck et al. 1994), although in the original case described in 1907 by Alzheimer, delusions of jealousy appeared early. The early appearance of hallucinations suggests Lewy body disease.

"He spent most of the day piling miscellaneous objects in one place and then transporting them to another spot in the house." The patient described by Alzheimer did the same thing. One interpretation of the repetitive activities is that Dementia patients become demoralized by failure, avoid difficult tasks, and begin to carry out repetitive activities that they have mastered.

"He became stubborn and querulous." Some knowledge of previous personality is useful in interpreting symptoms like these. Irritability is commonly seen in Alzheimer's disease in association with Mood Disorders and catastrophic reactions and can also be precipitated when a caretaker sets limits on the patient's behavior. Change of premorbid traits of personality is unpredictable. Aggressive individuals may become passive, and placid individuals may become aggressive.

"Eventually, he required assistance in shaving and dressing." After 3–4 years of illness, patients become apractic—that is, they lose the capac-

ity to perform learned motor movements. This symptom is sometimes reflected in the loss of capacity to write and copy drawings, as well as in the inability to carry out everyday tasks.

Examination

"When examined 6 years after the first symptoms had developed, the patient was alert and cooperative." The presence of alertness and presumably clear consciousness is helpful in ruling out Delirium as a cause of the impairment.

"He was disoriented with respect to place and time." Orientation to time is affected before orientation to place in Alzheimer's disease.

"He could not recall the names of four of five objects after a 5-minute interval of distraction." We are not told whether the patient was able to register all five words when they were initially presented. Testing registration, or working memory, is important because it is often affected. The completion of the registration task indicates the number of items that the patient has comprehended. In this example, the patient must have registered five items in order to be able to recall four of five. Asking the patient to report the objects immediately after they were presented to him tests the ability to quickly encode new matieral. The delay required for testing retrieval and recall of the information has not been clearly established. However, after the memory items have been successfully registered, the patient should be given tasks that prevent their rehearsal.

"He could not remember the names of his college and graduate school or the subject in which he had majored. He could describe his job by title only. In 1978 he thought that Kennedy was president of the United States. He did not know Stalin's nationality." Families often report that patients can remember distant personal events but do not remember what they did yesterday. The Hiker could recall neither past events nor recent events.

"His speech was fluent and well articulated..." Fluent, well-articulated speech and language are expected early in Alzheimer's disease but not in disorders with a subcortical Dementia presentation, such as vascular dementia, Parkinson's disease, hydrocephalus, acquired immunodeficiency syndrome, or depression. In subcortical Dementia, the speech can be slow and poorly articulated, and there may be long latencies between the examiner's question and the patient's answer.

"...but he had considerable difficulty finding words and used many long, essentially meaningless phrases. He called a cup a vase and identified the rims of glasses as 'the holders.'" The loss of the availability of words and their meanings creates what is called *empty speech*. Families are often troubled early in the course of the disease because the patient's language

deterioration interrupts dinner table conversation. After 3–4 years of illness, aphasia develops in patients with Alzheimer's disease. Patients have difficulty understanding complex commands and may use jargon.

"He performed simple calculations poorly." Calculations depend on arithmetical skills and also on attention and concentration. Loss of ability to handle money is an early sign of Alzheimer's disease, and it would certainly be expected at year 6.

"He could not copy a cube or draw a house." Loss of the ability to draw is a sign of apraxia and is sometimes associated with loss of daily living skills.

"His interpretation of proverbs was concrete…" Interpretation of proverbs and the recognition of similarities, such as how an apple and an orange are alike, are affected in patients with Alzheimer's disease. These tests are difficult to evaluate because of a range of correct answers and because performance is affected by culture and education.

"…and he had no insight into the nature of his disturbance." Patients with Alzheimer's disease usually declare that there is nothing wrong with them but may admit to having some memory trouble. This phenomenon has not been thoroughly studied, but it may represent an agnosia. Agnosia occurs in patients who have right parietal lesions. Such patients neglect their right side and deny any paralysis. The denial that anything is wrong could also represent the overconfidence that is typical of mania or the failure of self-evaluation in the presence of extreme apathy. It could also be interpreted as an attempt by the patient to maintain dignity and freedom.

"An elementary neurological examination revealed nothing abnormal, and routine laboratory tests were negative." The neurological examination in the differential diagnosis of Dementia can indicate the gait disorders and slow movement of the patient with subcortical dementia, adventitious movements of Huntington's disease, tremor of Parkinson's disease, asterixis of Delirium, and, rarely, myoclonus of Alzheimer's disease. Preservation of fine motor movement is the rule in Alzheimer's disease.

"A computed tomography (CT) scan, however, showed marked cortical atrophy." Cognitive impairment of Alzheimer's disease is due to the loss of synapses (Terry et al. 1994). Cortical atrophy is usually present but is often reported erroneously as an age-related change. The introduction of measurement of brain volumes and metabolism to the interpretation of head scans will enhance diagnostic accuracy and also provide a means to track decline. Changes in brain structure correlate with cognitive impairment (Aylward et al. 1996; Jobst et al. 1997). Abnormalities in blood flow detected by single photon emission computed tomography occur early and sometimes precede cognitive changes (Huang et al. 2002).

"This man's condition progressed, and he required admission to the hospital within a year of his initial assessment. Over the next year, he became essentially mute, and mental status testing was impossible." Patients with Alzheimer's disease do become mute late in the illness, but the presence of depression must always be considered, especially when patients lose weight.

"He had a tendency to pace back and forth constantly on the ward; on one occasion he managed to get out of the locked ward and was found some miles from the hospital." Periods of overactivity, wandering, and sleep disturbance are common late in the disease. Treatment with mood stabilizers like divalproex (Depakote) is sometimes helpful.

"His retained physical appearance was in striking contrast to his devastated intellectual capacities for a long time, but eventually he began to lose weight, took to his bed, and developed contractures (permanent muscular contractions). He died at age 72 of pneumonia." The 11-year duration of Alzheimer's disease is within the expected range that has been reported.

"Autopsy revealed cerebral atrophy and, microscopically, the plaques and tangles diagnostic of Alzheimer's disease." Autopsy is still important because the more recently differentiated varieties of Dementia, such as Lewy body disease, cannot be differentiated from Alzheimer's disease by brain scans. Autopsy studies indicate that clinical diagnosis prior to the patient's death is accurate 85%–90% of the time (Joachim et al. 1988).

Treatment and Management

Treatment and management for such a patient begin with taking a history from the patient and the family separately. Even if the patient is too impaired cognitively to provide much history, it is important to respect the patient's dignity and to listen to his or her view of the condition. The caretakers provide the details of the history and also need the physician's understanding and support; therefore, that the physician knows something of their story in relation to the patient is important. Careful inquiry is needed to reveal the presence of noncognitive symptoms, such as depression, delusions, and hallucinations. A structured tool such as the Dementia Symptoms Scale is helpful (Loreck et al. 1994). After taking the history and examining the patient, I ask the patient and the family what they want to know—they might want to know the diagnosis, prognosis, and etiology—and then I tell them. Most are worried about the potential inheritance of disease by the children of the patient. The general principles of genetic counseling are followed (Folstein and Folstein 1995, 1998).

I then recommend the two treatments that have, so far, been demonstrated to be effective in altering the course of the symptoms: a cholinesterase inhibitor and vitamin E. Three cholinesterase inhibitors—donepezil, galantamine, and rivastigmine—are used at dosages that vary for each drug. Side effects of cholinesterase inhibitors include tremor, nausea, gastrointestinal bleeding, and Delirium. The optimal dosage of vitamin E has not yet been established, but, in a published trial, 2,000 U/day were given (Sano et al. 1997). Noncognitive symptoms such as depression are treated empirically with mood stabilizers, antidepressants, and low doses of antipsychotics. Trazodone is useful in sleep regulation. Benzodiazepines during the day before stressful activities can help.

The patient and family also need a plan for day-to-day management. I help them to create a structured daily schedule so that the patient is stimulated but not unduly challenged and so that the caretakers are given periods of respite. This sometimes requires family meetings in which the patient's children, and sometimes grandchildren, are enlisted. Patients often do not want to burden their children and so do not ask for their help. Other aspects of the patient's interactions with society also need attention, including driving, financial management, and consideration of power of attorney. Follow-up visits with the family are scheduled frequently enough to answer questions about situations as they arise (e.g., "Should we take a vacation?") and to check for side effects of medications. I see families monthly at first and then quarterly. At each visit, I speak with the patient alone and ask about his or her concerns and then meet with the family separately. As in the initial evaluation, I conclude the visit by meeting with the family and patient together to summarize the results of the visit. These meetings usually require only a few minutes with each party.

Care for patients with Alzheimer's disease requires the collaboration of many professionals who, together, manage the disease, the patient's reactions to it, the behaviors that develop, and the personal situation that is confronted by the patient and family members.

References

Aylward EH, Rasmusson DX, Brandt J, et al: CT measurement of suprasellar cistern predicts rate of cognitive decline in Alzheimer's disease. J Int Neuropsychol Soc 2:89–95, 1996

Blacker D, Bertram L, Saunders AJ, et al: Results of a high-resolution genome screen of 437 Alzheimer's disease families. Hum Mol Genet 12(1):23–32, 2003

Braak H, Braak E: Neuropathological staging of Alzheimer-related changes. Acta Neuropathologica 82:239–259, 1991

Folstein MF, Whitehouse PJ: Cognitive impairment of Alzheimer disease. Neurobehav Toxicol Teratol 5(6):631–634, 1983

Folstein SE, Folstein MF: Genetic counseling for psychiatric disorders: teaching consultants about genotypes and phenotypes, in American Psychiatric Press Review of Psychiatry, Vol 14. Edited by Oldham JM, Riba M. Washington, DC, American Psychiatric Press, 1995, pp 425–458

Folstein SE, Folstein MF: Genetic counseling in Alzheimer's disease and Huntington's disease: principles and practice, in Neurobiology of Primary Dementia. Edited by Folstein MF. Washington, DC, American Psychiatric Press, 1998, pp 329–364

Goldstein K: The Organism. Boston, MA, Beacon Press, 1963, p 35

Huang C, Wahlund LO, Svensson L, et al: Cingulate cortex hypoperfusion predicts Alzheimer's disease in mild cognitive impairment. BMC Neurol 2(1):9, 2002

Joachim CL, Morris JH, Selkoe DJ: Clinically diagnosed Alzheimer's disease: autopsy results in 150 cases. Ann Neurol 24(1):50–56, 1988

Jobst KA, Barnetson LP, Shepstone BJ: Accurate prediction of histologically confirmed Alzheimer's disease and the differential diagnosis of dementia: the use of NINCDS-ADRDA and DSM-III-R criteria, SPECT, X-ray CT, and APO E4 medial temporal lobe dementias. The Oxford Project to Investigate Memory and Aging. Int Psychogeriatr 9 (suppl 1):191–222; discussion 247–252, 1997

Loreck DJ, Folstein MF: Depression in Alzheimer disease, in Depression in Neurological Disease. Edited by Starkstein SE, Robinson RG. Baltimore, MD, Johns Hopkins University Press, 1993, pp 50–62

Loreck DJ, Bylsma F, Folstein MF: The Dementia Symptoms Scale: a new scale for comprehensive assessment of psychopathology in Alzheimer's disease. Am J Geriatr Psychiatry 2(1):60–74, 1994

Maurer K, Volk S, Gerbaldo H: Auguste D and Alzheimer's disease. Lancet 349:1546–1549, 1997

Rovner BW, Broadhead J, Spencer M, et al: Depression and Alzheimer's disease. Am J Psychiatry 146(3):350–353, 1989

Sano M, Ernesto C, Thomas RG, et al: A controlled trial of selegiline, alpha-tocopherol, or both as treatment for Alzheimer's disease. The Alzheimer's Disease Cooperative Study. N Engl J Med 336(17):1216–1222, 1997

Terry RD, Masliah E, Hansen LA: Structural basis of the cognitive alterations in Alzheimer's disease, in Alzheimer Disease. Edited by Terry RD, Katzman R, Bick K. New York, Raven Press, 1994, pp 179–196

Zweig RM, Ross CA, Hedreen JC, et al: The neuropathology of aminergic nuclei in Alzheimer's disease. Ann Neurol 24(2):233–242, 1988 [Research done at the Neuropathology Laboratory, Johns Hopkins University School of Medicine, Baltimore, MD. Article also printed in Prog Clin Biol Res 317:353–365, 1989]

Suggested Reading

Folstein MF, Robinson R, Folstein SE, et al: Depression and neurological disorders: new treatment opportunities for elderly depressed patients. J Affect Disord Suppl 1:S11–S14, 1985

Close to the Bone

A 23-year-old woman from Arkansas wrote a letter to the head of a New York research group after seeing a television program in which he described his work with patients with unusual eating patterns. In the letter, which requested that she be accepted into his program, the woman described her problems as follows:

Several years ago, in college, I started using laxatives to lose weight. I started with a few and increased the number as they became ineffective. After 2 years I was taking 250–300 Ex-Lax pills at one time with a glass of water, 20 per gulp. I would lose as much as 20 pounds in a 24-hour period, mostly water and some food, [and would be] dehydrated so that I couldn't stand, and could barely talk. I ended up in the university infirmary several times with diagnoses of food poisoning, severe gastrointestinal flu, etc., with bland diets and medications. I was released within a day or two. A small duodenal ulcer appeared and disappeared on X rays in 1975.

I would not eat for days, then would eat something, and, overcome by guilt at eating, and hunger, would eat, eat, eat. A girl on my dorm floor told me that she occasionally forced herself to vomit so that she wouldn't gain weight. I did this every once in a while and discovered that I could consume large amounts of food, vomit, and still lose weight. This was spring of 1975. I lost nearly 50 pounds over a few months, to 90 pounds. My hair started coming out in handfuls, and my teeth were loose.

I never felt lovelier or more confident about my appearance: physically liberated, streamlined, close-to-the-bone. I was flat everywhere except my stomach when I binged, when I would be full-blown and distended. When I bent over, each rib and back vertebra was outlined. After vomiting, my stomach was once more flat, empty. The more I lost, the more I was afraid of getting fat. I was afraid to drink water for days at a time because it would add pounds on the scale and make me miserable. Yet I drank (or drink; perhaps I should be writing this all in the present tense) easily a half-gallon of milk and other liquids at once when bingeing. I didn't need the laxatives as much to get rid of food, and eventually stopped using them altogether (although I am still chronically constipated, I become nauseous whenever I see them in the drugstore).

I exercised for hours each day to tone my figure from the weight fluctuations, and joined the university track team. I wore track shoes all the time and ran to classes and around town, stick-legs pumping. I went to track practice daily after being sick, until I was forced to quit; a single lap would make me dizzy, with cramps in my stomach and legs.

At some point during my last semester before dropping out I came across an article on anorexia nervosa. It frightened me; my own personal obsession with food and body weight was shared by other people. I had not menstruated in 2 years. So, I forced myself to eat and digest healthy food. Hated it. I studied nutrition and gradually forced myself to accept a new attitude toward food—vitalizing—something needed for life. I gained weight, fighting panic. In a rigid, controlled way I have maintained myself nutritionally ever since: 105–115 pounds at 5′6″. I know what I need to survive and I eat it—a balanced diet with the fewest possible calories, mostly vegetables, fruits, fish, fowl, whole grain products, and so on. In 5 years I have not eaten anything like pizza, pastas or pork, sweets, or anything fattening, fried or rich without being very sick. Once I allowed myself an ice cream cone. But I am usually sick if I deviate as much as one bite.

It was difficult for me to face people at school, and I dropped courses each semester, collecting incompletes but finishing well in the few classes I stayed with. The absurdity of my reclusiveness was evident even to me during my last semester when I signed up for correspondence courses, while living only two blocks from the correspondence university building on campus. I felt I would only be able to face people when I lost "just a few more pounds."

Fat. I cannot stand it. This feeling is stronger and more desperate than any horror at what I am doing to myself. If I gain a few pounds I hate to leave the house and let people see me. Yet I am sad to see how I have pushed aside the friends, activities, and state of energized health that once rounded my life.

For all of this hiding, it will surprise you to know that I am by profession a model. Last year when I was more in control of my eating-vomiting I enjoyed working in front of a camera, and I was doing well. Lately I've been sick too much and feel out-of-shape and physically unself-confident for the discipline involved. I keep myself supported during this time with part-time secretarial work, and whatever unsolicited photo bookings my past clients give me. For the most part I do the secretarial work. And I can't seem to stop being sick all of the time.

The more I threw up when I was in college, the longer it took, and the harder it became. I needed to use different instruments to induce vomiting. Now I double two electrical cords and shove them several feet down into my throat. This is preceded by 6–10 doses of ipecac [an emetic]. My knees are calloused from the time spent kneeling sick. The eating-vomiting process takes usually 2–3 hours, sometimes as long as 8. I dread the gagging and pain and sometimes my throat is very sore and I procrastinate using the ipecac and cords. I sit on the floor, biting my nails, and pulling the skin off around my nails with tweezers. Usually I wear rubber gloves to prevent this somewhat.

After emptying my stomach completely I wash thoroughly. In a little while I will hydrate myself with a bottle of diet pop, and take a handful of Lasix [furosemide; a diuretic] 40 mg (which I have numerous prescriptions for). Sometimes I am faint, very cold. I splash cool water on my face, smooth my hair, but my hands are shaking some. I will take aspirin if my hands hurt sharply,…so I can sleep later. My lips, fingers are bluish and cold. I see in the mirror that blood vessels are broken. There are red spots over my eyes. They always fade in a day or two. There is a certain relief when it is over, that the food is gone, and I am not horribly fat from it. And I cry often…for some rest, some calm. It is foolish for me to cry for someone, someone to help me; when it is only me who is hiding and hurting myself.

Now there is a funny new split in my behavior, this honesty about my illness. Hopefully it will bring me more help than humiliation. Sometimes I feel an hypocrisy in my actions, and in the frightened, well-ordered attempts to seek out help. All the while I am still sick, night after night after night. And often days as well.

Two sets of logic seem to be operating against each other, each determined, each half-canceling the effects of the other. It is the part of me which forced me to eat that I'm talking about…which cools my throat with water after hours of heaving, which takes potassium supplements to counteract diuretics, and aspirin for torn hands. It is this part of me, which walks into a psychiatrist's office twice weekly and sees the liability of hurting myself seriously, which makes constant small efforts to repair the tearing-down.

It almost sounds as if I am being brutalized by some unrelenting force. Ridiculous to feel this way, or to stand and cry, because the hands that cool my throat and try to make small repairs only just punched lengths of cord into my stomach. No demons, only me.

For your consideration, I am

Gratefully yours,

Nancy Lee Duval

Ms. Duval was admitted to the research ward for study. Additional history revealed that her eating problems began gradually during her adolescence and had been severe for the past 3–4 years. At age 14, she weighed 128 pounds, and she had reached her adult height of 5'6". She felt "terribly fat" and began to diet without great success. At age 17, she weighed 165 pounds. Ms. Duval began to diet more seriously for fear that she would be ridiculed and went down to 130 pounds over the next year. She recalled feeling very depressed, overwhelmed, and insignificant. She began to avoid difficult classes so that she would never get less than straight As and lied about her school and grade performance for fear of being humiliated. She had great social anxiety in interacting with boys, which culminated in her transferring to a girls' school for the last year of high school.

When Ms. Duval left for college, her difficulties increased. She had trouble deciding how to organize her time—whether to study, date, or see friends. She became more desperate to lose weight and began to use laxatives, as she describes in her letter. At age 20, in Ms. Duval's sophomore year of college, she reached her lowest weight of 88 pounds (70% of ideal body weight) and stopped menstruating.

As Ms. Duval describes in her letter, she recognized that there was a problem and eventually forced herself to gain weight. Nonetheless, the overeating and vomiting she had begun the previous year worsened. Because she was preoccupied with her weight and her eating, her school performance suffered, and she dropped out of school midway through college at age 21.

Ms. Duval is the second of four children and the only girl. She comes from an upper-middle-class professional family. From the patient's description, it sounds as though the father has a history of alcoholism. There are clear indications of difficulties between the mother and the father and between the boys and the parents, but no other family member has ever had psychiatric treatment.

DSM-IV-TR Casebook Diagnosis of "Close to the Bone"

Ms. Duval has Anorexia Nervosa (DSM-IV-TR, p. 589), a disorder that was first described 300 years ago and was given its current name in 1868. Although theories about the cause of the disorder have come and gone, the essential features have remained unchanged. Ms. Duval poignantly describes these features.

She had an intense and irrational fear of becoming obese, even when she was emaciated. Her body image was disturbed in that she perceived herself as fat when her weight was average and "never lovelier" when, to others, she must have appeared grotesquely thin. She lost about 30% of her body weight by relentless dieting and exercising, self-induced vomiting, and use of cathartics and diuretics. She had not menstruated for the past 3 years.

She also has recurrent episodes of binge eating—rapid, uncontrolled consumption of high-calorie foods. These binges are followed by vomiting and remorse. Because of this pattern of recurrent binge eating and purging, the diagnosis of Anorexia Nervosa is qualified as the Binge-Eating/Purging Type.

Follow-Up

Ms. Duval remained in the research ward for several weeks, during which time she participated in research studies and, under the structure of the hospital setting, was able to give up her abuse of laxatives and diuretics. After her return home, she continued in treatment with a psychiatrist in psychoanalytically oriented psychotherapy two times a week, which she had begun 6 months previously. That therapy continued for approximately another 6 months, at which point her family refused to support it. The patient also felt that, although she had gained some insight into her difficulties, she had been unable to change her behavior.

Two years after leaving the hospital, she wrote that she was "doing much better." She had reenrolled in college and was completing her course work satisfactorily. She had seen a nutritionist and believed that form of treatment was useful for her in learning what a normal diet was and how to maintain a normal weight. She was also receiving counseling from the school guidance counselors, but she did not directly relate that to her eating difficulties. Her weight was normal, and she was menstruating regularly. She continued to have intermittent difficulty with binge eating and vomiting, but the frequency and severity of these problems were much reduced. She no longer abused diuretics or laxatives.

Discussion of "Close to the Bone"
by Katherine A. Halmi, M.D.*

Effective treatment of a patient with an Eating Disorder must begin with an organized and intelligent assessment of the Eating Disorder. After reading the dramatic, media-appealing letter of the patient, it was necessary for the treatment staff to obtain additional pertinent history, such as a height and weight history, in order to establish a feasible target—maintenance weight for the patient. At age 14, Ms. Duval achieved her adult height of 5'6" and weighed 128 pounds. A normal weight range at this height can be from 118 to 148 pounds, which corresponds with a body mass index (kilograms divided by height in square meters) from 19 through 24. Dieting is the most common stress factor that induces binge eating. This patient certainly engaged in overeating, if not binge eating, after periods of food restriction to reach a weight of 165 pounds at age 17. At that time, she was definitely overweight, with a body mass index of about 26.7. In setting a target weight, it is also helpful to know at what weight a patient's menses begins. Because this patient had been overweight, it is more reasonable to set a target weight in the middle to the upper end of a normal range, as it requires less stress to maintain a weight closer to a lifetime high weight.

The next category to assess is Eating Disorder symptoms. By the time she left for college, Ms. Duval had lost 35 pounds, and her dieting behavior was out of control. At college, she began her laxative abuse, which was followed by vomiting, and reached her lowest weight of 88 pounds while becoming amenorrheic. It is somewhat surprising that she survived the periods of losing 20 pounds over 24 hours with her excessive Ex-Lax pill abuse without requiring an emergency room visit for cardiac arrhythmias. As the weight loss progressed, so did the fear of becoming fat and the increased time spent exercising. Fear of the consequences of having Anorexia Nervosa forced the patient to main-

---

Dr. Halmi is Professor of Psychiatry at Cornell University Medical College and Director of the Eating Disorder Program. For the past 20 years, Dr. Halmi's research has primarily focused on eating behavior and Anorexia Nervosa and Bulimia Nervosa disorders. She has investigated the disorders with a broad perspective, including neuroendocrine studies, cognitive behavioral and pharmacological treatment studies, metabolic studies, investigations of comorbid psychopathology, studies of core Eating Disorder psychopathology, and longitudinal follow-up studies. She is well known internationally because of her published research.

tain a weight between 105 and 115 pounds, which is below the lowest acceptable weight for someone at a height of 5'6".

Usually, the longer the patient has been self-inducing vomiting, the easier it is to do so, but this apparently was not the case with Ms. Duval. The use of ipecac can be very dangerous because it may cause irreversible cardiac muscle damage, resulting in heart failure. The combination of ipecac use, diuretic abuse, and vomiting can lower the serum potassium level dangerously and create an environment for cardiac arrhythmias and sudden death. This patient's history calls for immediate, appropriate medical tests. Blood chemistry testing reveals the serum potassium level, which, if below 2.5 mEq/L, calls for hospitalization. With the strong history of potassium depletion behaviors, an electrocardiogram is an absolute necessity. Liver enzymes may be elevated, which is associated with malnutrition, and increased serum amylase levels are related to severity of self-induced vomiting. A complete blood count is necessary because a low white blood cell count is related to emaciation and malnutrition. Patients who binge and purge have a high association (30%–40%) of alcohol and substance abuse, which needs to be explored and verified with a urine toxicology screen (Halmi 2003).

A general psychiatric screen for common comorbid disorders, such as Major Depressive Disorder, and Anxiety Disorders (especially Obsessive-Compulsive Disorder, Social Phobia, and Posttraumatic Stress Disorder) is necessary to plan an effective treatment program. Special inquiry should be made into impulsive or self-injurious behaviors, which occur with the binge-eating/purging type of Anorexia Nervosa. Inquiries should also be made concerning suicidal preoccupation and past suicide attempts. An assessment of current level of functioning may provide further evidence for whether hospitalization is justified. The family history of such patients often reveals alcoholism, Mood Disorders, and Anxiety Disorders. It is not unusual for these families to be most chaotic in their interactions.

Treatment—Phase 1

Ms. Duval's out-of-control, life-threatening Eating Disorder behaviors required hospitalization in a specialized Eating Disorder treatment setting (Halmi 2003).

One of the most aggravating problems in treating patients with severe bulimic behaviors and laxative abuse is the failure of third-party payers to acknowledge the need for these patients to be hospitalized. In most cases, the patient's electrolytes must be severely deranged or the patient must have a markedly abnormal electrocardiogram for the managed care company to approve of hospitalization. For Ms. Duval, the only way she was able to get proper treatment was to be admitted to a state-financed research unit where treatment was free so long as she fit into a research protocol. Patients with severe binge eating and laxative abuse are unable to reduce or stop the behavior without inpatient therapy. Thus, patients continue on and on in outpatient therapy, and, subsequently, their behavior becomes more and more reinforced.

Treatment during this hospitalization will include 1) 24-hour surveillance for response-prevention of bingeing and purging; 2) individual cognitive-behavioral psychotherapy sessions; 3) multiple group therapy sessions for body image and eating behavior issues, self-esteem and self-efficacy, and assertiveness problems and specific female issues; 4) family counseling; and 5) appropriate medical treatment.

It is essential to stop the binge-purge behavior in order to treat the medical abnormalities (e.g., electrolyte imbalances and dehydration), as well as to reestablish normal eating behavior. The opportunity to binge is removed, and access to food is restricted to meal times and supervised snacks. A nutritionist should calculate the number of calories required for the patient to maintain her weight, and every few days the total calorie intake should be increased in order for the patient to gain weight if she is underweight. It is feasible for Ms. Duval to gain a minimum of 2–3 pounds per week. In the hospital, patients are observed during meals and for several hours after meals. Access to the bathroom is restricted or supervised to prevent surreptitious vomiting. The urge to binge may be extinguished with relaxation techniques or having the patient engage in a favorite activity.

To ensure adequate intake of all nutrients, including amino acids, minerals, vitamins, and fatty acids, and to allow a precise determination of daily caloric intake, the patient is given a liquid formula in six equal feedings throughout the day. When the patient is within 85% of her target weight range, food can be added, and if the patient continues to gain, she can be placed entirely on food provided on trays so that an accurate intake and output can be calculated. The patient should be weighed each morning after urinating, and generally it is beneficial to tell the patient her weight. Gradually, the preselected food trays should be removed—first breakfast, then lunch, and then dinner—so, eventually, she may have the experience of choosing her own foods before she is discharged from the hospital.

There are very few randomized, controlled trials for the treatment of Anorexia Nervosa to provide evidence-based treatment recommendations. There is evidence that selective serotonin reuptake inhibitors (SSRIs) are effective in reducing binge-purge behavior and perhaps are effective in preventing weight relapse in patients with Anorexia Nervosa (Fluoxetine Bulimia Nervosa Collaborative Study Group 1992; Kaye et al. 2000). For this reason, I would place Ms. Duval on an SSRI such as fluoxetine (Prozac) when she is within 85% of her target weight. SSRIs are not very helpful when a patient is below 80% of his or her target weight.

In a controlled inpatient environment, behavior therapy was found effective for inducing weight gain (Vitousek 2002). Behavior therapy includes contingency contracting, in which the patient and the therapist agree on rewards (e.g., visiting privileges, increased physical activity, and social activity) that the patient will receive when weight gain is achieved. Behavior therapy is used primarily to restore weight, which is necessary for two reasons. First, the state of emaciation causes irritability, depression, preoccupation with food, and sleep disturbance. Second, cognitive impairment is a common by-product of emaciation. It is exceedingly difficult to achieve behavioral change with psychotherapy in a patient who is experiencing the psychological and emotional effects of emaciation (Halmi 2003).

As Ms. Duval lost more weight, she became more perfectionistic and depressed. She also had increased social anxiety in interacting with boys and eventually became isolated from most of her peers. She had a rigid and extreme thinking style, especially on matters of weight and body image. She also had distorted thoughts about issues of self-esteem and self-adequacy and had a self-concept with pervasive feelings of ineffectiveness. These cognitive distortions are best dealt with in individual cognitive therapy. Cognitive therapy techniques for treating anorexia were first developed by Garner and Bemis (1985), and more recent refinement of these techniques is well described by Kleifield et al. (1996). Controlled clinical trials have shown cognitive-behavioral therapy (CBT) to be more effective than drug treatment or other forms of psychotherapy. In individual therapy sessions, Ms. Duval should be taught cognitive restructuring and problem-solving techniques. Cognitive restructuring is a method in which patients are taught to identify automatic thoughts and challenge their core beliefs. Patients become aware of specific negative thoughts, present arguments and evidence to support the validity of these thoughts, and then present arguments and evidence that cast doubt on the validity of the thoughts. Finally, patients form a reasoned conclusion based on the evidence. Problem solving is a method whereby patients learn to reason through dealing with difficult food-related and/or interpersonal situations and is especially relevant to events likely to trigger anorectic or bulimic behaviors. When patients learn to use these techniques effectively, they reduce their vulnerability to relying on anorectic behaviors as a means of coping.

For example, a cognitive restructuring exercise with Ms. Duval would be to have her state her distorted cognition that if she gains a few pounds, everyone will notice. She would list the evidence to support this idea and then the evidence against it. With the guidance of her therapist, she would realize that most people would be unaware that she had gained weight, and most people would find her equally, if not more, attractive. Ms. Duval would then reach the final logical conclusion that a drastic behavior such as refusing to go out of the house is ridiculous.

An example of problem solving would be to have Ms. Duval state her problem of binge eating. She would then think of different methods to use to stop binge eating. One possibility is that she could eat at regular 3- to 4-hour intervals to prevent extreme hunger. Another possibility is that she could engage in a series of alternative behaviors to binge eating. Ms. Duval would then decide on a strategy to use for the following week and practice it. At her next therapy session, she would discuss the effectiveness and/or problems with her chosen strategy.

Ms. Duval would also benefit from repeated exercises of cost-benefit analyses. These are especially useful at a time when the patient is tempted to engage in harmful Eating Disorder behaviors. In a cost-benefit analysis, Ms. Duval would list the costs of one of her behaviors, such as vomiting, on one side of a paper and the benefits on the other. The costs of vomiting would include the medical problems of dental injury and weakness from a low potassium level. Social costs would include isolation from friends. The benefits would include the escape from or avoidance of interpersonal problems or issues of maturity, such as independence.

Finally, Ms. Duval would benefit from some joint counseling sessions with her parents, both because there is evidence of multiple problems in their family relationships and she is highly dependent on her parents, who are financing her treatment.

Throughout hospitalization and before discharge, Ms. Duval should have counseling sessions with a nutritionist who can give her alternative food plans and help her understand what she should be eating to maintain her weight within a normal range. It is a common myth among educated laypeople and many uninformed therapists that discovering the "cause" will cure the patient with Anorexia Nervosa and will allow the patient to stop her bingeing and purging behavior. How can one, in reality, ever know what the true cause of the illness is and whether a single factor determines the illness? The patient, through psychodynamic psychotherapy, may become aware of certain relationships between events of the past and the development of her eating behavior, but that, in and of itself, does not provide evidence for a "cause" nor does this insight lead to behavior change, as Ms. Duval has found.

Treatment—Phase 2

After discharge from the inpatient setting, CBT should be continued. It is notable that 2 years after Ms. Duval left the research program in the hospital, she was still occasionally binge eating and vomiting, although less frequently. Outpatient cognitive-behavioral psychotherapy is effective in treating binge-purge behavior and would most likely be beneficial and effective for Ms. Duval (Fairburn et al. 1995). She noted that, although she gained some insight into her difficulties with post-hospitalization psychoanalytically oriented psychotherapy, she was unable to change her behavior. The techniques patients learn in cognitive therapy can also be applied to solving problems in interpersonal relationships and other stressful situations.

Because the relapse rate is high in both Anorexia Nervosa and Bulimia Nervosa (about 40%), it would most likely be a good idea to have three or four "booster" sessions in the course of 1 year to review the CBT techniques and strategies that were effective for Ms. Duval so that she can maintain weight and cease bingeing and purging behavior (Mitchell et al. 2001).

References

Fairburn CG, Norman PA, Welch SL, et al: A prospective study of outcome in bulimia nervosa and the long-term effects of three psychological treatments. Arch Gen Psychiatry 52:304–312, 1995

Fluoxetine Bulimia Nervosa Collaborative Study Group: Fluoxetine in the treatment of bulimia nervosa: a multicenter placebo-controlled double-blind trial. Arch Gen Psychiatry 49:139–147, 1992

Garner DM, Bemis KM: A cognitive-behavioral approach to anorexia nervosa, in Handbook of Psychotherapy for Anorexia Nervosa and Bulimia. Edited by Garner DM, Garfinkel PE. New York, Guilford Press, 1985, pp 107–146

Halmi KA: Eating disorders: anorexia nervosa, bulimia nervosa and obesity, in Textbook of Clinical Psychiatry. Edited by Hales RE, Yudolfsky SC. Washington, DC, American Psychiatric Publishing, 2003, pp 1001–1021

Kaye WH, Nagata T, Weltzin TE, et al: Double-blind placebo-controlled administration of fluoxetine in restricting and purging-type anorexia nervosa. Biol Psychiatry 49:644–652, 2000

Kleifield EI, Wagner S, Halmi KA: Cognitive-behavioral treatment of anorexia nervosa. Psychiatr Clin North Am 19:715–734, 1996

Mitchell JE, Peterson CB, Myers T, et al: Combining pharmacotherapy and psychotherapy in the treatment of patients with eating disorders. Psychiatr Clin North Am 24:315–323, 2001

Vitousek KB: Cognitive-behavioral therapy for anorexia nervosa, in Eating Disorders and Obesity. Edited by Fairburn CG, Brownell KD. New York, Guilford Press, 2002, pp 308–313

Time Traveler

I evaluated Robert Edwards, age 12, at the request of his parents, who were concerned about his long-standing social difficulties. Although Robert was a gifted student academically, he was increasingly isolated socially. Robert had been born at term after an uncomplicated pregnancy. His parents had no concerns about Robert in his first years of life. He was saying his first words by 1 year and spoke in sentences by 16 months. Bladder and bowel control were achieved between ages 3 and 4, although nighttime bladder control was not achieved until almost age 6. Although motorically somewhat awkward and clumsy, his parents reported that he was an early and avid reader who had seemed to learn to read through his interest in videotapes; for example, he was reading the Narnia Chronicles in kindergarten. Social difficulties were noted when Robert entered preschool at age 3. For example, he would inappropriately approach other children by coming up to them from behind and giving them a hug. He was transferred to a more structured, academically based preschool setting where he did somewhat better but was quickly seen as a rather eccentric child, in part because of his special interest in astronomy. This interest was quite intense and intruded on essentially all aspects of his life (e.g., in any conversation with peers he inevitably brought the conversation or play around to stars and planets). Over time, his interests came to include computer games—their rules, the programmers, and companies that produce them.

Robert was seen for occupational therapy evaluation at age 5 when he was noted to have low motor tone. A psychiatrist saw Robert at age 8, and a diagnosis of Anxiety Disorder was made—apparently in light of his significant anxiety in social situations. Play therapy was undertaken for approximately 1 year and then discontinued, as it appeared to be ineffective. Robert was enrolled in regular kindergarten and grade school. He was not identified as having any special educational needs until age 10. Psycholog-

---

This case is adapted from Volkmar FR, Klin A, Schultz RT, et al.: Asperger's disorder (clinical case conference). Am J Psychiatry 157(2):262–267, 2000, with permission.

ical testing was undertaken at age 10 years, 3 months, and at that time, on the Wechsler Intelligence Scale for Children, 3rd Edition (Wechsler 1987), his verbal IQ was 145; performance IQ, 119; and full scale IQ, 135. The split between his verbal and nonverbal abilities was statistically significant and relatively unusual. Achievement testing revealed a range of abilities. For example, his reading composite standard score was 134; writing, 125; math reasoning, 159; and written expression, 101 (with 100 being the norm average score for each test). He had significant difficulties with tasks that required visual-motor coordination, including handwriting. At that time, Robert's gross- and fine-motor problems included awkward gait and difficulties with riding a bike and writing; these difficulties were of sufficient concern to prompt occupational and physical therapy services. Robert's classroom teacher started to make some accommodations for him. In some areas, he did very well (e.g., he was enrolled in the gifted math program).

Apart from a history of recurrent croup and allergies, Robert had been in good general health. Robert had never had an electroencephalogram or magnetic resonance imaging scan; there had been no question of seizure disorder. His hearing was within normal limits. Robert's older brother had a history of some mild motor delays. There was a family history of depression and social difficulties in members of the extended family. There was no family history of autism.

Current Assessment

Robert, who had traveled some distance for the assessment, was seen over a period of several days. He was accompanied by his mother, who provided historical information as well as information on Robert's current functioning. Robert's social difficulties were readily apparent during the course of our contact. He responded to my greeting with an appropriate but abrupt response ("Hello—do you know what time it is?") and then turned to the side with a rather unmodulated smile, which he did not vary much for quite some time. He was inconsistent in responding to other people's facial expressions or gestures and often did not attend to social stimuli. Robert actively avoided eye contact and seemed to look through people. Most of the time, his emotional expressions—vocal as well as gestural—lacked variability and modulation. One notable exception involved a conversation about feelings of sadness and hurtful feelings in which he briefly commented on his difficulty talking about sadness with others and questioned whether doing so was worth the effort.

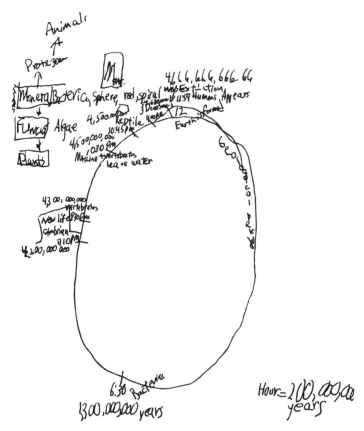

Drawing produced by "Robert" during the evaluation that illustrates his interest in time. The drawing shows the history of the universe from the moment of its creation (12 midnight), through geological time, the advent of bacteria (6:30), and so forth. The figure illustrates, on the one hand, the patient's profound interest (and knowledge) regarding this topic that tended to be all-encompassing and, on the other hand, his less developed fine-motor abilities.

Although somewhat quiet and reserved initially, he became much more animated as he felt more comfortable with me and the situation. At this time, he began to describe his interest in astronomy and, more recently, in time (see drawing) and engaged in a long monologue describing the history of the universe and the various time epochs illustrated in his drawing. After Robert started this topic, he pursued it

---

Autobiographical Statement

My name is Robert Edwards. I am an intelligent, unsociable but adaptable person. I would like to dispel any untrue rumors about me. I am not edible. I cannot fly. I cannot use telekinesis. My brain is not large enough to destroy the entire world when unfolded. I did not teach my long-haired guinea pig, Chronos, to eat everything in sight (that is the nature of the long-haired guinea pig).

---

with great intensity and vigor despite my repeated attempts to redirect the discussion. This interest also appeared repeatedly in his school work (e.g., in an autobiographical statement he had recently prepared; see above).

Robert described two children he considered his friends, although these relationships appeared to be based almost exclusively on their common interest in computers. His language was quite sophisticated but somewhat monotonic and pedantic. There were no indications of disorganized thinking. Robert denied vegetative signs of depression (e.g., problems with sleep or appetite), although his mood clearly was predominantly depressed. This seemed to be most evident when he discussed his feelings about school. He described himself as quite isolated and withdrawn in a novel group situation, although he mentioned that he was an excellent public speaker as long as the presentation was a formal one that he could rehearse and memorize in advance.

Robert was not overly preoccupied with extraneous stimuli, could focus on tasks with prompting, and did not exhibit unusual motoric behaviors (e.g., self-stimulatory behaviors or tics). He did attempt to reset my watch, which he said was 5 minutes too slow.

Robert's intellectual abilities were reassessed, and, again, there was a significant and very unusual discrepancy between his verbal and performance IQs, favoring the former. His visual-motor coordination skills were quite impaired, as were his planning, organization, and visual-spatial skills. Tests of expressive and receptive vocabulary revealed that he was functioning at more than 3 standard deviations above the mean. His communication style was quite formal and pedantic (e.g., when asked to provide another word for "call," Robert's response was "beckon" and for the word "thin," he provided "dimensionally challenged"). He had difficulty with tasks that required integration of nonverbal information (e.g., facial expressions, gestures, body proximity) in order to interpret another's perspective; thus, for example, he had very limited understanding of sarcasm or irony and took the literal meaning of what someone said without taking into account their tone of voice or facial expression. It was difficult for Robert to carry on a conversation except on topics of his choosing, and then he would not respond to cues from his conversational partner (e.g., signaling boredom or a desire to shift the topic of conversation). On a measure of adaptive behavior (Sparrow et al. 1984), his interpersonal skills were reported to be at the 2 years, 7 months level.

DSM-IV-TR Diagnosis of "Time Traveler"

Robert's problems were first noted when he entered preschool at age 3 and it became apparent that he was not developing age-appropriate peer relationships. During his evaluation at age 12, I noted a lack of social reciprocity (e.g., unmodulated smile, avoidance of eye contact, absence of variability in his voice and gestures), which had probably been present since his early years. His most striking symptom, however, is his abnormally intense preoccupation with astronomy. This combination of intense preoccupation with a narrow area of interest and impairment in social and emotional responsivity occurring in a child who does not show delays in cognitive development, language, or self-help skills is characteristic of Asperger's Disorder (DSM-IV-TR, p. 84). The condition is differentiated from Autistic Disorder by the normal—and often, as in this case, precocious—cognitive and language development. Children with Asperger's Disorder are significantly impaired in their social functioning, although they may perform well in a particular academic or occupational niche.

Discussion of "Time Traveler" by Fred Volkmar, M.D.*

Robert's case illustrates many of the clinical features associated with Asperger's Disorder. This condition, which was newly included in DSM-IV (American Psychiatric Association 1994), is defined on the basis of a patient's severe social disability (of the type observed in autism) but with well-preserved early language abilities. Consistent with Asperger's original description (Asperger 1944), parental concern usually arises first after age 3, in contrast to autism, which usually causes concern before age 2. Verbal abilities often serve as the child's way of connecting, in at least a limited way, with others. Although they are not technically required for the diagnosis, unusual circumscribed interests are typically present (i.e., technically, any of the restricted interests listed for Autistic Disorder are sufficient). These interests tend to be fact based and actually interfere with the child's development; they differ from the unusual abilities in autism (e.g., drawing, music, or calendar calculation), which tend to be more mechanical in nature and are usually seen in the context of overall Mental Retardation. Motor clumsiness is often an associated feature. As currently defined in DSM-IV-TR, the diagnosis of autism takes precedence over a diagnosis of Asperger's Disorder if criteria are met for both, but in Robert's case, the language difficulties characteristic of autism were not present, and the apparent *onset* of the disorder is after age 3.

Although Robert's diagnostic assignment is considered relatively straightforward, various controversies exist regarding this diagnostic concept. The term *Asperger's Disorder* has been used in very different ways to denote different types of a Pervasive Developmental Disorder (e.g., as synonymous with higher functioning autism, to adults with autism, or to Pervasive Developmental Disorder Not Otherwise Specified [PDD-NOS]) (Klin and Volkmar 2003). In addition, various other diagnostic concepts have been proposed for similar conditions—for

---

Dr. Volkmar is the Irving B. Harris Professor of Child Psychiatry, Pediatrics, and Psychology at Yale University. Dr. Volkmar has a long-standing interest in autism and related disorders. His interest in Asperger's Disorder was piqued by his work on the DSM-IV field trial for autism. He is a coeditor of the Handbook of Autism *(3rd Edition, in press) and co-author, along with Ami Klin and Sara Sparrow, of* Asperger Syndrome *(Klin et al. 2000). He is an associate editor of the* Journal of Autism and Developmental Disorders, *the* Journal of Child Psychology and Psychiatry, *and the* American Journal of Psychiatry.

example, semantic-pragmatic processing disorder (Bishop 1989), right hemisphere learning problems (Ellis et al. 1994), and nonverbal learning disability (Rourke 1989). Although these issues are not resolved, several lines of evidence suggest important differences between autism and PDD-NOS. In the DSM-IV field trial, for example, patients with clinical diagnoses of Asperger's Disorder were found to differ in several ways from patients with autism and PDD-NOS; the patients with Asperger's Disorder had a different pattern of verbal-performance IQ (favoring the former) compared to the patients with autism and, in contrast to the patients with PDD-NOS, had a significantly greater social impairment (Volkmar et al. 1994). Other studies have now suggested differences in terms of neuropsychological profiles (Klin et al. 1995), family history (Volkmar et al. 1998), and psychiatric comorbidity (Ghaziuddin et al. 1998). These differences may have important implications for treatment and research of patients with Asperger's Disorder.

Considerable interest has focused on the issue of comorbidity in Asperger's Disorder, with various case reports suggesting higher levels of psychosis or violent behavior (Ghaziuddin et al. 1998); controlled studies are lacking. In my experience, and in Robert's case, depression is the most common comorbid condition. Usually, the onset of depression begins in adolescence as the child is increasingly aware of, and frustrated by, his or her social disabilities. It is important not to overlook this depression, which can be treated with psychotherapy and medication (or both). Rourke (1989) has written extensively on the implications for the unusual profile of learning disabilities often seen in individuals with Asperger's Disorder.

Although the social disability in Asperger's Disorder and Autistic Disorder are defined in the same way, there are important differences in treatment. In Asperger's Disorder, in contrast to autism, the cognitive style is heavily biased toward verbal functioning. Although language skills are relatively preserved and serve as a *lifeline* for social interaction, there is often a significant discrepancy between the sophistication of linguistic form and structure on the one hand and social use of language on the other. Unfortunately, educators (and others) may be misled by the individual's verbal abilities and may attribute poor social skills and poor performance on nonverbal tasks to negativism or other volitional behaviors. As a result, these individuals may be viewed as behavior disordered or "socially, emotionally maladjusted" and then placed in classes for conduct-disordered children. This placement puts the child with Asperger's Disorder, a perfect victim, with perfect victimizers (Klin and Volkmar 1997). As a result of the child's growing social isolation, often in the face of some desire for social contact, it is not surprising that the child may become depressed.

In terms of intervention, the better verbal abilities associated with Asperger's Disorder suggest the utility of verbally mediated treatment programs not usually indicated in autism (e.g., very structured and problem-oriented psychotherapy and counseling may be indicated). Verbal skills can be used to teach problem-solving techniques that can be generalized from one situation to another. For example, the child can be taught a set of rules for identifying contextual cues such as location, facial expressions, body proximity, and gestures, which facilitate more appropriate comments, topic initiations, and social inferences. Robert, for example, could use explicit verbal approaches in solving social problems. Similar verbal problem-solving techniques can be implemented to help the child cope with more novel or emotionally charged situations (e.g., helping the child become more aware of anxiety in response to change or novelty and then using a set of verbal routines to elaborate rules for coping). Verbal cues can also be used to help children with Asperger's Disorder complete activities with more challenging motor demands by breaking down each task into specific steps and promoting verbal self-regulation. Vocational planning should encompass the individual's strengths and deficits (e.g., problems in visual-motor and visual-spatial integration may be important) (Klin and Volkmar 1997).

A number of interventions were helpful to Robert. These interventions included provision of information on Asperger's Disorder to his teachers, implementation of a social skills training program, and very focused psychotherapy that included reality-oriented, problem-solving therapy. This model is quite relevant to Robert, who has difficulties in social functioning, neuropsychological deficits on tests of drawing and copying ability, and deficits in face perception.

References

American Psychiatric Association: Diagnostic and Statistical Manual, 4th Edition, Text Revision. Washington, DC, American Psychiatric Association, 2000

Asperger H: Die "autistichen Psychopathen" im Kindersalter. Archive fur psychiatrie und Nervenkrankheiten 117:76–136, 1944

Bishop DV: Autism, Asperger's syndrome and semantic-pragmatic disorder: where are the boundaries (special issue: autism)? Br J Dis Comm 24(2):107–121, 1989

Ellis HD, Ellis DM, Fraser W, et al: A preliminary study of right hemisphere cognitive deficits and impaired social judgments among young people with Asperger syndrome. Eur Child Adolesc Psychiatry 3(4):255–266, 1994

Ghaziuddin M, Weidmer-Mikhail E, Ghaziuddin N: Comorbidity of Asperger syndrome: a preliminary report. J Intell Dis Res 42(Pt 4):279–283, 1998

Klin A, Volkmar FR: Asperger syndrome, in Handbook of Autism and Pervasive Developmental Disorders, 2nd Edition. Edited by Cohen DJ, Volkmar FR. New York, Wiley & Sons, 1997, pp 94–122

Klin A, Volkmar FR: Asperger syndrome—diagnosis and external validity. Child Adolesc Psychiatr Clin North Am 12(1):1–15, 2003

Klin A, Volkmar FR, Sparrow SS, et al: Validity and neuropsychological characterization of Asperger syndrome: convergence with nonverbal learning disabilities syndrome. J Child Psychol Psychiatry 36(7):1127–1140, 1995

Klin A, Volkmar FR, Sparrow SS (eds): Asperger Syndrome. New York, Guilford Press, 2000

Rourke BP: Nonverbal Learning Disabilities: The Syndrome and the Model. New York, Guilford, 1989

Sparrow S, Balla D, Cicchetti D: Vineland Adaptive Behavior Scales. Circle Pines, MN, American Guidance Service, 1984

Volkmar FR, Klin A, Siegel B, et al: Field trial for autistic disorder in DSM-IV. Am J Psychiatry 151(9):1361–1367, 1994

Volkmar FR, Klin A, Pauls D: Nosological and genetic aspects of Asperger syndrome. J Autism Dev Disord 28(5):457–463, 1998

Wechsler D: Wechsler Intelligence Scale for Children, 3rd Edition. San Antonio, TX, Psychological Corporation, 1987

Into Everything

At age 9, Eddie is referred to a child psychiatrist at the request of his school because of the difficulties he creates in class. He has been suspended for a day twice this school year. His teacher complains that he is so restless that his classmates are unable to concentrate. He is hardly ever in his seat. He roams around the class, talking to other children while they are working. When the teacher is able to get him to stay in his seat, he fidgets with his hands and feet and drops things on the floor. He never seems to know what he is going to do next and may suddenly do something quite outrageous. His most recent suspension was for swinging from the fluorescent light fixture over the blackboard. Because he was unable to climb down again, the class was in an uproar.

Eddie's mother says that his behavior has been difficult since he was a toddler and that, as a 3-year-old, he was unbearably restless and demanding. He has always required little sleep and wakes before anyone else. When he was small, "he got into everything," particularly in the early morning, when he would awaken at 4:30 A.M. or 5:00 A.M. and go downstairs by himself. His parents would awaken to find the living room or kitchen "demolished." When he was age 4, he managed to unlock the door of the apartment and wander off into a busy main street but, fortunately, was rescued from oncoming traffic by a passerby. He was not accepted into a preschool program because of his behavior; eventually, after a very difficult year in kindergarten, he was placed in a special behavioral program for first- and second-graders. He is now in a regular class for most of his subjects but spends a lot of time in a resource room with a special teacher. When Eddie is with his own class, he is unable to participate in games because he cannot wait for his turn.

Psychological testing has shown that Eddie is of average ability, and his achievements are only slightly below expected level. The psychologist describes his attention span as "virtually nonexistent."

He has no interest in television and dislikes games or toys that require any concentration or patience. He is not popular with other children, and at home he prefers to be outdoors, playing with his dog or riding his bike. If he does play with toys, his games are messy and destructive, and his mother cannot get him to keep his things in any order.

Eddie has been treated with a stimulant, methylphenidate, in small doses. While taking the drug, he was much easier to manage at school. He was less restless and, possibly, more attentive.

DSM-IV-TR Casebook Diagnosis of "Into Everything"

Eddie's behavior graphically demonstrates the characteristic inattention, impulsivity, and hyperactivity of Attention-Deficit/Hyperactivity Disorder (ADHD) (DSM-IV-TR, p. 92). He primarily shows symptoms of hyperactivity/impulsivity: He often has difficulty remaining seated, fidgets, runs about or climbs in situations where it is inappropriate, and has difficulty waiting his turn. He also displays some symptoms of inattention: He cannot sustain attention, he does not seem to listen to what is being said to him, and he strongly dislikes activities that require patience and concentration.

Discussion of "Into Everything" by Peter S. Jensen, M.D.*

What a handful this youngster is! Given his early difficulties running out of doors, it is a relief that he is still alive. Yet, in many ways, Eddie presents a classic picture of fairly severe ADHD. He shows evidence of significant impairment at home, where his parents truly have their hands full. At school, he is also impaired, less so in terms of actual academic achievement than in the area of classroom behavior and peer relations. Of note, his peer relationship difficulties and home-parenting problems often accompany ADHD (Hinshaw 2002), even though these characteristics are not part of the diagnostic criteria that define the disorder. Understanding the extent of these impairments is crucial, because it is these difficulties at home and school that often result in a pattern of accumulating comorbidities, particularly Oppositional Defiant Disorder and Conduct Disorder, as well as Mood and Anxiety Disorders. For example, we know that early behavioral difficulties often set in motion a pattern of reciprocal coercive behaviors between parents and children with the result that oppositional-defiant and conduct disorder–related problems often ensue. The parent may try to force good behavior from the child, whereas the child, in return, escalates the level of noncompliance and/or aggression. Similarly, the child who experiences school failure or rejection by his or her peers is more likely to go on to develop both internalizing and externalizing problems (Hinshaw 2002; Hinshaw et al. 2002). All of these difficulties finally culminate in quite problematic outcomes for many of these children (Biederman et

*Dr. Jensen is the Ruane Professor of Child Psychiatry and Director of the Center for the Advancement of Children's Mental Health at Columbia University. He began to study ADHD 20 years ago, shortly after finishing his child psychiatric residency. Inspired by the late Dennis Cantwell, M.D., he became quite interested in multimodal treatments of ADHD and set up an ADHD evaluation and treatment clinic while serving in the Army in Augusta, Georgia. Thereafter, he moved to the National Institute of Mental Health (NIMH), where, while serving as the chief of the Child and Adolescent Disorders Research Branch, he realized a long-standing ambition to facilitate the development and implementation of a large multisite clinical trial testing multimodal treatments for ADHD. This study, the NIMH Multimodal Treatment Study of Children With ADHD (the MTA study), has become the de facto standard for successful clinical trials within the field of child psychiatry. While at NIMH, Dr. Jensen spearheaded the 1998 National Institutes of Health Consensus Conference on ADHD. This conference led to the publication of his most recent edited volume with Jim Cooper, M.D., titled Attention Deficit Hyperactivity Disorder: State of the Science; Best Practices (Jensen and Cooper 2002).

al. 1991). From what we know about Eddie, he appears to be well on his way on this path of escalating adverse outcomes.

There is much we do not know about Eddie from this brief vignette: What is the actual nature of the parenting problems experienced by the parents? Such a child may well generate a pattern of harsh and/or coercive parenting, which, in turn, leads to patterns of increased aggression, anger, lowered self-esteem, lack of motivation, school failure, and association with peers with similar problems (Hinshaw et al. 2002). Do the parents agree on the diagnosis and treatment? Have they been able to institute appropriate behavior modification strategies at home? Does either or both of the parents have ADHD, which would make it hard for them to be consistent and follow-up on a behavioral plan for rewards and consequences for appropriate and inappropriate behavior at home? Does he get along with siblings (probably not well, I would guess)? If not, how might these problems magnify his other difficulties, in terms of his own feeling that things "aren't fair" and that his aggressive or acting-out behavior at home is justified?

How about the situation at school? The vignette tells us that earlier he had been placed in special education classroom settings and that he is now in the regular classroom, which suggests that earlier efforts in school may have been met by some degree of success in mitigating the severity of his behavior. Does he have a good relationship with his current teacher? Do the parents and teachers work together to shape his school behavior with appropriate home-based rewards? Is he cooperative and motivated to try to exert some control over his own behavior? Has the teacher been able to institute appropriate classroom behavior modification methods that can yield significant benefits and may even reduce medication requirements for such children? Is swinging from the classroom light fixture not merely "ADHD behavior" but also an attempt to generate some attention and admiration from his peers because most normal strategies do not seem to work for him?

We know that he has difficulties with peer relations, but does he have at least one friend that he can call his own? Does he have a skill that he is good at and that he himself feels good about? Success in these areas may offset his difficulties in school and at home. Unfortunately for Eddie, we read in the vignette that he does not have much going for him at home, at school, or with peers, but he likes animals and riding his bike. Might these interests be used as areas in which his skills and self-esteem could be enhanced, such as by having a pet and learning to take care of it, learning how to do stunts on his bike, participating in motocross bike races, or participating in other outdoor activities such as fishing, hiking, camping, etc.?

We know that Eddie "has been treated with a stimulant in small doses," but is he in treatment now? If not, why not? Frequently, parents have grave reservations about medication, in part because of frequent negative and biased reports about stimulants in the media (Jensen et al. 1999), but parents can also be reluctant to continue medication because they perceive changes in the child's personality, sleep, or appetite that others may not fully appreciate or take as seriously as do the parents (Greenhill et al. 2001). Working with the parents, clarifying misconceptions, and/or working to find a medication approach that is not only efficacious for symptoms but also acceptable in the context of family concerns and values are critical.

Why has he only been on "small doses" of medication? Recent evidence suggests that when optimal treatments are used, the goal of "normalizing" ADHD children's behaviors is within reach for about two-thirds of ADHD children (MTA Cooperative Group 1999a). Very frequently, clinicians stop short of an optimal dose, either because they are not fully comfortable with using the medications or are afraid of inducing side effects. Sometimes clinicians fail to move on to another medication after adequate doses of one medication have proved insufficient to achieve good functioning (MTA Cooperative Group 1999a, 1999b).

Starting first with Eddie, I like to make sure that Eddie and his family have an age-appropriate understanding of what ADHD is all about. Frequently, I tell such youngsters and their parents that having ADHD is like needing glasses: With ADHD, it is hard to focus and pay attention, even when one wants to. Thus, the treatments, whether medication or behavior therapy—the only two proven approaches—can assist a child so that it is not quite so hard to pay attention. I like to make sure that a child such as Eddie knows that he is still responsible for his own behavior and that the medication does not "make him be good." Like eyeglasses, the medication just makes it easier for him to focus and pay better attention to the things that are important so that he can do it "if he wants to."

How much self-control a child has is an issue that is easily misunderstood, because his parents may see that he is able to ride his bike for hours on end or play nonstop video games (i.e., "he could do it if he wanted to" is a frequent parental refrain). The parents and teachers alike need to understand that much of Eddie's behavior is not willful and that, in most (but not all) instances, he is not deliberately forgetting or not minding. It is just that these simple tasks that require sustained attention and keeping things in mind are much harder for him than for others. (The executive functions of the brain appear to be impaired in such children [Barkley 1997].) So, the trick for adults is to cut the kid a little slack, avoid punitive or harsh approaches (which often backfire with these kids), be patient in giving repeated and necessary reminders, and use positive approaches (e.g., a reward system for appropriate home or school behavior) and lots of praise when he shows appropriate behaviors. For most kids with ADHD, this strategy eventually sinks in, and it avoids the negative interactions between the child and adults that can result in escalating aggression and failure across an ever greater number of settings and situations.

Most children with ADHD—more than 90%—respond to one or more of several stimulant medications (Swanson 1993). For a child just starting medications, I will often choose one of the longer-acting agents, such as methylphenidate (Concerta; 18 mg) or Adderall XR (10 mg), gradually titrating upward every 3–5 days based on phone contact and updates from the parents regarding response and any possible side effects. Medications should be titrated upward to achieve either a point at which the child's functioning is comparable to most classroom peers (i.e., "no room for improvement") or a point at which side effects prohibit higher doses. If this strategy does not yield a good response, another stimulant class (e.g., switching from methylphenidate to an amphetamine compound) should be tried (Greenhill 2002). Substantial evidence supports the efficacy of the tricyclic antidepressants as well, and they should be considered when no stimulant has proved to be satisfactory (Biederman and Spencer 2002). Other agents also have good evidence for efficacy, including bupropion (Wellbutrin) and a selective norepinephrine reuptake inhibitor recently approved by the U.S. Food and Drug Administration, atomoxetine (Strattera). This latter agent has the advantages of once-daily dosing and of not being considered a controlled substance by the Drug Enforcement Agency, thus making prescription refills less problematic. Since 2000, we have also seen the advent of truly efficacious all-day (12-hour) preparations of the stimulants, thereby avoiding the need for in-school dosing as well as avoiding problems of giving medication in the later afternoon (Greenhill 2002).

Although medications are significantly more effective than behavior therapy for most children, many children obtain some additional benefits from behavioral modification programs in home and school settings (Hinshaw et al. 1998). The added behavioral components may be especially effective for children with multiple comorbidities (Jensen et al. 2001) and strongly valued by parents and teachers, who often feel somewhat helpless if all they have to offer is medication. Recent evidence suggests that the overall most effective strategy is the combination of medication and behavioral therapy (Hinshaw et al. 1998; Jensen et al. 2001).

Behavioral therapies (Hinshaw et al. 1998) include the parent (or teacher) working with the child to identify target behaviors that need to be encouraged (or eliminated) and then implementing a program of short- and long-term positive rewards for the child maintaining appropriate behaviors, as well as judicious and sparing use of negative consequences (e.g., loss of privileges, time out).

For example, in Eddie's case, it might be very sensible for the parents and teachers together to institute a program to encourage his on-task behavior at school, which would be supported by his parents providing a reward after school if his behavior has been appropriate. One typical method is for the teacher to fill out a short checklist (a daily behavioral "report card") of four to five behaviors that she or he wants to reinforce in Eddie. This report card is then tucked into his backpack and is brought home to his parents. If Eddie is able to perform a certain number of these behaviors (e.g., four of five), then he gets to choose from a menu of rewards that he and his parents have worked out ahead of time, such as the chance for some extra bike-riding time, or half an hour of video-game time, etc. Over time, as Eddie succeeds in meeting the goal, the frequency and difficulty of the daily target behaviors are increased, thereby gradually "shaping" his behavior into ever more appropriate patterns. Physicians without extensive experience in these therapies should find an expert colleague to whom the child can be referred, and/or they might obtain additional training in such methods via continuing medical education courses.

Academic remediation (e.g., making a tutor available for a child who is struggling in a given topical area) is often a very useful additional method. When significant conflict has arisen in the classroom or if the child and teacher have been unable to form a good relationship, a change of teachers is sometimes helpful to give the child a fresh start. Physicians should assist parents in obtaining special school resources and services when warranted, as is often the case, under the Individuals With Disabilities Education Act or under Section 504 of the Americans With Disabilities Act.

Because of media misinformation they may have heard, parents may be concerned about the possibility that stimulant treatments can lead to a long-term risk for substance abuse. However, most of the research evidence points in just the opposite direction—namely, well-delivered treatments reduce risk for later substance use (Wilens 2002). Likewise, parents may be concerned about the adverse effects of these medications on the child's developing brain. Here, again, there is little evidence to support such concerns, and the available evidence shows that untreated ADHD has quite significant effects not just for short-term but also for intermediate- and longer-term outcomes (Loney et al. 2002).

Despite persistent media focus on putative causes of ADHD, diet, food additives such as dyes, refined sugar, too much television, and trace minerals have not been shown to have any causal relationship with ADHD (Arnold 2002). Genetic factors, pre- and perinatal events, and head trauma have all been implicated as possible partial causes (Swanson and Castellanos 2002), but no complete understanding of the etiology of ADHD is yet available.

In many instances, ADHD is a gratifying disorder to treat, as treatment responses are often immediate and dramatic. Many of the longer-term problematic outcomes are thought to be related to the accumulation of comorbidities over time, which in and of themselves can be quite devastating (e.g., Conduct Disorder, substance use, and school failure). Helping children with ADHD often simply boils down to helping them survive the school years with enough pockets of strength and sufficient self-esteem and skill areas so that once they choose their own vocational area, they are not burdened by antisocial behavioral patterns, legal problems, substance use, or their own or their families' lowered expectations.

References

Arnold LEA: Treatment alternatives for attention deficit hyperactivity disorder, in Attention Deficit Hyperactivity Disorder: State of the Science; Best Practices. Edited by Jensen PS, Cooper JR. Kingston, NJ, Civic Research Institute, 2002, pp 13-1–13-29

Barkley RA: Behavioral inhibition, sustained attention, and executive functions: constructing a unifying theory of ADHD. Psych Bull 121:65–94, 1997

Biederman J, Spencer TJ: Non-stimulant treatments for ADHD, in Attention Deficit Hyperactivity Disorder: State of the Science; Best Practices. Edited by Jensen PS, Cooper JR. Kingston, NJ, Civic Research Institute, 2002, pp 11-1–11-16

Biederman J, Newcorn J, Sprich S: Comorbidity of attention deficit hyperactivity disorder with conduct, depressive, anxiety, and other disorders. Am J Psychiatry 148:564–577, 1991

Greenhill LL: Stimulant medication treatment of children with attention deficit hyperactivity disorder, in Attention Deficit Hyperactivity Disorder: State of the Science; Best Practices. Edited by Jensen PS, Cooper JR. Kingston, NJ, Civic Research Institute, 2002, pp 9-1–9-27

Greenhill LL, Swanson JM, Vitiello B, et al: Determining the best dose of methylphenidate under controlled conditions: lessons from the MTA titration. J Am Acad Child Adolesc Psychiatry 40:180–187, 2001

Hinshaw SP: Is ADHD an impairing condition in childhood and adolescence?, in Attention Deficit Hyperactivity Disorder: State of the Science; Best Practices. Edited by Jensen PS, Cooper JR. Kingston, NJ, Civic Research Institute, 2002, pp 5-1–5-21

Hinshaw SP, Klein RG, Abikoff H: Childhood attention-deficit hyperactivity disorder: nonpharmacologic and combination treatments, in A Guide to Treatments That Work. Edited by Nathan PE, Gorman JM. New York, Oxford University Press, 1998, pp 26–41

Hinshaw SP, Owens EB, Wells KC, et al: Family processes and treatment outcome in the MTA: negative/ineffective parenting practices in relation to multimodal treatment. J Abnorm Child Psychol 28:555–568, 2002

Jensen PS, Cooper JR (eds): Attention Deficit Hyperactivity Disorder: State of the Science; Best Practices. Kingston, NJ, Civic Research Institute, 2002

Jensen PS, Kettle L, Roper MS, et al: Are stimulants over-prescribed? treatment of ADHD in four U.S. communities. J Am Acad Child Adolesc Psychiatry 38:797–804, 1999

Jensen PS, Hinshaw SP, Kraemer HC, et al: ADHD comorbidity findings from the MTA study: comparing comorbid subgroups. J Am Acad Child Adolesc Psychiatry 40:147–158, 2001

Loney J, Kramer JR, Salisbury H: Medicated and unmedicated ADHD children—adult involvement with legal and illegal drugs, in Attention Deficit Hyperactivity Disorder: State of the Science; Best Practices. Edited by Jensen PS, Cooper JR. Kingston, NJ, Civic Research Institute, 2002, pp 17-1–17-16

MTA Cooperative Group: A 14-month randomized clinical trial of treatment strategies for attention deficit hyperactivity disorder. Arch Gen Psychiatry 56:1073–1086, 1999a

MTA Cooperative Group: Moderators and mediators of treatment response for children with attention-deficit/hyperactivity disorder. Arch Gen Psychiatry 56:1088–1096, 1999b

Swanson J: Effect of stimulant medication on hyperactive children: a review of reviews. Exceptional Child 60:154–162, 1993

Swanson JM, Castellanos FX: Biologic bases of ADHD: neuroanatomy, genetics, and pathophysiology, in Attention Deficit Hyperactivity Disorder: State of the Science; Best Practices. Edited by Jensen PS, Cooper JR. Kingston, NJ, Civic Research Institute, 2002, pp 7-1–7-20

Wilens TE: Attention deficit hyperactivity disorder and substance use disorders—the nature of the relationship, subtypes at risk, and treatment issues, in Attention Deficit Hyperactivity Disorder: State of the Science; Best Practices. Edited by Jensen PS, Cooper JR. Kingston, NJ, Civic Research Institute, 2002, pp 19-1–19-17

Roller Coaster

When Ernest Eaton's desperate wife finally convinced him to agree to a comprehensive inpatient evaluation, he was 37, was unemployed, and had been essentially nonfunctional for several years. After a week during which he was partying all night and shopping all day, his wife said that she would leave him if he did not check into a psychiatric hospital. The admitting psychiatrist found Mr. Eaton to be a fast-talking, jovial, seductive man with no evidence of delusions or hallucinations.

Mr. Eaton's troubles began 7 years earlier when he was working as an insurance adjuster and had a few months of mild, intermittent, depressive symptoms, anxiety, fatigue, insomnia, and loss of appetite. At the time, he attributed these symptoms to stress at work, and within a few months, he was back to his usual self.

A few years later, an asymptomatic thyroid mass was noted during a routine physical examination of Mr. Eaton. One month after removal of the mass (a papillary cyst), Mr. Eaton noted dramatic mood changes. Twenty-five days of remarkable energy, hyperactivity, and euphoria were followed by 5 days of depression, during which he slept a lot and felt that he could hardly move. This pattern of alternating periods of elation and depression, apparently with few "normal" days, repeated itself continuously over the following years.

During his energetic periods, Mr. Eaton was optimistic and self-confident but was also short tempered and easily irritated. His judgment at work was erratic. He spent large sums of money on unnecessary and, for him, uncharacteristic purchases, such as a high-priced stereo system and several Doberman pinschers. He also had several impulsive sexual flings. During his depressed periods, he often stayed in bed all day because of fatigue, lack of motivation, and depressed mood. He felt guilty about the irresponsibilities and excesses of the previous several weeks. He stopped eating, bathing, and shaving. After several days of this withdrawal, Mr. Eaton would rise from bed one morning feeling better and, within 2 days, be back at work, often working feverishly, although ineffectively, to catch up on work he had let slide during his depressed periods.

Although both Mr. Eaton and his wife denied any drug use, other than drinking binges during his hyperactive periods, Mr. Eaton had been dismissed from his job 5 years previously because his supervisor was convinced that his overactivity was due to drug use. Mrs. Eaton has supported him financially since then.

When he finally agreed to a psychiatric evaluation 2 years ago, Mr. Eaton was minimally cooperative and noncompliant with several medications that were prescribed, including lithium, neuroleptics, and antidepressants. His mood swings continued with few interruptions up to the current hospitalization.

In the hospital results of his physical examination, blood chemistry, blood counts, computed tomography scan, and cognitive testing were unremarkable. Thyroid function testing revealed some laboratory evidence of thyroid hypofunction, but he was without clinical signs of thyroid disease. After 1 week in the hospital, he switched to his characteristic depressive state.

DSM-IV-TR Casebook Diagnosis of "Roller Coaster"

The diagnosis of Bipolar I Disorder, Most Recent Episode Manic, is not difficult to make in this case (DSM-IV-TR, p. 389). In his energetic periods, Mr. Eaton had the characteristic symptoms of a manic episode: decreased need for sleep, overactivity, overtalkativeness, and excessive involvement in pleasurable activities without thinking of the consequences. In his depressed periods, he met the symptom but not the duration, which are criteria for major depressive episodes. Because he had had more than four episodes of mania in a 1-year period, separated by periods of depression, the Bipolar I Disorder is further qualified as With Rapid Cycling (DSM-IV-TR, p. 428).

Unlike Mr. Eaton, not all persons with rapid cycling experience predictable shifts from mania to depression without intervening periods of euthymia. Rapid cycling usually involves one or more manic or hypomanic episodes, as in this case, but is also diagnosed if all of the episodes are depressed, manic, or hypomanic, so long as they are separated by periods of remission (or switches to the opposite pole).

Follow-Up

After 3 weeks in the hospital, Mr. Eaton's mood was stabilized by the use of lithium and thyroxine, the latter being added for mood stabilization as opposed to treating the laboratory evidence of thyroid hypofunction. He left the hospital, very quickly found a new job, and did well for the following year. Because Mr. Eaton felt well, he decided that he did not need the medication and stopped taking the lithium. Within weeks, he became extremely manic and had to be hospitalized again.

Discussion of "Roller Coaster" by Gary S. Sachs, M.D.*

Mr. Eaton has Bipolar I Disorder and a history of rapid cycling. Once this diagnosis is established, treatment would be conducted in accordance with the Rapid Cycling Treatment Pathway used in our clinic, which organizes management of rapid cycling around seven main decision points. The first decision point in this general approach is to determine the need to treat an acute episode. As shown in this case, symptoms of acute mania generally warrant inpatient treatment.

---

*Dr. Sachs is Associate Professor in Psychiatry at Harvard Medical School, Clinical Assistant in Psychiatry and Director of the Bipolar Mood Disorder Program at Massachusetts General Hospital, and Director of the Partners Bipolar Treatment Center. Dr. Sachs earned his medical degree at the University of Maryland School of Medicine. He was an intern in family practice and psychiatry at the University of Maryland Hospital in Baltimore and was a resident in psychiatry and Chief Resident of the Acute Psychiatry Service at Massachusetts General Hospital in Boston. Dr. Sachs is the Principal Investigator of the National Institute of Mental Health Systematic Treatment Enhancement Program for Bipolar Disorder. He serves on the scientific advisory board of the National Depression and Manic Depression Association, is Co–Editor-in-Chief of Clinical Approaches to Bipolar Disorder, and is on numerous editorial boards. Dr. Sachs has authored more than 150 articles, abstracts, books, reviews, and book chapters.

Although rapid cycling was defined in reference to Mr. Eaton's poor response to lithium, his reported response to lithium and thyroxine made it reasonable to offer this treatment again during the acute manic phase. Given his previous excellent response to treatment, his prognosis after resumption of his prior treatment regimen appears to be quite good. It is not unusual for treatments that have been declared ineffective to prove beneficial when used consistently. Evidence supports the use of thyroxine at high doses for refractory rapid cycling. The thyroxine dose in this case is not stated, but its use requires monitoring. A more in-depth review of his current symptom acuity and cycle frequency over the last four episodes might well result in alternative or additional acute treatment, such as an atypical antipsychotic medication or benzodiazepine. Once a stable remission has been achieved, however, the focus of treatment shifts to prevention of recurrence and maximizing the patient's quality of life. The time when the patient is in remission offers an opportunity to review the decision about continuing thyroxine over the long term and whether there is need for additional endocrine workup.

The second decision point—evaluation of potential secondary factors—includes not only consideration of neuroendocrine status, psychoactive substance use, sleep habits, and comorbid general medical conditions but also management of interpersonal relationships and lifestyle issues such as occupational demands or travel that might undermine circadian stability.

Mr. Eaton's subclinical thyroid status adds a measure of uncertainty and complexity to the diagnostic formulation. Hypothyroidism is not considered an etiological factor in producing acute mania, so the occurrence of mania justifies the diagnosis of a primary bipolar Mood Disorder. Researchers have not consistently found the association of hypothyroidism with rapid cycling (Bauer et al. 1990; Cowdry et al. 1983; Kusalic 1992; Wehr et al. 1988). Therefore, diagnosing Mr. Eaton with Bipolar I Disorder is well established. The rapid cycling course of his illness, however, could arise either as part of his primary disorder or secondary to his thyroid status. His use of alcohol may not meet criteria for abuse, but binge drinking would nonetheless be an important issue to consider for treatment. A discussion with Mr. Eaton aimed at obtaining a negotiated commitment to an extended period of sobriety is important. Uncontrolled Bipolar Disorder and uncontrolled drinking are synergistic risk factors for suicide and other potentially disastrous outcomes. Disulfiram (Antabuse) would also be offered to help him sustain his resolve to manage his drinking (Isometsa 2001; Nilsson and Axelsson 1990).

Decision point three recommends a gradual taper of any standard antidepressants that might currently be in use. We know that Mr. Eaton is not taking any antidepressant medication.

Decision point four recommends optimizing or adding mood-stabilizing agents. Given Mr. Eaton's prior experience with lithium, it appears to be a good choice, presuming its success in the current acute phase is sustained, but it is important to determine whether Mr. Eaton finds lithium acceptable.

Mr. Eaton should be encouraged to participate in a review of medication, lifestyle, and psychotherapeutic options. In his case, once the acute symptoms permit productive discussion, it would be useful to work collaboratively with him and his family on a long-term treatment plan aimed at prevention of future recurrence. A decision to stop medication after 1 year of being well is quite common, particularly early in the course of bipolar illness. Discussion of this decision offers an opportunity for iterative improvement in the treatment plan.

If adverse effects of lithium played a substantial role in Mr. Eaton's decision to discontinue use, alternatives should be offered. The presentation of multiple options allows the patient to select treatments from a "menu of reasonable choices." Lamotrigine has been shown to be beneficial for patients with rapid cycling and also delays the recurrence of the episodes in non–rapid-cycling patients. Valproic acid (Valproate), carbamazepine, and atypical antipsychotic agents such as olanzapine are also evidence-based options for long-term treatment. Mr. Eaton and those who support him should be made aware of the side effect profile of each treatment option and learn simple strategies for good mood hygiene. Specific forms of psychosocial intervention, such as cognitive-behavioral therapy, family-focused therapy, and interpersonal social rhythm therapy, may also be helpful adjuncts to mood-stabilizing medication.

The decision to discontinue treatment often represents discordance between the patient's view of his or her condition and the view of care providers and significant others around the patient. There is frequent misunderstanding or disagreement about the nature of the patient's diagnosis. Hence, the period immediately after an acute episode is a time to focus on building concordance between the patient and care providers. Improving the level of agreement between care providers and the patient is a major objective of long-term treatment. The patient and family should understand that, by nature, Bipolar Disorder is a chronic recurrent condition. In this context, it is often helpful to have the patient describe and name his or her condition. Although desirable, agreement on whether to label the condition "Bipolar Disorder" or "rapid cycling" should not be made an obstacle to dispensing treatment. Treatment decisions for Mr. Eaton can be discussed in reference to his relative youth and his history of occupational accomplishment. People do sometimes make bad choices for themselves, but a collaborative approach in which patients are presented reasonable choices and a realistic appraisal of their prognosis can lead to better treatment adherence, because most patients are more likely to behave in accordance with plans that reflect their input and personal preferences.

The level of concordance—the degree to which clinicians and patients are in agreement on the appropriate diagnosis and treatment—fluctuates as a function of three main factors: current clinical status, therapeutic alliance, and accumulated individual experience. It is helpful to explicitly recognize the interplay between mood symptoms and the ability to sustain a treatment plan made during a period of euthymia. The tendency for treatment plans to be honored during periods of wellness is reassuring; however, even long-standing plans are easily cast aside when illness distorts judgment. Patients often discontinue medication as a means by which to demonstrate their wellness. In a written collaborative care plan, the patient can describe early signs of impending episodes and establish directives for specific interventions by family members and care providers. By distributing their plan for managing foreseeable contingencies to their closest supports, patients retain autonomy during periods of wellness but empower others to act on their behalf in times when illness impairs their judgment. Many patients will understand this as a process similar to constitutional provisions for a vice presidency.

The fifth decision point—evaluate treatment outcome—establishes the feedback loop between intervention and assessment. Ongoing management includes systematic clinical assessments of mood state, laboratory monitoring, management of adverse effects, encouragement of good mood hygiene, sobriety, and daily mood charting. These can be used specifically to assess the benefit of each intervention. It is reasonable to evaluate treatment outcome over a period of three cycle lengths or 6 months, whichever is longer. Few patients enjoy full resolution of cycling over the first year of treatment, but longitudinal records in the chart indicating that episodes are becoming fewer, briefer, and/or milder encourages continuation of the treatment plan.

Lack of improvement, however, brings the patient to the sixth decision point: add additional mood-stabilizing interventions. Although the order in which agents are implemented should again reflect collaboration with the patient, the most benign agents with proven efficacy, such as those mentioned earlier, are offered before unproved agents or those with substantial risk for intolerable adverse affects.

Patients who experience years of sustained rapid cycling in the absence of a secondary factor are often poorly responsive to treatment. These patients may face health risks due to the accumulation of an excessive number of ineffective medications. Thus, it is reasonable to discontinue a treatment when an intervention has had no benefit or has contributed to apparent worsening.

The seventh decision point is as follows: At each follow-up visit, consider the possibility that the priority of treatment will need to shift back to treatment of an acute episode. This recommendation does not conflict with the general approach already described when the episode is mixed, manic, or hypomanic, but depressive symptomatology may necessitate periods of antidepressant use. The determination to use potentially destabilizing interventions should be made in light of the need to maintain patient safety and the patient's individual tolerance for dysphoria.

References

Bauer MS, Whybrow PC, Winokur A: Rapid cycling bipolar affective disorder, I: association with grade I hypothyroidism. Arch Gen Psychiatry 47(5):427–432, 1990

Cowdry RW, Wehr TA, Zis AP, et al: Thyroid abnormalities associated with rapid-cycling bipolar illness. Arch Gen Psychiatry 40(4):414–420, 1983

Isometsa ET: Psychological autopsy studies—a review. Eur Psychiatry 16(7):379–385, 2001

Kusalic M: Grade II and grade III hypothyroidism in rapid-cycling bipolar patients. Neuropsychobiology 25(4):177–181, 1992

Nilsson A, Axelsson R: Lithium discontinuers, I: clinical characteristics and outcome. Acta Psychiatr Scand 82(6):433–438, 1990

Wehr TA, Sack DA, Rosenthal NE, et al: Rapid cycling affective disorder: contributing factors and treatment responses in 51 patients. Am J Psychiatry 145(2):179–184, 1988

Suggested Reading

American Psychiatric Association: Diagnostic and Statistical Manual of Mental Disorders, 4th Edition, Text Revision. Washington, DC, American Psychiatric Association, 2000

Bauer M, McBride L: Structured Group Psychotherapy for Bipolar Disorder: The Life Goals Program. New York, Springer Publishing Company, 1996

Bauer MS, Whybrow PC: Rapid cycling bipolar affective disorder, II: treatment of refractory rapid cycling with high-dose levothyroxine: a preliminary study. Arch Gen Psychiatry 47(5):435–440, 1990

Bowden CL, Calabrese JR, Sachs G, et al: A placebo-controlled 18-month trial of lamotrigine and lithium maintenance treatment in recently manic or hypomanic patients with bipolar I disorder. Arch Gen Psychiatry 60(4):392–400, 2003

Cole DP, Thase ME, Mallinger AG, et al: Slower treatment response in bipolar depression predicted by lower pretreatment thyroid function. Am J Psychiatry 159:116–121, 2002

Coryell W, Endicott J, Keller M: Rapid cycling affective disorder: demographics, diagnosis, family, and course. Arch Gen Psychiatry 49:126–131, 1992

Dunner D, Fieve R: Clinical factors in lithium carbonate prophylaxis failure. Arch Gen Psychiatry 30:229–233, 1974

Frank EK, Kupfer DJ, Ehlers CL, et al: Interpersonal and social rhythm therapy for bipolar disorder: integrating interpersonal and behavioral approaches. Behav Therapist 17:143–149, 1994

Miklowitz D: Psychotherapy in combination with drug treatment for bipolar disorder. J Clin Psychopharmacol 16(suppl 1):56S–66S, 1996

Sachs GS, Thase MT: Bipolar Disorder: A Systematic Approach to Treatment. London, Dunitz Press, 2000

Sachs GS, Thase M: Bipolar disorder therapeutics: maintenance treatment. Biol Psychiatry 48:573–581, 2000

Strakowski SM, DelBello MP, Fleck DE, et al: The impact of substance abuse on the course of bipolar disorder. Biol Psychiatry 48:477–485, 2000

Still a Student

Ellen Waters's psychotherapist referred her for a medication consultation because of her continuing depressed mood and panic attacks. She is a 37-year-old part-time graduate student who lives alone and supports herself by working as a home health aide. She completed the course work for a Ph.D. in sociology 3 years ago but has not yet begun her thesis.

Ellen is indeed an unhappy-looking woman, and she describes herself as being unhappy through much of her life, with no long periods of feeling really good. Her father had a history of alcohol problems, and there was always a great deal of strife in her parents' marriage. She denies sexual or physical abuse but feels that her parents were "emotionally abusive" to her. She was first referred for treatment after she made a suicide attempt at age 14, and there have been many times over the years during which her usual low-level depression has become considerably worse, but she has not sought treatment.

Two years ago, when she had been seeing her current boyfriend for about 4 years, it became clear to her that he was unwilling to marry her or live with her. She began to get more depressed and to experience acute panic attacks; it was at that time that she entered psychotherapy.

Ellen says she was depressed most of the time during the month before the consultation. She had gained about 10 pounds because she was constantly nibbling on chips or cookies or making herself peanut butter sandwiches. She often awakened in the middle of the night, was unable to go back to sleep for hours, and then overslept the following day, often sleeping up to 18 hours. She says she feels like dead weight, her legs and arms are heavy, and she is always tired. She ruminates about her own failures and cannot concentrate on any serious reading. Although she often wishes to be dead, she has not made any recent suicide attempts.

Ellen's mood is clearly reactive to favorable events. Small attentions from her therapist or her boyfriend can cause her to feel really good for hours at a time. She has an equally extreme reaction to any sort of rejection. If a friend does not return a call, or if someone appears romantically interested and then withdraws, then she feels devastated to the point where she cannot work. She then stays at home, overeats, and avoids people.

Ellen's academic and vocational histories have been erratic. She has a master's degree in psychology and worked as a counselor for a while but found this work too upsetting. She then began a Ph.D. program in sociology and completed her course work but interrupted her studies to train in physical therapy. She has never worked in one job for more than a few years and has spent much of her adult life as a student. Her current romance is the longest she has sustained. She lived with a man once, but this relationship was brief and tumultuous. Boyfriends have described her as "needy and clinging," and it appears that her current boyfriend fears her neediness.

Although Ellen reports chronic depression, when she is asked about "high" periods, she describes many episodes of abnormally elevated mood that have lasted for several months. During these times, she would function on 4 or 5 hours of sleep a night, run up huge telephone bills, and feel that her thoughts were racing. She was able to get a lot done, but her friends were obviously concerned about the change in her behavior, urging her to "slow down" and "calm down." She has never gotten into any real trouble during these episodes.

DSM-IV-TR Casebook Diagnosis of "Still a Student"

Ellen's long history of mild depressive symptoms suggests the diagnosis of Dysthymic Disorder. However, her many episodes of elevated mood, decreased sleep, increased activity, and racing thoughts clearly indicate Hypomanic Episodes (DSM-IV-TR, p. 368), which rules out a diagnosis of Dysthymic Disorder in favor of a diagnosis of Bipolar II Disorder (DSM-IV-TR, p. 397). Because she currently has a Major Depressive Episode (weight gain, insomnia, trouble concentrating, self-deprecation, suicidal ideation), it would be further specified as Current Episode Depressed.

Whereas most patients with a Major Depressive Episode have trouble sleeping and loss of appetite, Ellen often sleeps 18 hours and has an increase in appetite. These features, often referred to as "reverse vegetative symptoms," in the presence of rejection sensitivity and depressed mood that brightens in response to positive events, warrant the additional specification of With Atypical Features. This clinical picture has been demonstrated to be associated with good response to monoamine oxidase inhibitors and poorer response to traditional tricyclic antidepressant medications.

Ellen also complains of "panic attacks." We suspect that she has the characteristic symptoms of panic attacks and concern about their recurrence but that she does not have agoraphobic symptoms. If this were the case, we would add the diagnosis of Panic Disorder Without Agoraphobia (DSM-IV-TR, p. 440).

Discussion of "Still a Student" by Mark Bauer, M.D.*

When Ellen was a child, psychiatry in America was in the throes of a serious identity crisis. The previously solid psychoanalytic basis for much of psychiatry, so strongly laid down in the post–World War II years, had become progressively enfeebled by its inability to address major theoretical and clinical issues empirically. Meanwhile, Szasz, Laing, Bateman, and the like were claiming that all mental disorders were

---

*Dr. Bauer received his B.A. from the University of Chicago and his M.D. from the University of Pennsylvania. He is currently Associate Professor of Psychiatry at Brown University and on staff at the Providence (RI) Veterans Affairs Medical Center. He has served as Principal Investigator on federal grants each year since residency and has received awards for research, teaching, administration, and clinical care, including twice being named Exemplary Psychiatrist by the National Alliance for the Mentally Ill. Dr. Bauer's scientific contributions have included use of high-dose thyroid hormone treatment for rapid-cycling Bipolar Disorder, as well as advances in assessment, phenomenology, and course in Bipolar Disorder. Since 1991, his focus has been on developing and testing methods to improve treatment delivery for manic-depressive disorder, particularly using collaborative practice approaches. Two books by Dr. Bauer outline the collaborative practice approach discussed here—one in great detail for Bipolar Disorder (Bauer and McBride 2003) and the other in summary form for use in general clinical practice with various disorders (Bauer 2003a).

products of psychosocial factors—some going so far as to claim that serious mental disorders like schizophrenia were the only sane response to an insane society. On the other hand, Klein, Fieve, Dunner, Rickels, Prien, Goodwin, Emrich, and other fathers of modern psychopharmacology were providing incontrovertible evidence that complex behavioral disorders could be eradicated and normal function could be restored to many by the administration of simple pharmaceutical compounds. Less astute minds used these important advances to suggest that psychiatry should slough off its psychosocial roots and become a medical subspecialty.

George L. Engel stepped into the fray with his landmark article in *Science*, articulating a biopsychosocial model for all of medicine, including psychiatry (1977). In effect, Engel said that psychiatry is positioned exactly where it should be, with practitioners and theoretical bases that can address both the biological and psychosocial roots of clinical problems. Medicine and surgery should follow us in taking a biopsychosocial approach to all the problems they treat, even those as acute and seemingly purely biological as acute myocardial infarction. There's likely to be a psychosocial root to all these problems…and even if there's not, psychosocial factors must be addressed in assessing individuals with these problems and in planning treatment for them.

Let's now take a biopsychosocial look at assessment and treatment planning for Ellen. First, there are four assessment principles that will guide us to the appropriate diagnostic thought processes (Bauer 2003a):

1. *A symptom does not make a syndrome.* What are Ellen's main presenting symptoms? The symptoms are depression, panic, and her intriguing mood reactivity and rejection sensitivity. It is easy to jump from any of these symptoms to a syndrome or diagnosis—easy but fraught with error. One could err in assuming the problem was a personality disorder or an adjustment disorder and consign Ellen to years of general supportive psychotherapy. One could also err by assuming she simply has a major depressive disorder or panic disorder and blithely prescribe medications because of how (putatively) safe they have become of late. More information is needed, and, had it been obtained, Ellen might have been saved a number of years of suffering. In fact, it is typical for individuals like Ellen to go 7 years with the disorder before the appropriate diagnosis is made (Lish et al. 1994).

2. *Diagnosis drives treatment.* Just as in other fields of medicine, the diagnosis determines the treatment. If we skip the step of diagnosis and, say, toss a "safe" selective serotonin reuptake inhibitor Ellen's way to treat her panic and her depressive symptoms, we are liable to get her into trouble. How?

3. *Psychiatric disorder is longitudinal as well as cross-sectional.* Even if we demonstrate that Ellen has a current major depressive episode, even one with atypical features, this does not yet give us an accurate diagnosis. If we look at Ellen's case longitudinally, we see that she has also had what appear to be mild hypomanic episodes. Clearly, giving antidepressants alone to an individual with Bipolar II Disorder without providing close follow-up and good education is perilous because of the ability of antidepressants to precipitate hypomania (e.g., Joffe et al. 2002).

4. *All behaviors have a differential diagnosis.* All behaviors, not just symptoms, have a differential diagnosis. As we identify Ellen's hypomanic symptoms, although they may fulfill DSM criteria, we must still ask, "Should these symptoms be a focus of treatment? Or, are they acceptable behaviors to her?" We should recall that the *sine qua non* for a DSM diagnosis is that the symptoms must cause dysfunction or subjective suffering. What if Ellen builds her life around these hypomanic periods? What if she does not want to give them up? This issue will need to be addressed in a collaborative practice framework.

So here we have Ellen: She has Bipolar II Disorder and is now depressed with atypical features and panic attacks. The solution is to pull out the medications and give her some basic education and coping-with-living advice, right? Is that all?

First, let's turn to the issue of medications. This issue is the easy part. There is no shortage of clinical practice guidelines to help us, including the evidence-based guidelines of the American Psychiatric Association (2002), Canadian Psychiatric Association (Haslam et al. 1997), U.S. Department of Veterans Affairs (Bauer et al. 1999), and the Texas Department of Mental Health and Mental Retardation (Suppes et al. 2002) or the expert survey–based Expert Consensus Guidelines (Sachs et al. 2000)—albeit each is supported by the same modest amount of empirical data (Bauer and Mitchner 2004). From my perspective, I might propose lithium or perhaps lamotrigine (Lamictal) because these have the best documented efficacy for acute depressive episodes during Bipolar Disorder. If conditions were favorable—and we will see about this as we think biopsychosocially and collaboratively below—I might suggest monoamine oxidase inhibitors, such as tranylcypromine (Parnate) or phenelzine (Nardil), which have been shown to be quite effective in a couple of controlled trials in patients with depressive episodes with atypical features in Bipolar Disorder (Himmelhoch et al. 1991; Thase et al. 1992), as well as in patients with atypical depression with panic attacks (Quitkin et al. 1990). Serotonin reuptake inhibitors are also an option because they have a more benign safety profile, although there are few controlled trial efficacy data for their use in atypical depressive episodes.

But let's first find out what Ellen thinks. Why? It is certainly a good thing to approach the individuals who present to us for help as key players in their own treatment simply by virtue of basic human dignity considerations, but it also makes good clinical sense:

- In an assessment, we are likely to obtain the best information from Ellen if she knows that we are trying to understand her own point of view of the symptoms and their impact on her.
- In terms of treatment, it is critical to collaborate and identify a list of target symptoms or a problem list that is prioritized based on the individual's values and needs.
- Similarly, to maximize adherence, we need to identify those side effects (pharmacologic but also psychotherapeutic) that Ellen wants most to avoid, and all treatments have costs as well as benefits (see Bauer 2003a).

Our role in this collaborative approach is to be less of a paternalistic clinician and more of a "coach" who seeks to assist Ellen in living with her specific difficulties. We bring to bear our professional expertise and experience but not necessarily our values.

What bothers Ellen most? Undoubtedly, she is bothered most by the depression and the panic. Depression is what causes most of the dysfunction in Bipolar Disorder, and even subsyndromal levels of depression cause dysfunction (reviewed in Bauer et al. 2001).

So, at least the depression and panic need treatment. Now, if we consider psychosocial aspects of her illness, we begin to ask more questions about the person who has the illness. Is Ellen intelligent and motivated enough to manage her illness with some degree of independence? Can she relate her typical pattern of symptoms during episodes and, of critical importance, recognize and report her early warning symptoms? Can she identify triggers to episodes? Can she appropriately access care between sessions? What are her own coping patterns when she is having trouble with symptoms? Does she withdraw? Does she "play with pain"—that is, can she continue to function in her various roles despite her depressive symptoms? Does she drink or take drugs? And what are the costs and benefits of each individual response (i.e., there are costs and benefits for every coping response, however apparently ill-advised or socially acceptable)? Finally, does she reside within a social nexus that supports her in symptom monitoring and treatment compliance, or are there likely to be impediments?

So, if Ellen is a sufficiently astute manager of her illness and if her hypomanias are not too destructive, we may be able to utilize tranylcypromine or phenelzine alone, as long as she can identify early warning symptoms; she has others who can help her do so, preferably; and she has adequate access to her providers. Otherwise, management with lithium or lamotrigine might be a safer first bet; an antidepressant could be added if response was insufficient.

Here's another point at which our professional expertise will likely play a key role. Ellen says depression is the problem, but we know from our professional experience that hypomania can also be quite disruptive to relationships, work, etc. Moreover, the inconsistency in relationships and the swings themselves between manic and depressive symptoms confer a measure of morbidity: How do spouses, coworkers, and children react, act, and plan when they do not know whether "Dr. Jekyll" or "Ms. Hyde" will show up? So, we need to evaluate and educate around this issue.

Overall, it's quite likely that Ellen is not as astute an observer of her symptom profile, early warning signs, triggers, and coping responses as she could be. We can help her identify and work with these responses by using any of several psychosocial approaches, because these tasks appear to comprise the core of most psychosocial interventions for Bipolar Disorder (reviewed in Chapter 5 of Bauer and McBride 2003). It would be better if a formal psychotherapy were available to her, but if not, the same collaborative principles can be applied in any office-based setting by any trained clinician.

So, compared to these psychosocial factors, the biological choice of lithium versus lamotrigine versus tranylcypromine versus some combination seems relatively simple. It is the psychosocial factors—and the collaborative approach to them—that will make or break Ellen's biological treatment. In fact, a collaborative approach to helping such individuals with their "medical model" serious mental disorders might be considered to be a response, some 25 years later, to Engel's challenge to understand and intervene across the entire spectrum of biopsychosocial aspects of illness.

References

American Psychiatric Association: Practice guideline for the treatment of persons with bipolar disorder (revision). Am J Psychiatry 159(suppl):1–50, 2002

Bauer MS: The Field Guide to Psychiatric Assessment and Treatment. Philadelphia, PA, Lippincott Williams & Wilkins, 2003a

Bauer MS: Bipolar (manic-depressive) disorder, in Psychiatry. Edited by Tasman A, Kay J, Lieberman AJ. Philadelphia, PA, Saunders, 2003b, pp 1237–1270

Bauer MS, McBride L: Structured Group Psychotherapy for Bipolar Disorder: The Life Goals Program, 2nd Edition. New York, Springer, 2003

Bauer MS, Mitchner L: What is a "mood stabilizer?" an evidence-based response. Am J Psychiatry 161:3–18, 2004

Bauer MS, Callahan A, Jampala C, et al: Clinical practice guidelines for bipolar disorder from the Department of Veterans Affairs. J Clin Psychiatry 60:9–21, 1999

Bauer MS, Kirk G, Gavin C, et al: Correlates of functional and economic outcome in bipolar disorder: a prospective study. J Affect Disord 65:231–241, 2001

Engel GL: The need for a new medical model: a challenge for biomedicine. Science 129:186–196, 1977

Haslam D, Kennedy S, Kusumakar V, et al: The treatment of bipolar disorder: review of the literature, guidelines, and options. Can J Psychiatry 42:67S–99S, 1997

Himmelhoch J, Thase M, Mallinger A, et al: Tranylcypromine versus imipramine in anergic bipolar depression. Am J Psychiatry 148:910–916, 1991

Joffe RT, MacQueen GM, Marriott M, et al: Induction of mania and cycle acceleration in bipolar disorder: effect of different classes of antidepressant. Acta Psychiatr Scand 105:427–430, 2002

Lish J, Dime-Meenan S, Whybrow P, et al: The National Depressive and Manic Depressive (DMDA) survey of bipolar members. J Affective Disord 31:281–294, 1994

Quitkin FM, McGrath PJ, Stewart JW, et al: Atypical depression, panic attacks, and response to imipramine and phenelzine: a replication. Arch Gen Psychiatry 47:935–941, 1990

Sachs GS, Printz DJ, Kahn DA, et al: The Expert Consensus Guideline Series: Medication Treatment of Bipolar Disorder, 2000. Minneapolis, MN, Postgraduate Medicine, 2000

Suppes T, Dennehy EB, Swann AC, et al: Report of the Texas Consensus Conference Panel on Medication Treatment of Bipolar Disorder 2000. J Clin Psychiatry 63:288–299, 2002

Thase M, Mallinger A, McKnight D, et al: Treatment of imipramine-resistant recurrent depression, IV: a double-blind crossover study of tranylcypromine for anergic bipolar depression. Am J Psychiatry 149:195–198, 1992

Elephant Man

Chris is a shy, anxious-looking 31-year-old carpenter who has been hospitalized after making a suicide attempt by putting his head in a plastic bag. He asks to meet with the psychiatrist in a darkened room. He is wearing a baseball cap pulled down over his forehead that is partially covering his eyes. Looking down at the floor, Chris says he has no friends, has just been fired from his job, and was recently rejected by his girlfriend. When the psychiatrist asks Chris to elaborate, he replies, "It's really hard to talk about this, Doctor. I don't know if I can. It's too embarrassing. Well, I guess I should tell you...after all, I'm in the hospital because of it. It's my nose." "Your nose?" the psychiatrist asks. "Yes, these huge pockmarks on my nose. They're grotesque! I look like a monster. I'm as ugly as the Elephant Man! These marks on my nose are all I can think about. I've thought about them every day for the past 15 years. I even have nightmares about them. And I think that everyone can see them and that they laugh at me because of them. That's why I wear this hat all the time. And that's why I couldn't talk to you in a bright room...you'd see how ugly I am."

The psychiatrist couldn't see the huge pockmarks that Chris was referring to, even when she later met him in a brightly lit room. Chris is, in fact, a handsome man with normal-appearing facial pores. The psychiatrist says, "I see no ugly pockmarks. Is it possible that your view of your appearance is distorted, that maybe the pockmarks are just normal-looking facial pores?"

"That's a hard question to answer," Chris replies. "I've pretty much kept this preoccupation a secret because it's so embarrassing. I'm afraid people will think I'm vain. But I've told a few people about it, and they've tried to convince me that the pores really aren't visible. Sometimes I sort of believe them. I think I probably am distorting and that they're not so bad. Then I look in the mirror and see that they're huge and ugly, and I'm convinced that people laugh at them. Then no one can talk me out of it. When people try to, I think they just feel sorry for me and that they're trying to make me feel better. This has affected me in a lot of ways, Doctor," Chris adds. "It may be hard for you to believe, but this problem has ruined my life. All I can think about is my face. I spend hours a day looking at the marks in the mirror. But I just can't resist. I started missing more and more work, and I stopped going out with my friends and my girlfriend. I got so anxious when people looked at me that I started staying in the house most of the time. Sometimes when I did go out, I went through red lights so I wouldn't have to sit in my car at the light where people might be staring at me. The hat helped a little, but it didn't cover all the marks. I tried covering them with makeup for a while, but I thought people could see the makeup so that didn't really help. The only time I really felt comfortable was when I wore my nephew's Batman mask on Halloween. Then no one could see the marks. I missed so much work that I was fired. My girlfriend stuck it out with me for a long time, but she finally couldn't take it anymore. One thing that was really hard for her was that I started asking her about 50 times a day whether I looked okay and whether she could see the marks. I think that was the last straw. If I had a choice, I'd rather have cancer. It must be less painful. This is like an arrow through my heart."

Chris went on to discuss the fact that he had seen a dermatologist to request dermabrasion but was refused the procedure because "the dermatologist said there was nothing there." He finally convinced another dermatologist to do the procedure but thought it did not help. Eventually, he felt so desperate over the supposed marks that he made two suicide attempts. His most recent attempt occurred after he looked in the mirror and was horrified by what he saw. He told the psychiatrist, "I saw how awful I looked, and I thought, I'm not sure it's worth it to go on living if I have to look like this and think about this all the time." His first suicide attempt had also led to hospitalization, but, because Chris was so ashamed of his concern and thought it would not be taken seriously, he had kept it a secret and told the staff only that he was depressed.

DSM-IV-TR Casebook Diagnosis of "Elephant Man"

Chris looks normal but is preoccupied with a supposed defect in his appearance. This preoccupation has clearly caused him much distress and has significantly interfered with his functioning. Although this is a fairly severe case of Body Dysmorphic Disorder (BDD) (DSM-IV-TR, p. 510), it is not atypical; occupational, social, and other important areas of functioning may be severely impaired, and suicide attempts are not uncommon. However, the degree of distress and dysfunction associated with this disorder spans a spectrum of severity; some people with this disorder—although distressed and perhaps not functioning up to their capacity— nevertheless cope relatively well.

Discussion of "Elephant Man" by Katharine A. Phillips, M.D.,* and Rocco Crino, Ph.D.**

Chris has a severe—although not atypical—case of BDD (Phillips 1996, 2001). Like many other patients do, Chris initially told the hospital staff only that he was depressed, because he worried that if he mentioned his concern about his appearance, he would be considered silly or vain. Before BDD can be effectively treated, it must be appropriately diagnosed (Phillips 1996, 2001). Diagnosis is critically important because untreated BDD can cause severe impairment in functioning, hospitalization, and even suicide. A number of studies have documented that clinicians underrecognize and underdiagnose BDD (Phillips 2001). The patient may not volunteer the symptoms because of embarrassment and shame, and

*Dr. Phillips is Professor of Psychiatry at Brown Medical School and Director of the Body Dysmorphic Disorder and Body Image Program at Butler Hospital in Providence, Rhode Island. Dr. Phillips has been doing research and treating patients with BDD since 1990, which has involved approximately 800 individuals with this disorder. Her pioneering work, which has focused largely on BDD's psychopathology and pharmacological treatment, has brought this disorder to the attention of the public and professionals alike. She has written and edited several books on BDD and body image, including The Broken Mirror: Understanding and Treating Body Dysmorphic Disorder (Phillips 1996).
**Dr. Crino is Senior Lecturer in the School of Psychiatry at the University of New South Wales and Director of the Anxiety Disorders Unit at St. Vincent's Hospital in Sydney, Australia. Since 1988, Dr. Crino has worked extensively in the treatment of Obsessive-Compulsive Disorder and related conditions. In 1999, he established a cognitive-behavioral treatment program for BDD. He has published papers in the area of anxiety and related disorders and is coauthor of The Treatment of Anxiety Disorders (Cambridge University Press, 1994).

the clinician may not ask. If BDD symptoms are elicited, they may be misdiagnosed as depression, Obsessive-Compulsive Disorder, Social Phobia, Agoraphobia, Avoidant Personality Disorder, Psychotic Disorder NOS, or even Schizophrenia. If these disorders—rather than BDD—are targeted in treatment, the treatment may fail.

Some patients who present for psychiatric treatment are well informed about BDD (and may even have to convince a skeptical clinician that this is the correct diagnosis!). Others, however, are reluctantly dragged to treatment by distraught family members. Still others begrudgingly see a psychiatrist at the behest of a wary dermatologist or surgeon, and they do so only because the patient views the psychiatric consult as a ticket to a desired cosmetic procedure. Regardless of the patient's motivation, it is important to provide education about BDD, explaining that it is a relatively common and treatable body image disorder. Many patients welcome the diagnosis and the information that BDD can be treated, whereas others (typically those with poor or absent insight) reject the diagnosis and treatment. It can help to focus on the potential for psychiatric treatment to decrease the excessive preoccupation with the perceived appearance flaws, to diminish suffering, and to improve functioning and quality of life. It is usually fruitless to extensively discuss or argue over whether the defect is "real." It may instead help to explain that people with BDD versus other people have quite different views of how the BDD sufferer looks for reasons that are not well understood. Then the patient can be encouraged to focus on the potential for treatment to improve his or her life.

Our general approach to patients who want dermatologic treatment, surgery, or other nonpsychiatric treatment (e.g., electrolysis) is to say that no one can predict how an individual patient will respond to such treatment, but as best we know it is usually ineffective for BDD and can even worsen the appearance concerns (Phillips 1996, 2001). We have seen many patients who seriously regret having had such treatment. (Patients who damage their skin by picking at it, however, may require dermatologic as well as psychiatric care.) We explain that psychiatric treatment is much less risky, does not make patients think they look worse, is likely to help them feel better and improve their life, and is worth a try.

We would start treating Chris with a serotonin reuptake inhibitor (SRI) and cognitive-behavioral therapy (CBT). Although research on these two treatments is still limited, they are the best studied and appear efficacious for a majority of BDD patients (Neziroglu and Khemlani-Patel 2002; Phillips 2002). It isn't known which treatment is more effective or whether the combination is better than either treatment alone. Based on our clinical experience, we would recommend always treating a severely ill patient like Chris with an SRI. He is too depressed and too high a suicide risk to go without one. Furthermore, some BDD patients are too severely depressed, anxious, delusional, or unmotivated to do the work that CBT requires. Treating such patients with an SRI may diminish their BDD symptoms to the point that they can meaningfully participate in CBT. A reasonable treatment for patients with symptoms of moderate severity is use of an SRI or CBT, or both. For mild BDD, it may be preferable to start with CBT. For moderate or mild BDD, however, it is important to also consider other factors, such as comorbidity, the patient's preference, and the availability of CBT therapists knowledgeable about BDD, when choosing treatment.

Two controlled studies, three open-label trials, and case reports and series indicate that SRIs are often efficacious for BDD (Hollander et al. 1999; Phillips 1996, 2002; Phillips et al. 2001, 2002). Response to an SRI usually results in decreased distress and decreased time spent being preoccupied with the "defect," improved functioning (such as return to work or school), improvement in depressive symptoms, decreased repetitive behaviors (e.g., mirror checking), and improvement in insight and referential thinking. Importantly, SRIs appear more effective than other medications, including non-SRI antidepressants. An intriguing and clinically important finding is that studies indicate that SRIs alone are efficacious for patients with delusional BDD (i.e., those who are completely convinced that they look abnormal and cannot be convinced otherwise [Hollander et al. 1999; Phillips 2001, 2002]). This approach might sound counterintuitive, as psychotic symptoms in other disorders are typically treated with antipsychotics. Unfortunately, very few data are available on the efficacy of antipsychotics for BDD, but these data (which are largely retrospective) suggest that antipsychotics alone are not effective, even for delusional patients (Phillips 2002).

It is very important to use a high enough SRI dose for a long enough time (Phillips 2001, 2002). Although no studies have compared different SRI doses, clinical experience indicates that patients with BDD usually require higher doses than those typically used for depression. In the first author's clinical practice, the mean SRI doses have been fluoxetine (Prozac), 66.7 ± 23.5 mg/day; fluvoxamine (Luvox), 308.3 ± 49.2 mg/day; paroxetine (Paxil), 55.0 ± 12.9 mg/day; sertraline (Zoloft),

202.1 ± 45.8 mg/day; clomipramine (Anafranil), 203.3 ± 52.5 mg/day; citalopram (Celexa), 71.4 ± 27.3 mg/day; and escitalopram (Lexapro), 30.4 ± 10.1 mg/day, all of which are at the upper end of, or even exceed, the recommended dose range (Phillips et al. 2001). It's also important that the SRI trial is long enough. Most studies (which used fairly rapid titration schedules) have reported an average time to response in the range of 6–9 weeks, with some patients requiring as long as 12, or occasionally even 16, weeks to respond. We commonly see unimproved patients who have previously received many brief (e.g., 4–8 weeks) trials of low-dose SRIs; often, such patients have been diagnosed with depression while BDD was missed.

There is no one-size-fits-all formula for dose titration; it will depend on a number of factors, including illness severity (with quicker titration generally advisable for sicker patients, especially those who are suicidal), medication tolerability, and patient preference. A reasonable goal, however, is to reach the maximum dose recommended by the manufacturer (if a lower dose does not work) by 5–9 weeks from the start of treatment, if tolerated. This approach may result in a higher dose than necessary (although the dose can always be lowered subsequently, if desired), but it has the advantage of not missing a response because of undertreatment, and it also prevents an unnecessarily protracted treatment trial, which could result from slower upward titration.

Clinical experience suggests that, with continued SRI treatment, relapse is rare and many patients further improve. Although formal medication discontinuation studies have not been done, it appears that most patients relapse when an effective SRI is discontinued (Phillips et al. 2001). Therefore, we would treat a patient with severe BDD for years and would consider treating a patient like Chris with an SRI for the rest of his life. Typically, we continue an effective SRI for a minimum of 1–2 years. If the patient wishes to discontinue the medication, we plan this carefully, ideally selecting a time of minimal stress and tapering the SRI slowly over many months. It is unknown whether treatment with CBT may decrease the risk of relapse when an SRI is discontinued; this question is important and needs to be studied.

If Chris doesn't respond to the first SRI (e.g., a 12- to 14-week trial of citalopram reaching 60 mg/day by weeks 5–6), there are several options (Phillips 1996, 2002). One option is to increase the SRI dose (excluding clomipramine) above the maximum recommended dose (e.g., reaching 80–100 mg/day of citalopram or paroxetine). After an initial 12-week trial, 2–3 weeks on a higher-than-maximum dose is usually adequate to see whether the higher dose will work. We do not use this approach routinely but may use it when the patient has partially but inadequately responded to the maximum recommended dose and is tolerating the medication well. This approach is even more appealing if a number of SRIs have not been useful for the patient, in which case the remaining options are diminishing. Another option is to switch to another SRI and to conduct sequential trials of all of the SRIs, if necessary. A substantial percentage of patients who do not respond to an initial SRI trial will respond to a subsequent SRI (Phillips et al. 2001).

Yet another option is to add an augmenting medication to the SRI. Potentially effective choices include buspirone, an atypical antipsychotic; clomipramine; or another antidepressant (e.g., bupropion [Wellbutrin], venlafaxine [Effexor]) (Phillips 2002; Phillips et al. 2001). If clomipramine is combined with an SRI, the clomipramine level must be carefully monitored. Augmentation may make more sense for patients who have partially responded to an SRI, but it can also be tried if there has been only a minimal SRI response or no response. Combining an atypical antipsychotic with an SRI, although virtually unstudied, is particularly appealing for a delusional patient. It is not known which augmentation strategy is most effective or whether it is better to augment or switch to another SRI. Augmentation strategies are more appealing if there is a high risk of serious consequences due to relapse, which could occur when switching a patient from a partially effective SRI. Very anxious, agitated, and distressed patients may benefit from the addition of a benzodiazepine to the SRI (although we are reluctant to do this for patients with a history of substance abuse). For patients for whom multiple SRIs have failed, venlafaxine or a monoamine oxidase inhibitor (e.g., phenelzine [Nardil] or tranylcypromine sulfate [Parnate]) is worth trying.

CBT has also been shown to be efficacious for BDD (Neziroglu and Khemlani-Patel 2002; Phillips 1996). Evidence of the efficacy of CBT comes from case series (Marks and Mishan 1988) as well as two randomized studies in which BDD was compared to a no-treatment waiting-list control (Rosen et al. 1995; Veale et al. 1996). One study consisted of patients quite different from Chris, in that all were women who appeared to have relatively mild BDD, and many of them were concerned with weight and body shape (Rosen et al. 1995). Other reports, however, contained men as well as women and included patients with more severe and typical BDD symptoms (Marks and Mishan 1988; Neziroglu and Khemlani-Patel 2002; Veale et al. 1996).

When starting CBT with Chris, we would begin by thoroughly assessing his BDD symptoms. This assessment would include determining his beliefs about his looks; supporting evidence for such beliefs; and his checking behaviors (e.g., mirror checking), reassurance-seeking behaviors, camouflaging behaviors (e.g., wearing a hat and makeup), and avoidance behaviors (e.g., going through red traffic lights, not allowing people in close proximity, avoiding brightly lit rooms). To engage him in treatment, we would focus discussion on the time-consuming, distressing, and impairing nature of his preoccupations. We would educate him about the CBT model and develop an individualized case conceptualization to generate a treatment plan and emphasize how his behaviors reinforce his preoccupations and beliefs.

We would do an initial response prevention to decrease these reinforcing behaviors, explaining that bringing the behaviors under control will minimize his preoccupation and distress. We would make a list of these behaviors and rate each of them in terms of how much anxiety would be provoked if that particular behavior were controlled (e.g., "How anxiety-provoking would it be if you didn't wear a hat when you leave the house?"). Once anxiety ratings are established, the patient would decrease (ideally, stop) each behavior in a hierarchical fashion—starting from the least and moving toward the most anxiety-provoking situations. Checking mirrors and other reflective surfaces (e.g., windows, backs of spoons) is one of the most important behaviors to control. Most BDD patients check so excessively and closely that they are likely to obtain a very distorted view of themselves. Chris stands several inches from the mirror for hours a day intensely staring at and examining his pores, which no doubt makes them appear larger than they actually are. Similarly, checking other reflective surfaces will only further reinforce his distorted image because such surfaces (e.g., car bumpers, shiny plastic or chrome surfaces) provide a distorted reflection. Although mirror checking is difficult to totally control, a realistic goal would be to have Chris stand several feet from the mirror when brushing his hair or doing normal grooming and to have him not approach the mirror at any other time. Some experts would also recommend "mirror retraining," in which patients learn to objectively (rather than negatively) describe their entire body (not just disliked areas) while looking in the mirror. Such retraining is done only at specified times of the day and must not include excessive checking (i.e., ritualizing).

We would also have Chris do behavioral experiments. These would be designed to test his appearance-related beliefs and provide him with disconfirming evidence of his beliefs. For example, setting up a simple but carefully planned task with a specific hypothesis could test his belief that others take special notice of and are horrified by his "disfigurement." The hypothesis could be that if he walks into a shop to purchase something, 80% of people will recoil from him with a look of horror on their face and move away from him within 5 seconds. Another hypothesis might be that if he walks down a crowded sidewalk, 75% of people approaching him will cross to the other side of the street before passing him because he is so ugly. Such tasks are carried out by the patient and are best conducted (at least initially) with the clinician, who would also look for evidence of whether the hypothesis is true. After the experiment, the patient and clinician discuss whether the expected outcome occurred and what the patient learned from the task. This process not only begins to expose Chris to his feared situations (i.e., exposure) but also allows the clinician to gently challenge some of his beliefs on the basis of the experiment's results. Like standard exposure, behavioral experiments are conducted in a hierarchical fashion (from easier to more difficult). In designing such tasks, it is important to clearly spell out the task before it is conducted and to have a very concrete hypothesis, which the patient formulates with the clinician's help. The behaviors that Chris expects from others need to be clearly defined so that he does not misinterpret normal looks or smiles from others. For example, he should determine how many people actually laugh at him, stare at him intently, or move away from him with a clear look of horror or disgust. Such behavioral experiments would be expanded to include previously avoided situations, such as social gatherings, outings, being in close proximity to others or under bright lights, and waiting at traffic lights. Repeated exposure to such situations would provide evidence contrary to his beliefs and would also assist Chris in habituating to these previously anxiety-provoking situations.

We would also do cognitive restructuring, as developed by Beck, for depression and anxiety disorders. In cognitive restructuring, the patient identifies negative automatic thoughts (e.g., "Everyone here thinks I look deformed"), underlying core beliefs (e.g., "I'll always be alone because of how I look"), and cognitive errors (e.g., mind reading, fortune telling, catastrophizing). The therapist helps the patient examine the evidence for and against these beliefs and generate more accurate and helpful beliefs. Because most patients have poor or absent insight, as well as prominent depressive symptoms, we generally recommend using cognitive approaches in the form of cognitive restructuring and/or behavioral experiments in addition to standard behavioral techniques, such as exposure and response prevention. In our experience, the combination of behavioral experiments, cognitive restructuring, and exposure and response prevention is essential in the cognitive-behavioral treatment of BDD. It is also important for the clinician to assign homework so that the patient practices these CBT approaches between sessions to maximize gains beyond the sessions.

References

Hollander E, Allen A, Kwon J, et al: Clomipramine vs desipramine crossover trial in body dysmorphic disorder: selective efficacy of a serotonin reuptake inhibitor in imagined ugliness. Arch Gen Psychiatry 56:1033–1039, 1999

Marks IM, Mishan J: Dysmorphophobic avoidance with disturbed bodily perception: a pilot study of exposure therapy. Br J Psychiatry 152:674–678, 1988

Neziroglu F, Khemlani-Patel S: A review of cognitive and behavioral treatment for body dysmorphic disorder. CNS Spectrums 7:464–471, 2002

Phillips KA: Body dysmorphic disorder, in Somatoform and Factitious Disorders (Review of Psychiatry Series, Volume 20, Number 3). Edited by Phillips KA. Washington, DC, American Psychiatric Publishing, 2001, pp 67–94

Phillips KA: Pharmacologic treatment of body dysmorphic disorder: review of the evidence and a recommended treatment approach. CNS Spectrums 7:453–460, 2002

Phillips KA: The Broken Mirror: Understanding and Treating Body Dysmorphic Disorder. Revised and expanded edition. New York, Oxford University Press, 2004

Phillips KA, Albertini RS, Siniscalchi J, et al: Effectiveness of pharmacotherapy for body dysmorphic disorder: a chart-review study. J Clin Psychiatry 62:721–727, 2001

Phillips KA, Albertini RS, Rasmussen SA: A randomized placebo-controlled trial of fluoxetine in body dysmorphic disorder. Arch Gen Psychiatry 59:381–388, 2002

Rosen JC, Reiter J, Orosan P: Cognitive behavioral body image therapy for body dysmorphic disorder. J Consulting Clin Psychol 63:263–269, 1995

Veale D, Gournay K, Dryden W, et al: Body dysmorphic disorder: a cognitive behavioral model and pilot randomized controlled trial. Behav Res Ther 34:717–729, 1996

Disco Di

Diana Miller, age 25, entered a long-term treatment unit of a psychiatric hospital after a serious suicide attempt. Alone in her enormous suburban house with her parents away on vacation, she was depressed and desperately lonely; she made herself a Valium and Scotch cocktail, drank it, and then called her psychiatrist.

Diana had been a tractable child with a mediocre school record until she turned age 12. Then, her disposition, which had been cheerful and outgoing, changed drastically: She became demanding, sullen, and rebellious, shifting precipitously from a giddy euphoria to tearfulness and depression. She took up with a "fast" crowd, became promiscuous, abused marijuana and hallucinogens, and ran away from home at age 15 with a 17-year-old boy. Two weeks later, having eluded the private investigators her parents had hired, they both returned. She reentered school, but she dropped out for good in her junior year of high school. Her relationships with men were stormy and full of passion, unbearable longing, and violent arguments. She craved excitement and would get drunk, dance wildly on tabletops in discos, leave with strange men, and perhaps have sex in their cars. If she refused their sexual advances, she was sometimes put out onto the street. After one such incident, at age 17, she made her first suicide attempt, cutting her wrist severely, which led to her first hospitalization.

After her first hospitalization, Diana was referred to a therapist for intensive, twice-weekly dynamic psychotherapy, for which she had little aptitude. She filled up most of her sessions with a litany of complaints against her family, from whom she expected "100% attention." She called her therapist several times a day about one "crisis" or another.

During her long period of unsuccessful outpatient treatment, punctuated by several brief hospitalizations, she had many symptoms. She was afraid to travel even to her doctor's office without one of her parents. She was depressed, with suicidal preoccupations and feelings of hopelessness. She drank excessively and used up to 40 mg/day of Valium (diazepam). She had eating binges followed by crash diets to get back to her normal weight. She was obsessed with calories and with the need to have her food cut into particular shapes and arranged on her plate in a particular manner. If her mother failed to comply with these rules, she had tantrums, sometimes so extreme that she broke dishes and had to be physically restrained by her father.

Diana has never worked except for a few months as a receptionist in her father's company. She has never had an idea of what she wants to do with her life, apart from being with a "romantic man." She has never had female friends, and her only source of solace is her dog. She has often been "eaten alive" with boredom.

Efforts by her therapist to set limits have had little effect. She refused to join Alcoholics Anonymous or attend a day program or vocational rehabilitation center because she regarded these as "beneath" her. Instead, she languished at home, grew more depressed and agoraphobic, and escalated her Valium use to 80 mg/day. It was a serious suicide attempt this time that led to her current (seventh) psychiatric hospitalization.

DSM-IV-TR Casebook Diagnosis of "Disco Di"

Diana's history of many different symptoms over many years suggests several Axis I disorders. The depression and suicide attempt that prompted the last hospitalization suggest a diagnosis of Major Depressive Disorder or Dysthymic Disorder, or both. Because this case was presented to us several years after the hospitalization, we have insufficient information to choose between these diagnoses.

Her escalating dosage of Valium (with the resulting development of tolerance) and continued use despite its negative effect on her life suggest a diagnosis of Valium Dependence (DSM-IV-TR, p. 285). Her binge eating may have been frequent enough to warrant the additional diagnosis of binge-eating disorder (DSM-IV-TR, p. 787).

Her chronically chaotic life, her pervasive pattern of instability in mood and relationships, and her impulsivity are striking. These suggest an Axis II personality disorder as the primary disturbance, specifically, Borderline Personality Disorder (BPD) (DSM-IV-TR,

p. 710). Diana demonstrates at least five of the characteristic symptoms of this disorder. She certainly has unstable and intense interpersonal relationships, and the "violent arguments" suggest an alternation between extremes of idealization and devaluation. She has an identity disturbance (no goals in life), impulsive behavior in many areas (sex, substance abuse, eating), recurrent suicidal behavior, affective instability (sudden shifts of mood), and inappropriate and intense anger, and we suspect that her being "eaten alive" with boredom is evidence of chronic feelings of emptiness.

As is commonly the case in people with severe personality disorders, features of several other personality disorders are also present: Narcissistic (Alcoholics Anonymous was "beneath" her), Histrionic (craving excitement), Obsessive-Compulsive (rigidity about food), and Dependent (inability to manage without her family).

Follow-Up

In the hospital, Diana complained that the nurses were "cruel" to her and that other patients "hated" her. Many sessions were spent with her parents, counseling them to resist her pleas to return home. She was exquisitely sensitive to the slightest decrement in her Valium level, so that she could be weaned only 1 mg at a time. It took 3 months before she was "off" the drug. Afterward, her progress was unexpectedly good. Her disposition became cheerful. She grew cooperative toward the staff and friendly toward other patients. She learned secretarial skills in a hospital rehabilitation program and became less fearful of going outside and less fussy about food. By the end of her 10-month stay, she had developed a friendship with another convalescing patient, and the two arranged to share an apartment. Both found part-time work, and Diana continued therapy once a week as an outpatient.

Diana responded primarily to a supportive mode of psychotherapy—one that emphasized education, exhortation, encouragement, and limit setting. She was too anxious and too action prone to benefit from a psychodynamic approach that requires introspection and reflection. Brief hospitalizations could not stem the tide of her multiple and intense symptoms, of which her substance abuse was the most threatening. For Diana, what seemed

to work best was a long-term hospitalization, in which the substance abuse could be properly addressed and vocational rehabilitation could take hold. The enforced separation from her parents
helped her and her mother realize that each of them could survive without the other.

During 7 years of follow-up, Diana has held her ground, continues to work and live with the same roommate, and is able to visit
her parents with regularity without falling back into the old pattern of mother–daughter interdependence. Sensation seeking remains a noticeable part of her adaptation—she likes flashy clothes,
discos, and rock concerts—but she is less impulsive, abstains from
alcohol, and no longer places herself in jeopardy with strange men.

*Note: This case is discussed first by Dr. John Gunderson and then by Drs.
Kathryn E. Korslund and Marsha M. Linehan.*

Discussion of "Disco Di"
by John Gunderson, M.D.*

The issue of differential diagnosis is not particularly complicated in Diana's case. Her precipitous mood changes, including "euphoria," might
suggest an atypical Bipolar Disorder, but this diagnosis would overlook
the interpersonal sources of her mood changes. The fact that her
"progress was unexpectedly good" after being withdrawn from Valium
could be interpreted as evidence of a substance-induced Mood Disorder, but this would overlook the ways in which her problems preceded
her substance abuse. Diana presents most of the prototypic aspects of
the BPD diagnosis (i.e., labile and rapidly shifting affects, intense unsta-

**Dr. Gunderson is Professor of Psychiatry at Harvard Medical School and Director of
The Borderline Center at McLean Hospital in Belmont, Massachusetts. Dr. Gunderson's
research helped define BPD and has subsequently shown that its variable course is often
related to the variability in the treatments received by patients with BPD. His clinical
experience has spanned all levels of care and all treatment modalities. His textbook,* Borderline Personality Disorder: A Clinical Guide *(Gunderson 2001), combines his
extensive clinical experience with an appreciation for the lessons obtained from research.*

ble relationships, and self-defeating and potentially self-destructive behaviors). Having noted her prototypicality, it's worth adding that
Diana had features of BPD when she began treatment at age 17, which
would place her in the better prognosis subgroup for patients with this
disorder. These features were her history of involvement in romantic
relationships (marked by active and positive feelings [i.e., "passion"
and "longing"]), the ongoing involvement by her family and their support for her treatment (families being "overinvolved" is a good prognostic sign for BPD) (Hoffman and Hooley 1998), and the financial
wherewithal to make high-quality treatment an option.

Treatment Issues: Ages 12–17, Adolescence

The fact that Diana's behavior became rebellious and dangerous only
after the age of 12 implicates the conflicts attendant to her entering adolescence—the prospect of separation from her family; the need to
"own" her sexuality and establish primary relationships with peers;
and, in an achievement-oriented family, the prospect of being measured by her competitive success. The excesses of her adolescent behaviors (i.e., promiscuity, drugs, and running away) represent maladaptive
efforts to master these issues and, consciously or unconsciously, also
represent "cries for help." In this case, her parents' responses to her behavioral problems are registered only insofar as they had hired private
investigators to retrieve her when, at age 15, she ran away. It is unclear
whether her parents, or school authorities, were hesitant to invoke psychiatric help or the patient simply refused to comply with appropriate
admonitions. In any event, she began to see a psychotherapist only in
the aftermath of her first hospitalization at age 17.

Why Diana was so vulnerable to the stresses of adolescence remains
unclear. What is clear is that Diana lacked an environment in which
she felt secure with her own impulses and feelings and felt protected
from outside dangers. The need for this environment starts within her
home. Efforts to help this family create such an environment (i.e., to
change their responses to Diana) were critically needed. Interventions
with the parents are where Diana's treatment should have begun. Parents are usually much more motivated and ready to make changes
than are their adolescents. Parents generally welcome education about
BPD, feeling greatly reassured by knowing that there is a body of
knowledge about this disorder, and they are quite ready to recognize
that their ways of coping have not worked. Guidelines have been developed to help parents stay involved, avoid fights, and establish a

more consistent set of responses that do not reinforce the borderline offspring's dysfunction (Gunderson 2001). A recent study documents how situational changes that diminish stress and increase support can sometimes bring about dramatic resolutions in borderline psychopathology (Gunderson et al. 2003). A family intervention, with or without Diana's participation, could have made a critical difference in whether she developed the sustained behavioral problems that subsequently identified her as having BPD.

Treatment Issues: Ages 17–25

After entering treatment at age 17, Diana developed a regressive relationship—marked by a depressive, clinging, and bored dependency—with her therapist (recurrent crises with daily calls) and also, it would seem, with her parents. Imagine what it must have been like for the parents to have an adult daughter who "needed" to be driven to psychotherapy and "to have her food cut in particular shapes." The desperate behavioral problems outside the home that had marked her earlier adolescence were now replaced by equally maladaptive behaviors within the home. She withdrew from her peers and from competition, and her inability to regulate her behaviors now was manifest in alcohol and Valium abuse, bingeing, and obsessive-compulsive symptoms. Again, in this case description, little is said about the family's response to these dysfunctional behaviors. Still, it is clear that neither parent could set limits on Diana's behaviors, and there are suggestions that her mother may have unwittingly been reinforcing some of these behaviors. I would infer that Diana held both parents hostage. Very little is revealed about the therapist's responses to Diana during this period. The therapist seems to have found Diana unresponsive to limits and to have "little aptitude" for insight. Despite five additional hospitalizations, the patient languished in this manner, refusing additional treatments when they were recommended, until, at the age of 25, she made a serious suicide attempt.

The combination of psychotherapy and psychopharmacology that Diana received is characteristic of the usual outpatient treatments offered to patients with BPD. It can often be helpful and sometimes even sufficient. From ages 17–25, for someone like Diana, it was inappropriate. Missing from this combination, essential for Diana, are the sociotherapies—therapies directed at observable problems with social adjustment and competence. Such "rehabilitative" therapies are particularly important for young BPD patients who typically externalize or act out. Patients like Diana need to learn to sit still and think, to be confronted about their efforts to externalize problems, to listen to others' problems without trying to escape or solve them, to object when unfairly criticized without flight or raging, and to "own" their feelings and know these feelings are "normal." Such learning experiences can occur by education, example, corrective experiences, direction, reinforcement, and expectations. The social skills training package that is central to dialectical behavior therapy and the interpersonal skills that are central to interpersonal group therapy exemplify modalities that—like the social learning experiences an earlier generation of borderline patients could sometimes obtain from therapeutic communities in hospital or residential settings—offer learning opportunities that can overcome developmentally established social handicaps. As noted already, for an adolescent or young adult who is living at home, the simplest and most direct sociotherapy involves "customizing" the home environment by working with the parents. If Diana's family, or her school authorities, had somehow failed to perceive Diana's need for help until her first hospitalization at age 17, it was still critical to involve—change—the family in the aftermath of that major event.

For someone like Diana, it was unfortunate to have her treatment depend on the benefits from psychodynamically oriented outpatient psychotherapy. Psychodynamic training is invariably helpful in understanding borderline patients, but when such patients live in an unstructured setting, are subjectively very distressed, and/or are unable or unwilling to control their behaviors, they cannot be expected to involve themselves—and change—from introspection and insight (i.e., the distinguishing characteristics of psychodynamic psychotherapy). The initial interventions should be directed toward creating a "holding environment," and then at the subjective distress and the behavioral problems. A dynamically skilled case manager who would work with the patient's environment (i.e., Diana's family and school system) and who would give priority to Diana's subjective distress and behavioral dyscontrol would have been far more helpful. The types of interventions identified as subsequently being provided by her "supportive" therapist after the 10-month hospitalization (i.e., "education, exhortation, encouragement, and limit setting") were needed during this phase of her treatment—if not before.

The other arm of Diana's outpatient treatment—pharmacotherapy—also seems to have been poorly implemented. The abundant subjective distress experienced by most borderline patients can be helpfully addressed by medications—with partial and inconsistent success. The usual starting point for patients with BPD is a selective serotonin reuptake inhibitor. This class of medications might have usefully diminished both Diana's emotional intensity and her impulsivity (Soloff 1998). We do not know the rationale or the source of her escalating dosages of Valium. A psychopharmacologist who is knowledgeable about BPD would be cautious about misuse of medications and, specifically, would be aware of the high risk for dependency and abuse with benzodiazepines (Cowdry and Gardner 1988). If the Valium was prescribed by her therapist, this escalation might easily be an extension of the same misanthropic difficulties the therapist had in managing phone calls or in otherwise "setting limits" on Diana. (In this regard, it's worth noting that Diana must have been very persuasive. Even the extended period required in the hospital to eventually wean Diana from her Valium—4 months—seems unlikely to have been purely pharmacologically driven.) A clinician who is not trying to provide psychodynamic psychotherapy can more safely prescribe medications. A skilled psychopharmacologist who is experienced with BPD can work with a psychotherapist to provide "holding," which can help prevent such patients from dropping out of treatment when they are frustrated.

Treatment Issues: Ages 25 and 26

The patient's involvement in an extended hospitalization (10 months) provided an "enforced separation" from her mother that helped both realize that they "could survive without each other." The hospitalization also allowed a gradual weaning from her Valium dependency (as commented on earlier), diminished both her agoraphobic and bingeing behaviors, provided training in secretarial skills, and reinvolved her with peers.

It would be a serious mistake, in my judgment, to conclude from this case description that long-term hospitalization was necessary for Diana's improvement, and, by inference, that its unavailability in our current managed care environment compromises the likelihood of successful treatment. As noted, I strongly believe that the ineffectiveness of Diana's treatment prior to this long-term hospitalization—up to age 25—reflects a lack of knowledge about the treatment of BPD. It should be noted that this case dates back to the 1980s, when long-term hospitalizations and intensive psychoanalytic psychotherapies were considered optimal treatments. In my experience, long-term hospitalizations could occasionally prove to be useful owing to the social rehabilitative aspects of the therapeutic community (as was the case with *Girl, Interrupted*) (Kaysen 1994), but, more often, such hospitalizations contained unnecessary constraints that invoked hostile control struggles or regressions and, in either case, often led to prolonged impasses. Most patients with this disorder can be successfully treated by the thoughtful deployment of interventions that are far less intensive than long-term hospitalization. Residential, day care, or even intensive outpatient levels of care are generally more satisfactory (Gunderson 2001). The general principle that should guide such placements is to utilize the borderline patient's strengths and to diminish the secondary gains from being dysfunctional (e.g., being taken care of and made the center of attention). Of course, the effectiveness of any level of care or treatment modality for borderline patients depends on its being provided by clinicians who are knowledgeable and appropriately enthusiastic about working with these patients.

With respect to the benefits from Diana's hospitalization, it is notable that many sessions were spent counseling the parents to resist Diana's pleas to come home. This counseling, I believe, is critical in understanding Diana's improvement. By saying "no" to her—with the support of hospital staff—the parents were for the first time letting their judgment about Diana's welfare take priority over her wishes (i.e., demands) and, by inference, were putting her welfare above their own discomfort with her anger and recriminations. They were finally providing the "holding" Diana needed. This "weaning" from the family—for which the weaning from Valium was adjunctive—set the stage for the social rehabilitative benefits of establishing primary relationships with peers and for her long overdue vocational training. With improved social (i.e., peer and vocational) skills in place, Diana might now have an aptitude for psychodynamic psychotherapy that was previously thought to be absent.

As a footnote to the issue of Diana's individual psychotherapy, I would note that both borderline patients and psychotherapists vary in their interest and aptitude. Psychodynamic psychotherapy can be invaluable for those borderline patients who are capable of attending sessions reliably, who can withstand the inherent frustrations, and who take an interest in introspection (Waldinger and Gunderson 1989). With respect to Diana, she may have become a suitable candidate for this modality after leaving the hospital and having established a stable living and work situation. The psychodynamic therapist with whom she worked from ages 17–25 seems, in retrospect, to have had little aptitude or enthusiasm for such work with Diana. Thus, Diana's failure to progress when she had received that psychotherapy cannot be assumed to reflect the patient's lack of aptitude, nor should it be generalized to reflect a failure of this modality.

References

Cowdry RW, Gardner DL: Pharmacotherapy of borderline personality disorder: alprazolam, carbamazepine, trifluoperazine, and tranylcypromine. Arch Gen Psychiatry 45(2):111–119, 1988

Gunderson JG: Borderline Personality Disorder: A Clinical Guide. Washington, DC, American Psychiatric Press, 2001

Gunderson JG, Bender D, Sanislow C, et al: Plausibility and possible determinants of sudden "remissions" in borderline patients. Psychiatry 66(2):111–119, 2003

Hoffman PD, Hooley JM: Expressed emotion and the treatment of borderline personality disorder. In Session 4(3):39–54, 1998

Kaysen S: Girl, Interrupted. New York, Vintage Books, 1994

Soloff PH: Algorithm for pharmacological treatment of personality dimensions: symptom-specific treatments for cognitive-perceptual, affective and impulsive-behavioral dysregulation. Bull Menninger Clin 62:195–214, 1998

Waldinger RJ, Gunderson JG: Effective psychotherapy with borderline patients: case studies. Washington, DC, American Psychiatric Press, 1989

Discussion of "Disco Di"
by Kathryn E. Korslund, Ph.D.,*
and Marsha M. Linehan, Ph.D.**

The development and evaluation of effective treatments for BPD, both pharmacological and psychotherapeutic, is woefully inadequate, especially when the number of treatment trials for BPD is compared to the num-

*Dr. Korslund is a Research Scientist in the Department of Psychology at the University of Washington and is the Associate Director of the Behavioral Research and Therapy Clinics. She is a research psychologist and Dialectical Behavior Therapy supervisor and consultant.

**Dr. Linehan is the Director of the Behavioral Research and Therapy Clinics and Professor of Psychology and Psychiatry at the University of Washington. Dr. Linehan is the developer of DBT and is the author of Cognitive-Behavioral Treatment of Borderline Personality Disorder (Linehan 1993a) and Skills Training Manual for Treating Borderline Personality Disorder (Linehan 1993b).

bers for other disorders. To date, at least two treatments—dialectical behavior therapy (DBT) and psychodynamically based partial hospitalization—have empirical support for their efficacy. The usual outpatient treatments available in the community are marginally effective at best. Even the best treatments, however, are useless unless they reach those who need them. In this respect, Disco Di has shared a fate similar to that of many BPD patients who come to the attention of mental health professionals.

Diana's history is likely familiar to clinicians who treat patients with BPD. Frequent hospitalizations and prolonged misery characterized by emotional dysregulation, impulsive behavior, tumultuous relationships (including with therapists), and suicide attempts are hallmarks of the disorder. In fact, BPD is the only DSM-IV-TR diagnosis for which parasuicidal acts (i.e., suicide attempts and other intentional, nonfatal, self-injurious behaviors) are criteria.

The diagnosis of BPD, however, is frequently missed in clinical practice. As can be seen in Diana's case, the diagnosis was made only after several hospitalizations. BPD is characterized by intense and aversive emotions. The biosocial theory set forth by Linehan (1993a, 1993b) suggests that persons with BPD have an exquisite sensitivity to emotional stimuli; they are easily aroused to emotionally evocative cues (both within person and in the environment), experience emotion intensely, and have a delayed return to baseline emotional levels. The result is the experience of intense, overlapping aversive emotions.

From this model, suicidal behaviors (suicide, attempted suicide, nonsuicidal self-injury) and other maladaptive BPD criterion behaviors either function to reduce (or, in the case of suicide, end) painful emotional states or are themselves a consequence of dysregulated emotion. Thus, BPD can be conceptualized as a disorder of pervasive emotion dysregulation. The emotion system itself—mood-dependent action and action urges, cognitive processing, sensations and feelings, verbal and physical expressivity, biochemistry, etc.—are dysregulated across both positive (e.g., love, interest) and negative emotions. From this perspective, it is easy to understand why patients with BPD are sensitive and reactive to even slight changes in their environment, including the behavior of family, friends, and therapists. It also gives insight into why their lives are so painful.

In light of Diana's problems with alcohol and Valium, diagnostically one questions whether her case is an instance of BPD-like symptoms that are actually secondary to substance abuse. As she did not take Valium until she started treatment, it is unlikely that it is a substance-induced disorder. This result, however, reflects what often happens in treating BPD patients—when providers treat with pills rather than skills, and medication is used as palliative care to reduce the patient's (and often provider's) distress. Individuals with BPD are extremely difficult to treat, and, when grappling with problems of cognition and perception, dysphoria, anxiety, mood instability, and behavioral dyscontrol, it is not uncommon for the overwhelmed prescriber to proffer several medications from multiple drug classes (i.e., benzodiazepines, antidepressants, mood stabilizers, neuroleptics) in an attempt to achieve symptom relief.

It is virtually a miracle that Diana discontinued the Valium. The 3-month time frame is very reasonable, as it is not uncommon for BPD patients to have an exquisite sensitivity to medication and to require very gradual decrements in dosing. In part, she likely improved after discontinuing the Valium owing to an enhanced sense of self-efficacy gained by overcoming her reliance on the medication. As appears to be true in Diana's case, it is typical that patients worsen after addition of medications such as Valium. Therefore, the word to the wise clinician is to practice distress tolerance skills, as it is best to resist medicating in this manner.

Is there, then, no approach to medication that is effective for patients such as Diana? On the contrary, medication can be quite useful if it makes the person more likely to benefit from therapy. Unfortunately, haphazard polypharmacy and medications such as Valium do not help the patient. Instead, one might want to consider an empirically based medication algorithm designed to target the specific symptom domains reflective of BPD, such as antipsychotic medication for cognitive-perceptual problems (i.e., suspiciousness, dissociation, transitory stress-related hallucinations, and paranoid ideation) and antidepressant medication or mood stabilizers for affective dysregulation (i.e., labile mood; anxiety, dysphoria, depression; irritability and anger) and impulsive behavior (i.e., parasuicidal behaviors, impulsive-aggression, binge behaviors [with drugs, alcohol, sex, or food]) (Soloff 2000).

Although major, widespread, randomized controlled trials of this approach have not yet been conducted, preliminary results argue in its favor. Whatever the medication plan, one caveat applies: Potentially lethal individuals should not be given potentially lethal drugs. Thus, it may be necessary to dispense medications in small quantities or to avoid certain medications altogether.

Dropout rates from pharmacotherapy, however, tend to be very high, and compliance is often problematic. In clinical practice, about

half of patients and most therapists report medication misuse by patients, including taking other than prescribed dosages and overdoses
(Kelly et al. 1992). This is illustrated by Diana's story, wherein she increased her dose of Valium to twice the recommended daily limit, combined it with alcohol, and attempted suicide.

That Diana has sought out treatment on multiple occasions (and
likely from multiple providers) is congruent with what is seen in clinical practice. One study (Skodol et al. 1983) found that over their lifetime, 97% of patients with BPD presenting for treatment received
outpatient treatment from an average of 6.1 therapists (Perry et al.
1990; Skodol et al. 1983); 95% of patients received individual therapy,
56% group therapy, 42% family or couples psychotherapy, 37% day
treatment, 72% psychiatric hospitalization, and 24% treatment in a
halfway house (Bender et al. 2001).

Diana's treatment experience is unusual in that she improved with
long-term inpatient hospitalization. Often, inpatient hospitalization is
instituted after a suicide attempt. This move is usually made to allay
the legal fears of the treating clinician or in hopes of "stabilizing" the
patient such that the suicidal crisis will pass. There is no empirical evidence, however, that hospitalization is at all effective in preventing suicide or even increasing life expectancy. In fact, there is reason to believe
(as is illustrated in Diana's case) that the short-term "fix" most often
has devastating consequences.

First, inpatient psychiatric units have few, if any, expectations for
patients; are often overly nurturing (one patient seen at our clinic reported that the nursing staff peeled individual orange slices and fed
them to her); and essentially provide a level of nurturing that the patient does not have elsewhere in his or her life. Unfortunately, this nurturing is contingent on "mental patient" behaviors of sufficient
severity to trigger inpatient admission. Second, such positive attention
ordinarily increases in response to escalating suicidal behavior or communication and decreases in response to effective coping, thus reinforcing the very behaviors that brought the client to treatment. (Even
in outpatient therapy, it is not unusual for patients to lose access to
treatment if they cease suicidal behaviors.) Third, the very act of hospitalization removes the patient from an aversive or demanding environment, which can be a very powerful negative reinforcer (i.e., escape
conditioning) that serves to launch the "revolving door" phenomenon
of inpatient treatment so common to this patient population. The other
serious disservice of hospitalization is that by taking the patient out of

his or her environment, he or she has lost an opportunity to learn how to cope effectively in crisis, which is undoubtedly the time that effective coping is most needed!

Can hospitalization ever be helpful? Yes, but it is likely not the hospitalization per se that is effective. Bateman and Fonagy (2001) have developed an 18-month partial hospitalization program that has been shown to be effective, with treatment gains being maintained posttherapy when individual psychotherapy is continued after the hospital stay (Bateman and Fonagy 1999). Their study is also the only randomized clinical trial evaluating a psychoanalytically oriented treatment for BPD. The treatment provided was once-weekly individual therapy, thrice-weekly group therapy, once-weekly expressive therapy, once-weekly community meetings, once-monthly meetings with a case administrator, and once-monthly meetings to review medications. What is unclear from this study is whether the active ingredient stems from hospitalization, psychoanalytic treatment orientation, or provision of highly structured treatment.

Similar to the Bateman and Fonagy (1999) finding, recent research by Bohus and colleagues (in press) suggests that an inpatient 3-month treatment that targets psychoeducation, behavioral skills, contingency management of suicidal behaviors, and management at discharge produced significantly superior outcomes across a broad range of psychopathology variables as compared to a nonspecific treatment condition. What is common across these two studies is that the effective treatments were specific, intensive, and multifaceted. Thus, contrary to the rationale presented in the vignette, Diana's progress during her 10-month hospitalization was likely due to the highly structured and specific nature of the treatment, which, loosely translated, included many elements of the two treatments discussed earlier.

It is not surprising that Diana did not fare well with outpatient psychodynamic therapy, as there is currently no evidence to support this intervention. Outpatient psychoanalytically oriented and psychodynamic therapies have not been systematically tested. The only psychosocial treatment that has been tested is DBT. This, of course, is not to say that other treatments may not prove to be helpful. Fortunately, clinical trials of other therapy approaches for BPD (both cognitive-behavioral and psychodynamic object-relations) are currently under way. The jury, however, is out until the data come in.

At present, DBT is the best researched psychosocial treatment and the only one with more than one randomized controlled trial demonstrating efficacy across a range of target areas with this patient population. To date, there are six published randomized controlled trials of DBT for BPD by five independent research teams (Koons et al. 2001; Linehan et al. 1991, 1999, 2002b; Turner 2000; Verheul 2003). Results across these studies suggest that DBT is effective at reducing problematic behavioral patterns associated with BPD, including reduced frequency and severity of parasuicide (i.e., potentially lethal intentional, nonfatal, suicide attempts and/or other self-injurious behaviors), especially suicide attempts; reduction of substance dependence when it is targeted directly; increased maintenance in and compliance with treatment; reduced general psychopathology and enhanced general and social functioning; and decreases in emotional dysregulation (e.g., depression, anxiety, anger). A recent large randomized controlled trial (Linehan 2002a) found that, with seriously suicidal and out-of-control patients, outpatient DBT is more effective than outpatient nonbehavioral therapy, even when the nonbehavioral therapy is provided by peer-nominated expert psychotherapists paid to provide, with no restrictions whatsoever, the program of psychotherapy they believe is best for the client.

DBT is a cognitive-behavioral, comprehensive, principle-driven outpatient treatment program developed for chronically suicidal women with BPD (Linehan 1993a, 1993b). It has subsequently been adapted for BPD patients with problems other than suicidal behaviors and has been extended to other disorders involving problems of emotion regulation. On a fulcrum of dialectical philosophy, the treatment balances a focus on change with that of acceptance. The "technology of change" employs techniques from cognitive-behavioral therapy such as behavioral chain analysis (a moment-to-moment examination of the factors leading up to, following, and influencing a specific instance of the problem behavior, the ultimate goal of which is to understand the factors eliciting, maintaining, and interfering with resolution of the problem), exposure and response prevention, behavioral skills training, contingency management, and cognitive modification. Acceptance strategies come from Eastern mindfulness practice and principles of radical acceptance (the complete and genuine acknowledgment of reality as it is). Letting go of fighting reality is not easy for patients like Diana (and some therapists), as they often have difficulty with the distinction between recognition and approval of life's painful moments or mistakenly believe that acceptance precludes change. However, acceptance is required for change and is the only "solution" available when problems cannot be solved (e.g., emotional pain associated with a lifetime history of trauma).

From the case vignette, we are led to believe that Diana was a recalcitrant patient who worked actively against her therapist and for whom "setting limits" was ineffective. It should not surprise us so! Setting limits is often a euphemism for applying aversive contingencies (i.e., punishment), which, in the absence of a caring, genuine relationship, is not only unlikely to be effective in changing behavior but ultimately may be harmful to the therapist's efforts to develop a therapeutic connection or foster the client in creating a life worth living. That therapists push clients to change their behavior is no wonder, particularly when that behavior is life threatening. In the absence of a validating environment, however, intense emotional arousal interferes with cognitive processing, and no learning or behavior change takes place.

In DBT, limits are not set for the patient. Instead, the therapist works collaboratively, from a vantage point of genuine interest and caring. The therapeutic relationship is an authentic one between equals, one of whom happens to have the expertise required for getting the other to his or her goals. Reinforcing and aversive contingencies are openly applied to shape client behavior, and the client is taught about the role of contingencies in establishing and maintaining all forms of behavior. Didactic instruction and orientation to treatment rationales permeate the treatment. In this way, the DBT clinician is like a magician who performs all his or her tricks in plain view for the audience to see.

The case vignette notes that Diana made frequent telephone calls to her therapists. This sort of between-session contact is typical in treating individuals with BPD. For many clients, telephone contact with the therapist is extremely helpful. However, such contact should not be used indiscriminately. Instead, we advocate a telephone protocol aimed at increasing clients' skillfulness and generalizing what is learned in therapy to the natural environment. In this way, the therapist functions as a coach "calling in a play" to the client who is poised on the line of scrimmage. Such contact can also foster a sense of connectedness to the therapist and facilitate any necessary relationship repair after particularly difficult or painful sessions.

The DBT telephone protocol ties directly to the biosocial theory of the disorder—namely, that suicide behaviors function to solve the problem of intense and painful emotion. From this perspective, calls to the therapist after a suicide attempt are nonsensical, as the client has already "solved" the problem and therefore is not in need of help to generate or implement an effective solution. Diana, feeling "desperately lonely," drank a Valium and Scotch cocktail and then called her psychiatrist. Calls to the therapist after engaging in this type of maladaptive problem-solving behavior are assessed for potential of lethality. If the client requires medical attention, he or she would be directed to go to the emergency room. If he or she were unable to make arrangements him- or herself (or if the therapist has reason to believe that plans would not be followed), then help would be offered (e.g., arranging transportation with a friend, calling 911).

If the assessment revealed low lethality risk, the therapist would direct the client to get rid of any potentially lethal means and end the call, the theory being that there is nothing further the therapist can do, as the problem has essentially been solved. Any therapist attention at this time risks reinforcing suicide-related behavior as problem solving. At the next session, however, the therapist would conduct a painstakingly detailed analysis of the situation to determine 1) what led up to Diana's problem behavior in terms of vulnerability factors (e.g., being alone, feeling depressed and lonely, possession of potentially lethal medication); 2) what set off the problem (i.e., what was the cue); 3) the events, thoughts, actions, and emotions that linked the cue to the problem behavior (often, this is a painful emotion and there are beliefs that it will never go away or that it cannot be tolerated); and 4) the consequence of the behavior (both immediate and long term).

Diana's pattern of mood and behavioral instability across treatment is normal among BPD patients, and treatment alone is unlikely to beat it. A few hours a week of any therapy cannot simply overcome the pain and tremendous problems in the rest of these patients' lives. Treatment success of any orientation hinges on increasing the client's structured activities.

At the close of treatment, Diana had achieved behavioral control. Commenting that Diana still engaged in "sensation seeking" constitutes "pathologizing" normal behavior. This sort of vocabulary, so often used in describing BPD patient's motivations and behavior, is steeped in bias. At best, such terms are inaccurate; at worst, they communicate disdain for the client. At its core, the therapeutic relationship is one of respect, care, and service. As such, we encourage treatment providers to search for phenomenologically empathic descriptions of behavior.

From the description of the 7-year follow-up, it's evident that Diana has learned to adapt to her circumstances and surroundings but is not living a rich and full life. From a DBT perspective, we would say that she is now ready for Stage II treatment, in which the focus shifts from targeting behavioral control to increasing nontraumatic emotional experiencing. Essentially, after learning strategies to regulate her behavior when emotionally aroused, she now has the requisite skills to turn to introspection, reflection, and building a life that she values. For many clients like Diana, behavioral control can be reached after 1 year of DBT. Building a life that is cherished may not be an easy project, however, and the chance of the patient returning to old ways of coping is not abolished. For most of us, however, success is not measured by freedom from falls but by the skillfulness and speed with which we right ourselves.

References

Bateman A, Fonagy P: Effectiveness of partial hospitalization in the treatment of borderline personality disorder: a randomized controlled trial. Am J Psychiatry 156:1563–1569, 1999

Bateman A, Fonagy P: Treatment of borderline personality disorder with psychoanalytically oriented partial hospitalization: an 18-month follow-up. Am J Psychiatry 158:36–42, 2001

Bender DS, Dolan RT, Skodol AE, et al: Treatment utilization by patients with personality disorders. Am J Psychiatry 158:295–302, 2001

Bohus M, Haaf B, Simms T, et al: Effectiveness of inpatient dialectical behavioral therapy for borderline personality disorder: a controlled trial. Behav Res Ther (in press)

Kelly T, Soloff PH, Cornelius J, et al: Can we study (treat) borderline patients? attrition from research and open treatment. J Personal Disord 6:417–433, 1992

Koons CR, Robins CJ, Tweed JL, et al: Efficacy of dialectical behavior therapy in women veterans with borderline personality disorder. Behav Ther 32(2):371–390, 2001

Linehan MM: Cognitive-Behavioral Treatment of Borderline Personality Disorder. New York, Guilford Press, 1993a

Linehan MM: Skills Training Manual for Treating Borderline Personality Disorder. New York, Guilford Press, 1993b

Linehan MM, Armstrong HE, Suarez A, et al: Cognitive-behavioral treatment of chronically parasuicidal borderline patients. Arch Gen Psychiatry 48:1060–1064, 1991

Linehan MM, Schmidt H III, Dimeff LA, et al: Dialectical behavior therapy for patients with borderline personality disorder and drug-dependence. Am J Addict 8:279–292, 1999

Linehan MM, Comtois KA, Brown MZ, et al: Dialectical behavior therapy versus nonbehavioral treatment-by-experts in the community: clinical outcomes. Research symposium presented at the Association for Advancement of Behavior Therapy, 36th Annual Convention, Reno, NV, November 2002a

Linehan MM, Dimeff LA, Reynolds SK, et al: Dialectical behavior therapy versus comprehensive validation plus 12-step for the treatment of opioid dependent women meeting criteria for borderline personality disorder. Drug Alcohol Depend 67:13–26, 2002b

Perry JC, Herman JL, van der Kolk BA, et al: Psychotherapy and psychological trauma in borderline personality disorder. Psychiatr Ann 20:33–43, 1990

Skodol AE, Buckley P, Charles E: Is there a characteristic pattern to the treatment history of clinic outpatients with borderline personality? J Nerv Ment Dis 171:405–410, 1983

Soloff PH: Psychopharmacology of borderline personality disorder. Psychiatr Clin North Am 23:169–192, 2000

Turner RM: Naturalistic evaluation of dialectical behavior therapy–oriented treatment for borderline personality disorder. Cognitive and Behavioral Practice 7:413–419, 2000

Verheul R, van den Bosch LMC, Koeter MWJ, et al: Dialectical behaviour therapy for women with borderline personality disorder—12-month, randomised clinical trial in The Netherlands. Br J Psychiatry 182:135–140, 2003

Cocaine

Al Santini, a 39-year-old restaurant owner, is referred by a marriage counselor to a private outpatient substance abuse treatment program for evaluation and treatment of a possible "cocaine problem." According to the counselor, attempts to deal with the couple's marital problems have failed to produce any signs of progress over the past 6 or 7 months. The couple continues to have frequent, explosive arguments, some of which have led to physical violence. Fortunately, neither spouse has been seriously injured, but the continuing chaos in their relationship has led to a great deal of tension at home and appears to be contributing to the acting-out behavior and school problems of their two children, ages 9 and 13.

Several days ago, Al admitted to the counselor and to his wife that he had been using cocaine "occasionally" for at least the past year. The wife became angry and tearful, stating that if her husband failed to obtain treatment for his drug problem, she would separate from him and inform his parents of the problem. He reluctantly agreed to seek professional help, insisting that his cocaine use was "not a problem" and that he felt capable of stopping his drug use without entering a treatment program.

During the initial evaluation interview, Al reports that he is currently using cocaine, intranasally, 3–5 days a week, and that this pattern has been continuing for at least the past 2 years. On average, he consumes a total of 1–2 g of cocaine weekly, for which he pays $80 per gram. Most of his cocaine use occurs at work, in his private office or in the bathroom. He usually begins thinking about "coke" while driving to work in the morning. When he arrives at work, he finds it nearly impossible to avoid thinking of the cocaine vial in his desk drawer. Although he tries to distract himself and postpone using it as long as possible, he usually snorts his first "line" within an hour of arriving at work. On some days, he may snort another two or three lines over the course of the day. On other days, especially if he feels stressed or frustrated at work, he may snort a line or two every hour from morning through late afternoon. His cocaine use is sometimes fueled by offers of the drug from his business partner, whom the patient describes as a more controlled, infrequent user of the drug.

Al rarely uses cocaine at home, and never in the presence of his wife or children. Occasionally, he snorts a line or two on weekday evenings or weekends at home when everyone else is out of the house. Al denies current use of any other illicit drug but reports taking 10–20 mg of an antianxiety drug, Valium (diazepam) (prescribed by a physician friend), at bedtime on days when cocaine leaves him feeling restless, irritable, and unable to fall asleep. When Valium is unavailable, he drinks two or three beers instead.

He first tried cocaine 5 years ago at a friend's party. He enjoyed the energetic, euphoric feeling and the absence of any unpleasant side effects, except for a slightly uncomfortable "racing" feeling in his chest. For nearly 3 years thereafter, he used cocaine only when it was offered by others and never purchased his own supplies or found himself thinking about the drug between episodes of use. He rarely snorted more than four or five lines on any single occasion of use. During the past 2 years his cocaine use escalated to its current level, coincident with a number of significant changes in his life. His restaurant business became financially successful, he bought a large home in the suburbs, he had access to lots of cash, and the pressures of a growing business made him feel entitled to the relief and pleasures offered by cocaine.

He denies any history of alcohol or drug abuse problems. The only other drug he has ever used is marijuana, which he smoked infrequently in college but never really liked. He also denies any history of other emotional problems and, except for marriage counseling, reports that he has never needed help from a mental health professional.

During the interview, Al remarks several times that although he thinks that his cocaine use "might be a problem," he does not consider himself to be "addicted" to it and is still not sure that he really requires treatment. In support of this view, he lists the following evidence: 1) his current level of cocaine use is not causing him any financial problems or affecting his standard of living; 2) he is experiencing no significant drug-related health problems that he is aware of, with the possible exception of feeling lethargic the next day after a day of heavy use; 3) on many occasions, he has been able to stop using cocaine on his own, for several days at a time; and 4) when he stops using the drug, he experiences no withdrawal syndrome and no continuous drug cravings. On the other hand, he does admit the following: 1) he often uses much more cocaine than intended on certain days; 2) the drug use is impairing his functioning at work because of negative effects on his memory, attention span, and attitude toward employees and customers; 3) even when he is not actively intoxicated with cocaine, the aftereffects of the drug cause him to be short-tempered, irritable, and argumentative with his wife and children, leading to numerous family problems, including a possible breakup of his marriage; 4) although he seems able to stop using cocaine for a few days at a time, somehow he always goes back to it; and 5) as soon as he starts to use cocaine again, the craving and the preoccupation with the drug are immediately as intense as before he stopped using it.

At the end of the interview, Al agrees that although he came for the evaluation largely under pressure from his wife, he can see the potential benefits of trying to stop using cocaine on a more permanent basis. With a saddened expression, he explains how troubled and frightened he feels about the problems with his wife and children. He says that although marital problems existed before he started snorting cocaine, his continuing drug use has made them worse, and he now fears that his wife might leave him. He also feels extremely guilty about not being a "good father." He spends very little time with his children and often is distracted and irritable with them because of his cocaine use.

DSM-IV-TR Casebook Diagnosis of "Cocaine"

Al's use of cocaine illustrates the core concept of psychoactive substance dependence, a cluster of cognitive, behavioral, and physiologic symptoms indicating that the person has impaired control of psychoactive substance use and continues use of the substance despite adverse consequences. Al cannot stop himself from taking the first hit of cocaine in the morning, he uses it more often than he plans to, he keeps returning to it after stopping for a few days, he experiences withdrawal symptoms (lethargy), and he has reduced important social activities with his family because of mood changes caused by his taking cocaine. Therefore, the diagnosis is Cocaine Dependence, With Physiological Dependence (DSM-IV-TR, p. 242).

Follow-Up

Al entered the outpatient treatment program. His treatment included individual, group, and marital counseling combined with supervised urine screening and participation in a self-help group (Cocaine Anonymous). He initially had difficulty in fully acknowledging and accepting the seriousness of his drug dependency problem. He harbored fantasies about returning to "controlled" cocaine use and disputed the program's requirement of total abstinence from all mood-altering substances, arguing that because he had never experienced problems with alcohol, he saw no reason to deny himself an occasional drink with dinner or at social gatherings. During the first 3 months of treatment, he had two short "slips" back to taking cocaine, one of which was precipitated by drinking a glass of wine, which led to an intense craving for cocaine.

Subsequently, Al remained completely abstinent for the duration of the program (12 months) and became increasingly committed to maintaining a drug-free lifestyle. His relationships with his wife and children improved considerably. The violent arguments had stopped immediately with the cessation of cocaine use, and spending more time with his children became much easier without the negative influence of cocaine on his mood and mental state.

Three years later, Al was still abstinent. He was no longer in treatment but continued to attend Cocaine Anonymous meetings at least two or three times every week. If he were diagnosed at this time, the Cocaine Dependence would be specified as Sustained Full Remission because of the absence of any of the signs or symptoms of Cocaine Dependence for more than 12 months.

Discussion of "Cocaine" by Edward Nunes, M.D.*

The interviewer who evaluated Al has already carried out the first and most critical therapeutic intervention—namely, helping the patient acknowledge that he has a problem with cocaine. From there on, Al's clinical course and treatment proceed smoothly. It could have gone the other way, because cocaine-dependent patients, like those with other substance dependencies, frequently resist accepting that they have a problem or resist taking action, such as entering treatment (as Al, in fact, did). Thus, how the initial clinical encounter and diagnostic evaluation are carried out is important.

Several lines of empirical evidence are helpful in guiding a clinician's initial approach to diagnostic evaluation and treatment planning. First, brief advice from a physician to quit the abuse can, by itself, be an effective intervention (Bien et al. 1993). The impact of brief advice has been established mainly with respect to alcohol but is likely to generalize to other substances such as cocaine. The take-home message here is that it is always important to inquire about alcohol or drug use, consider how drugs or alcohol may be contributing to the patient's presenting symptoms, and advise abstinence if appropriate. Al did not present initially for consultation about his cocaine use. Al and his wife went to a counselor for help with marital problems. Could they have been spared 6 months of unproductive marital therapy had the significance of the cocaine abuse been recognized from the start?

Al's temper; propensity to arguments; distractibility; irritability with his children; and his feelings of fear, self-doubt, and guilt are consistent with the kinds of mood symptoms that can result from cocaine intoxication or withdrawal. That these disturbing symptoms cleared up immediately after cessation of cocaine use confirms the impression that these are direct consequences of his cocaine use. In the realm of diagnosis, substance use disorders can be viewed as "great pretenders,"

*Dr. Nunes is Associate Professor of Clinical Psychiatry at Columbia University College of Physicians and Surgeons and Research Psychiatrist at New York State Psychiatric Institute in New York City. His research focuses on treatment of drug dependence, including identification and treatment of comorbid psychiatric disorders, such as depression among substance-dependent patients, and combinations of behavioral and pharmacologic treatments. He also directs 1 of 17 Nodes of the National Institute on Drug Abuse Clinical Trials Network, focused on testing the effectiveness of evidence-based treatments in real-world practice settings.

mimicking a wide range of symptoms, including those of Mood and Anxiety Disorders, Sleep Disorders, psychosis, and Personality Disorders, as well as engendering physical ailments. Patients are often unaware that the substance(s) they are using may be contributing to the symptoms for which they seek help. Simple patient education and advice to quit, in this context, can be a powerful and gratifying intervention. It is a useful exercise to review the symptoms of intoxication and withdrawal due to various substances, as enumerated in DSM-IV-TR (American Psychiatric Association 2000), in order to be alert to possible substance-related symptoms and syndromes.

How the advice is delivered makes a difference. Individuals with substance use disorders are typically ambivalent about giving up their substance(s). This ambivalence is illustrated by Al's experience in the treatment program, where he first resisted acknowledging the seriousness of his problem and wanted to continue cocaine and alcohol use in a "controlled" fashion. How, then, can the clinician help a patient like Al resolve his ambivalence and take action? Here, the technique of motivational interviewing (Miller and Rollnick 2002) is extremely valuable. It is supported by substantial efficacy studies (Miller and Rollnick 2002), and all clinicians should learn about it. Clinicians, perhaps especially as physicians, often find themselves telling patients what to do ("I'm the doctor, and you should quit taking cocaine and drinking"), expecting them to follow the advice. Of course, patients often don't follow the advice in many realms—from substance abuse to compliance with blood pressure medication. Motivational interviewing sidesteps the authoritarian posture, which may only strengthen resistance to change, and instead encourages empathic listening on the part of the clinician and a collaborative discussion aimed at helping the patient to think it through and decide for him- or herself that he or she needs to quit. In Al's case, the initial diagnostic interview was successful in helping him connect his fear and sadness about what was happening to him and his family with the cocaine use, generating genuine motivation to quit.

Al's case also illustrates the valuable effects that family members or concerned significant others can have on a treatment course for substance-dependent patients. The fact that Al's wife took a stand that she would leave him if he would not seek treatment for his cocaine use was clearly instrumental in his motivation and was a critical first step in his treatment. Often, one or several people in a patient's life can exert this kind of "leverage," and patients such as Al should be encouraged to allow them to participate in the treatment. The clinician will want to avoid the appearance of taking sides with the significant others—ganging up on the patient—but instead should help the patient listen to the concerns of the people he or she is close to and decide how to respond to them. Several family or couple therapy techniques have been tested for treatment of substance-dependent patients in controlled trials and have been found to demonstrate solid evidence of efficacy (Liddle et al. 2001; Stanton and Shadish 1997; Szapocznik and Williams 2000). Such techniques are based on family systems theory—examining the disruptions in family systems brought about by a substance-abusing family member. From this perspective, Al's cocaine habit can be viewed as having caused him to abdicate his parental role, becoming instead like a difficult, angry child who his wife is left to manage by herself. Their children's school problems are further evidence of the disrupted family system—a response to the loss of the positive discipline and role modeling exerted by their "good father" before he became addicted. An effective family therapy or couples therapy can address not only the drug problem but also the larger couple or family problems because the drug use is viewed as one component of the disrupted family system. Thus, it is notable that Al's treatment program included ongoing marital counseling.

In the treatment of cocaine or other substance dependencies, it is important to identify and treat other co-occurring psychopathology. Having a drug or alcohol problem increases the risk of a range of disorders, including Mood Disorders, both unipolar and bipolar, Anxiety Disorders, Attention-Deficit/Hyperactivity Disorder (ADHD), Eating Disorders, and Personality Disorders, especially Borderline and Antisocial, not to mention other substance use disorders. ADHD often goes unrecognized in adults, and the stimulant properties of cocaine may attract such patients. Impatience and anger are frequent adult symptoms of ADHD, particularly in response to being frustrated or kept waiting. If Al's anger had not resolved so thoroughly after he quit using cocaine, it would have been important to examine whether the irritability might have been related, at least in part, to a Mood Disorder or ADHD and treated accordingly. Placebo-controlled trials of antidepressant medication for treatment of co-occurring depression among alcoholics and opiate addicts have yielded mixed results but on balance support efficacy of such treatment. Few such studies have been conducted among cocaine abusers, but results also appear encouraging (Nunes and Quitkin 1997). Few studies have examined treatment of co-occurring disorders other than depression, but it seems a safe general principle to treat other disorders when they are present. Such treatment will not cure the addiction by itself, but it may contribute to the success of a larger treatment plan.

Al enters a treatment program that includes individual and group therapy, marital counseling, urine screening, and self-help group participation, and he does beautifully. What makes a good treatment program? Does the therapeutic orientation or the various components matter? Would Al have been just as well off being seen in an individual therapist's office? Programs vary in quality, and it is important to pick good ones. Urine screening for cocaine and other drugs is essential; a good program should collect urines routinely and have procedures to supervise the collection (i.e., a staff member watches the patient urinate) if there is concern that the patient is hiding drug use by substituting fake urine. Most patients are frank about their use to clinicians if the clinician's stance is nonjudgmental and negative consequences are not tied to admissions of use. Patients are more likely to obfuscate if they fear consequences (e.g., disapproval by staff, anger or retaliation by spouse or family member, legal or employment issues). In general, it is best to create a trusting atmosphere. It is also important to be aware that some substances, such as alcohol or the high-potency benzodiazepines (e.g., Xanax [alprazolam]) or narcotics (e.g., fentanyl), are often not detected in urine.

Most substance abuse treatment programs in the United States today are oriented toward "12-step" self-help groups, such as Alcoholics Anonymous or Cocaine Anonymous, in which Al was encouraged to participate. The emphasis of self-help groups is on complete abstinence (note that Al was pressured to quit drinking alcohol, too), concrete strategies for maintaining abstinence, and following the 12 steps. Many patients do not feel comfortable in such groups, but those who take to them often do very well, as Al did. It is thus important, as a clinician, to continue to encourage patients to attend the group sessions and work through their resistance. This "traditional" approach found support in the largest controlled study of outpatient therapy for Cocaine Dependence to date—the National Institute on Drug Abuse's Collaborative Study (Crits-Christoph 1999)—which sought to embody such standard drug counseling interventions in treatment manuals. The study found that the combination of individual drug counseling and group drug counseling conducted by experienced counselors was more effective in reducing cocaine use at follow-up compared to group drug counseling alone or group drug counseling plus either of two psychotherapeutic techniques (cognitive therapy or supportive-expressive therapy). In fact, drug coun-

seling can be viewed as having contained many of the essential components of both of the psychotherapies, including an empathic stance,
building of the treatment alliance, and concrete advice on how to cope
with various challenges of abstinence, and it may have been delivered by
clinicians who were more experienced treating Cocaine Dependence.

Several other behavioral methods have been tested in controlled
trials and found to be efficacious in treating Cocaine Dependence. Cognitive-behavioral relapse-prevention therapy (Carroll et al. 1994) uses
cognitive and behavioral techniques to avoid or manage lapses in substance use. Contingency management (Higgins et al. 1994) provides
positive reinforcement (material or monetary) contingent on the patient demonstrating abstinence by producing cocaine-negative urine
tests. Despite much effort and many clinical trials, no medications can,
as yet, be recommended for treatment of Cocaine Dependence, other
than medications used to treat co-occurring disorders, as noted earlier.

Any treatment modality or style needs to deal with the fact that Al
is confronted with a close co-worker who is a cocaine user. In 12-
step–oriented treatment, this situation would be referred to as one of
those "persons, places, and things" that threaten sobriety. In cognitive-
behavioral relapse prevention, this would be a "high-risk situation"
that may serve as a "trigger." Offers of drugs from such persons, particularly if the drug itself or paraphernalia are waved under the patient's nose, may likely produce powerful cravings and lead to lapse or
relapse. Patients are generally encouraged to avoid such situations,
and relapse prevention therapy teaches various skills both for avoidance and for coping when confronted with the situation. A co-worker
can be particularly hard to avoid. Cash businesses, such as Al's restaurant business, can also be set-ups for relapse, and cash itself "in the
pocket" can also become a powerful trigger for drug use. Sometimes a
co-worker can be confronted by a patient and asked to cease and desist. As Al is apparently the boss, he may be in a good position to do so.
Sometimes the offending co-worker can be successfully shunned. Regarding money, it is often helpful to have someone else handle it, so
that it is not "burning a hole" in the patient's pocket. In any case, his
therapist would need to help Al problem solve these issues.

What about the issue of "controlled use" versus complete abstinence? Al, at the outset of treatment, wants to return to the controlled
use that he remembers from his first few years of dabbling in cocaine.
This is usually a mistake. Patients may sound quite persuasive on this
point, but it is best not to give in. For someone who has become depen-

dent on a substance, the substance itself is the most powerful "trigger" there is. Use of the substance will almost inevitably lead to relapse and to the full-dependence syndrome. On the other hand, lapses and relapses are to be expected. Al has a trouble-free course once he enters treatment, but many patients do not have such a smooth course. Substance dependence is a chronic, relapsing illness, and it is important that clinicians do not become discouraged or believe the relapse to represent a total failure. Rather, the relapse should be viewed as an opportunity to learn from mistakes, shore up the treatment plan, recommit to abstinence, and move ahead! Smoking cessation is illustrative of this point. Most smokers who try to quit fail, on any given attempt, to achieve sustained abstinence. However, most of those who keep trying to quit eventually succeed.

As a clinician, how do you choose the best treatment program for your particular patient? What treatment plan would I have chosen for Al? As noted earlier, a variety of treatment approaches have shown evidence of efficacy for treatment of Cocaine Dependence, both the traditional 12-step–oriented approach and newer cognitive, behavioral, family, and motivational approaches. However, there is little empirical evidence to guide treatment matching. For one thing, treatment-matching hypotheses are more difficult to test because they involve detecting an interaction between treatment and some matching factor (statistically a low-power proposition requiring larger sample sizes), whereas most efficacy studies are only powered with sufficient sample size to detect the main effect of treatment. Furthermore, deliberate efforts to detect matching have often come up empty handed, the most famous example being Project MATCH (Kadden 1996). This multisite trial with ample sample size was designed to test a variety of hypotheses about features that would predict which alcohol-dependent patients would do best with motivational treatment, as compared to a 12-step facilitation treatment, versus cognitive-behavioral relapse prevention. Yet, virtually none of these matching hypotheses was supported.

In the end, choosing the right treatment program depends on clinical judgment and a willingness to switch gears if the first approach chosen is not working. One thing I am clear on is that I would prefer not to treat Al by myself in my private office. I would rather share his treatment with an outpatient substance abuse treatment program or conduct it in the context of a psychiatric clinic offering specialized services for substance abusers. It is good to know what programs are available in your community and to establish collaborative relationships with the best ones. Ultimately, the best treatment programs are those that offer a variety of modalities; tailor treatment to each individual's needs, including his or her co-occurring disorders; and train and supervise clinical staff to effectively deliver the various evidence-based treatments discussed earlier.

References

American Psychiatric Association: Diagnostic and Statistical Manual of Mental Disorders, 4th Edition, Text Revision. Washington, DC, American Psychiatric Association, 2000

Bien TH, Miller WR, Tonigan JS: Brief interventions for alcohol problems: a review. Addiction 88:315–335, 1993

Carroll KM, Rounsaville BJ, Nich C, et al: One-year follow-up of psychotherapy and pharmacotherapy for cocaine dependence: delayed emergence of psychotherapy effects. Arch Gen Psychiatry 51:989–997, 1994

Crits-Christoph P, Siqueland L, Blaine J, et al: Psychosocial treatments for cocaine dependence: National Institute on Drug Abuse Collaborative Cocaine Treatment Study. Arch Gen Psychiatry 56(6):493–502, 1999

Higgins ST, Budney AJ, Bickel WK, et al: Incentives improve outcome in outpatient behavioral treatment of cocaine dependence. Arch Gen Psychiatry 51:568–576, 1994

Kadden RM: Project MATCH: treatment main effects and matching results. Alcohol Clin Exp Res 20(suppl 8):196A–197A, 1996

Liddle HA, Dakof GA, Parker K, et al: Multidimensional family therapy for adolescent drug abuse: results of a randomized clinical trial. Am J Drug Alcohol Abuse 27(4):651–688, 2001

Miller WR, Rollnick S: Motivational Interviewing: Preparing People for Change, 2nd Edition. New York, Guilford Press, 2002

Nunes EV, Quitkin FM: Treatment of depression in drug dependent patients: effects on mood and drug use. NIDA Res Monogr 172:61–85, 1997

Stanton MD, Shadish WR: Outcome, attrition, and family-couples treatment for drug abuse: a meta-analysis and review of the controlled, comparative studies. Psychol Bull 122(2):170–191, 1997

Szapocznik J, Williams RA: Brief strategic family therapy: twenty-five years of interplay among theory, research and practice in adolescent problem behavior. Clin Child Fam Psychol Rev 3(2):117–134, 2000

Unfaithful Wife

A woman in her late 40s took an overdose of drugs. When she re-covered, she confided to her family doctor that during the previous 18 months, her husband, Jeff, had been increasingly jealous and accusatory. Recently, his accusations had become totally irrational, and he was say-ing that she had multiple lovers, that she got out of bed at night to go to them, and that she was communicating with them by lights and mir-rors. Wrong-number telephone calls were "evidence" that men were contacting her, and he believed that cars passing the house at night flashed their headlights as a signal to her. He put tape on the windows and doors, nailed doors shut, and closely measured the location of ev-ery piece of furniture. Any change resulted in a tirade about her un-faithfulness. He refused to accept any food or cigarettes from her. During this time, her husband did not physically assault her, and their sexual activity remained at its usual level; however, he appeared in-creasingly distressed and haggard and lost 15 pounds.

The wife felt so wretched about her husband's behavior that she considered leaving him, but she was afraid he might become violent. She admitted her overdose was a "cry for help."

Jeff was referred for psychiatric assessment and complied will-ingly. He gave an account similar to his wife's but with total convic-tion about her infidelity. Despite his vehemence and his belief in all the various pieces of "evidence," he seemed to have some awareness that something was wrong with him. An interview with a daughter who lived at home corroborated her mother's innocence and her fa-ther's irrationality.

The marriage had been stable until the onset of this problem, al-though Jeff drank heavily as a young man and sometimes assaulted his wife. His heavy drinking and violent behavior had ceased in his mid-30s, and he had generally been a good husband and provider. He had never used street drugs at any time. His wife described him as al-ways being "pig-headed," but he was not normally unduly argumen-tative and had never previously evinced jealousy. He had attended school up to grade 7; he was probably of low-average intelligence. His family history included many relatives with alcoholism but no other mental disorders.

DSM-IV-TR Casebook Diagnosis of "Unfaithful Wife"

All of Jeff's difficulties stem from his unfounded belief that his wife has been unfaithful. It hardly needs to be stated that this is not a bizarre delusion. The persistence of a nonbizarre delusion of jealousy with behavior that is otherwise unremarkable, in the absence of other psychotic symptoms (e.g., prominent hallucinations, disorganized speech), a Mood Disorder, or a general medical condition that could account for the disturbance, indicates the diagnosis of Delusional Disorder, Jealous Type (DSM-IV-TR, p. 329).

Follow-Up

Jeff was unexpectedly agreeable to treatment and was started on a neuroleptic antipsychotic drug, Orap (pimozide), which he continues to take 3 years later. On two occasions, this drug has been withdrawn, but after 1 or 2 weeks he reports, "I'm beginning to get funny ideas about the wife again," and he voluntarily resumes the medication. Not long after commencing treatment with the neuroleptic, he had an episode of depression, which responded to a tricyclic antidepressant in addition to the Orap. The antidepressant was subsequently withdrawn, and the depression has not recurred.

Discussion of "Unfaithful Wife" by Lewis A. Opler, M.D., Ph.D.*

Delusional Disorder is rare, with population prevalence estimated to be about 0.03% (American Psychiatric Association 2000). Family studies by Kendler and colleagues (1985) suggest that Delusional Disorder is distinct from other psychotic disorders (e.g., it is not a Schizophrenia spectrum disorder). Because persons with Delusional Disorder lack insight but function adequately in most social situations, mental health professionals usually become involved only when the patient's non-bizarre delusions lead to behavior troubling to others.

Characteristically, it is the patient's family that first seeks and then encourages the patient to obtain psychiatric help. Uncharacteristically, Jeff offers little resistance to seeing a psychiatrist and readily agrees to take antipsychotic medications. Usually, such patients agree to take an anxiolytic such as Valium (diazepam) or Xanax (alprazolam) but, at least initially, refuse and often are affronted if an antipsychotic is suggested.

---

*Dr. Opler received his B.A. from Harvard University and both his Ph.D. in Pharmacology and his M.D. from the Albert Einstein College of Medicine. Dr. Opler is currently Clinical Professor of Psychiatry at the New York University School of Medicine, Lecturer in Psychiatry at the College of Physicians and Surgeons of Columbia University, and Director of the Research Division of the New York State Office of Mental Health. Dr. Opler was among the first clinical investigators to demonstrate that negative symptoms in Schizophrenia respond to novel treatment approaches. In carrying out this research, Dr. Opler developed (along with Drs. Kay and Fiszbein) the Positive and Negative Syndrome Scale, or PANSS, now used worldwide in clinical trials. In addition to his work on the assessment and treatment of symptoms in Schizophrenia and other psychotic disorders, Dr. Opler has carried out psychosocial research on the etiology and prevention of homelessness in persons with serious mental illness.

An outspoken advocate for the mentally ill, Dr. Opler has received several awards from the National Alliance for the Mentally Ill, as well as writing the "Ask the Doctor" column for the National Alliance for the Mentally Ill of New York State newsletter. In addition to his nearly 200 publications in scholarly journals, Dr. Opler has written two books to educate a broader audience: Prozac and Other Psychiatric Drugs (Pocket Books 1996) demystifies and destigmatizes the role of medication, and Resurrection and Redemption: Overcoming Mental Illness and Regaining Dignity (PublishAmerica 2003) discusses recovery from serious mental illness. In addition to his research and advocacy work, Dr. Opler is a highly respected clinician, having been chosen as one of the Best Doctors in America by his colleagues for several years.

Because Jeff is so amenable to taking an antipsychotic, this window of opportunity must be seized and managed skillfully! Given decades of clinical experience suggesting that Delusional Disorder responds quickly and effectively to low doses of Orap (pimozide) (Opler et al. 1995; Opler and Feinberg 1991), this underutilized antipsychotic remains the treatment of choice for this understudied psychotic disorder. Despite being a potent D_2-dopamine antagonist, pimozide, at the modest doses of 2–6 mg/day, is usually effective in treating Delusional Disorder. At these low doses, pimozide is well tolerated and offers the advantage of causing little or no sedation. Because pimozide is a weak calcium-channel antagonist, it is capable of causing QT_c prolongation (indicating a prolongation in cardiac conduction), which, when severe, can lead to heart block and even sudden death. I would obtain an electrocardiogram (ECG) before starting Jeff on 2 mg/day of pimozide, and I would monitor the ECG as I increase the dose of pimozide by 2 mg/week until I began to see clinical improvement. Usually, improvement is seen within 2 weeks, so it is unlikely that I would need to exceed 4–6 mg/day of pimozide, and, at these doses, pimozide rarely causes QT_c changes requiring that it be decreased or discontinued. Specifically, pimozide should be lowered or discontinued if the QT_c interval on ECG either increases 25% from baseline or is equal to or greater than 520 milliseconds.

As we learn from the case report, Jeff responds to pimozide, but, when he discontinues the medication on his own, he starts to get "funny ideas about the wife again." This is the point at which I would discuss the need to remain on maintenance medication. I would also now discuss trying one of the second-generation antipsychotics (SGAs) for maintenance pharmacotherapy, with the understanding that if the "funny ideas" do not go away again or if they get worse, then he will need to restart pimozide.

The presently available SGAs are Clozaril (clozapine), Zyprexa (olanzapine), Risperdal (risperidone), Geodon (ziprasidone), Seroquel (quetiapine), and Abilify (aripiprazole). They are often called "atypical antipsychotics," but I prefer to refer to them as SGAs because they are not a single class of drugs but, rather, differ significantly from one another in ways we are just beginning to understand. In Schizophrenia and psychotic Mood Disorder, most of the SGAs have been shown to be effective in treating positive, negative, and mood symptoms, while causing little or no clinically significant extrapyramidal symptoms. In addition, quetiapine, ziprasidone, and aripiprazole appear to cause little or no elevation in serum prolactin, a hormone involved in lactation, which is often abnormally elevated as a side effect of taking antipsychotic medication. In the maintenance phase of Delusional Disorder, I would treat Jeff with quetiapine because it is a well-tolerated medication with a relatively benign side-effect profile. In addition, recent evidence suggests that quetiapine may have efficacy in treating Delusional Disorder. Specifically, ratings on PANSS (Kay et al. 2000) were obtained for patients with a variety of psychotic disorders enrolled in the Quetiapine Experience With Safety and Tolerability study, a large-scale multicenter prospective study that included patients with a variety of psychotic disorders, including Delusional Disorder (Mullen et al. 2001). When PANSS scores were analyzed for patients with a DSM-IV diagnosis of Delusional Disorder, quetiapine treatment was associated with statistically significant improvement on the PANSS Total, Positive Scale, and Delusions item scores (Opler et al. 2003).

So, in summary, I would treat patients like Jeff initially with pimozide. I would switch to quetiapine at the point of remission of nonbizarre delusions or at any time if QT_c prolongation called for discontinuation of pimozide. I would stress to the patient and, if available, to his or her family the need for ongoing treatment. Although we can manage symptoms with pharmacotherapy, we do not know how to cure Delusional Disorder. The seriousness of delusional jealousy is often underappreciated because patients function adequately in most areas. And, yet, it is precisely the absence of cognitive and social decline that makes persons with delusional jealousy capable of planning and executing complex revenge scenarios (Silva et al. 1998, 2000). Convinced that his wife is unfaithful, Jeff, if untreated, could, like Shakespeare's Othello, become threatening and dangerous to his wife and her imagined lovers. Unlike Othello, however, these patients do not require Iago to fuel irrational jealousy, thus making long-term follow-up and treatment essential.

References

American Psychiatric Association: Diagnostic and Statistical Manual of Mental Disorders, 4th Edition, Text Revision. Washington, DC, American Psychiatric Association, 2000

Kay SR, Opler LA, Fiszbein A: The Positive and Negative Syndrome Scale (PANSS) Manual. Toronto, Multi-Health Systems Inc, 2000

Kendler KS, Masterson CC, Davies KL: Psychiatric illness in first degree relative of patients with paranoid psychosis, schizophrenia and medical illness. Br J Psychiatry 147:524–531, 1985

Mullen J, Jibson MD, Sweitzer D: A comparison of relative safety, efficacy, and tolerability of quetiapine and risperidone in outpatients with schizophrenia and other psychotic disorders: the quetiapine experience with safety and tolerability (QUEST) study. Clin Ther 23:1839–1854, 2001

Opler LA, Feinberg SS: The role of pimozide in clinical psychiatry: a review. J Clin Psychiatry 52:221–233, 1991

Opler LA, Klahr DM, Ramirez PM: Pharmacologic treatment of delusions. Psychiatr Clin North Am 18:379–391, 1995

Opler MG, Opler LA, Mullen J: Quetiapine in the treatment of delusional disorder. Presented at 55th Annual Institute on Psychiatric Services, Boston, MA, 2003

Silva JA, Ferrare MM, Leong GB, et al: The dangerousness of persons with delusional jealousy. J Am Acad Psychiatry Law 26:607–623, 1998

Silva JA, Derecho DV, Leong GB, et al: Stalking behavior in delusional jealousy. J Forensic Sci 45(1):77–82, 2000

Melancholy or Malarky?

Mr. Dennis O'Malley is a small, bent, disheveled 63-year-old man with a very faint Irish accent. He was referred for psychiatric evaluation when he attended the medical clinic where he was being treated for diabetes and maintenance of a colostomy that he had had for 5 years as a result of ulcerative colitis. He told his doctor that he was upset because he had been hearing voices and was promptly sent to the psychiatry clinic for an evaluation.

Mr. O'Malley is interviewed by a psychiatrist and begins telling his chief complaint, in traditional Irish fashion, with a story. A few weeks ago—he is not quite sure when—he took a fellow home from church and, feeling tired, lay down on the fellow's bed to take a nap. He awoke to find the fellow "on top of" him and raced out the door as fast as he could go. At this point, he is not sure whether it really happened or it was a dream or a hallucination. In any case, it was followed some time later by an experience on the street in which a strange man called him "an Irish fag." This upset him a great deal, and he has been brooding about it ever since. He remembers that about a year ago, the owners of a new car wash in the neighborhood called him a fag, and he wonders if these things are related. Two weeks ago, he began to hear voices calling him a fag and saying other derogatory things about him, and his "whole system dropped down." He knows he is not homosexual and understands at some level that what is happening is "in my mind." Nevertheless, he feels that everyone in the neighborhood believes that he is homosexual. He has been very nervous and shaky and has gone to his priest, who tells him that it is his imagination and he should ignore it. He is apparently still hearing the voices during the interview.

Mr. O'Malley describes his mood as "lousy" and "nervous and shaky." He does not volunteer that he is feeling depressed, but he says that he has not been interested in seeing friends or doing anything since his mood deteriorated. He also says that he has no appetite and has lost weight, but he denies changes in his sleeping. Although he does not acknowledge feeling guilty about things he has done, he says he feels guilty about "the blasphemous words" the voices are saying. When asked specifically about suicide, he says that he is Catholic and he would not go to heaven if he committed suicide, so therefore he would not kill himself; however, he says he has thought that he would be better off if something just happened to him to make his heart stop.

Mr. O'Malley had a similar experience 12 years ago when he heard blaspheming voices and became preoccupied with religious "scruples." He was treated as an outpatient for several months and took some kind of medication, the name of which he does not remember. He went back to work as a cab driver and continued driving until his deteriorating physical condition caused him to go on disability 5 years ago. He lives with his wife and a 25-year-old son and spends a good deal of time in church-related activities and playing the saxophone for various community affairs. He has not had a drink containing alcohol in 30 years.

When questioned about memory problems, he describes making the wrong turn once on a highway and a few other instances of forgetting whether he had turned off the gas stove in his kitchen.

The following day, the psychiatrist on the ward to which he had been admitted interviewed Mr. O'Malley's wife. She reported that he had always tended to exaggerate slights and was quick to take offense and to read criticism into the remarks of others. She saw his distress of the past few weeks as simply an exaggeration of his nature. She noticed that he had been "listless" for a few days and thought maybe he had a "virus." She described the episode 12 years earlier as similar to this one in that he had become increasingly nervous and suspicious and had begun hearing "voices."

DSM-IV-TR Casebook Diagnosis of "Melancholy or Malarky"

The first diagnostic question is whether the "voices" that call Mr. O'Malley an "Irish fag" are hallucinations or obsessions. The symptom has several features that suggest an obsession: They are recurrent, intrusive, and stereotyped. However, the patient does not experience them as products of his own mind but as accusations from other people, which he then elaborates to include everyone in the neighborhood. Therefore, the voices appear to be true hallucinations that are delusionally elaborated.

Are the delusions and hallucinations symptomatic of a Mood Disorder? He does say that he has not been interested in anything since this all began and that he has lost considerable weight and feels guilty about the blasphemous voices. He has recurrent thoughts of death even though he denies suicidal thoughts. We think there probably are enough symptoms to justify a diagnosis of Major Depressive Disorder (DSM-IV-TR, p. 376). We suspect that the prior episode was similar, so we add Recurrent to the diagnosis. Because the hallucinations and delusions are persecutory and the patient does not feel guilty about the things of which he is accused (as in a typical depressive delusion), we add also With Mood-Incongruent Psychotic Features (DSM-IV-TR, p. 413).

Follow-Up

Mr. O'Malley was treated with antipsychotic medication in an inpatient unit. The treating psychiatrists were not impressed with the depressive symptoms and therefore did not include antidepressant medication until some weeks later, when the voices diminished and the patient became more obviously depressed, at which point he was given nortriptyline, a tricyclic antidepressant. A full neurological examination, including a computed tomography scan, was negative. He left the hospital in 4 weeks, at which time he was much improved. The voices, although still present, were not as upsetting to him, and his wife was competent and willing to supervise his medication.

His outpatient psychiatrist, who began treating him when he left the hospital, was impressed with a new symptom: Mr. O'Malley's obsessive requests for reassurance that he had not disobeyed church rules, such as having thrown the communion wafer into the toilet, although he recognized that he had not done this. The outpatient psychiatrist gradually reduced his antipsychotic medication and changed his antidepressant to a selective serotonin reuptake inhibitor (SSRI), thinking that it might also be useful in the treatment of his obsessive-compulsive symptoms. While taking this medication, Mr. O'Malley slowly improved and, a year later, was free of symptoms and had returned to his baseline functioning.

Discussion of "Melancholy or Malarky" by Max Fink, M.D.*

Poor Mr. O'Malley! He is offered conventional antipsychotic medicines without attention to his depression; then, he is treated with an SSRI antidepressant (presumably to address his possible Obsessive-Compulsive Disorder symptoms) without attention to his delusions. He labors until his remitting illness resolves and "a year later, was free of symptoms and had returned to his baseline functioning." Does this approach to treatment differ from that offered by the nineteenth-century masters of psychopathology—Kraepelin, Bleuler, Kahlbaum, and Hoch? Hardly, for they too offered palliatives and sedatives but mainly hoped that time would allow the few patients who remitted to heal. Is there a better course of treatment available today? Was a year of Mr. O'Malley's illness avoidable?

Major Depressive Disorder With Psychotic Features (DSM-IV-TR, 296.34), commonly referred to as "psychotic depression," is the best diagnosis for Mr. O'Malley's illness. But such a diagnosis is often difficult to make because florid psychotic symptoms conceal the depression. Notice the fiddling by the psychiatrists assessing his behavior. Even at leading academic hospitals, the few such patients who are referred for electroconvulsive therapy (ECT) present after medication trials have proved inadequate (Mulsant et al. 1997). Of 52 patients referred in one study, only two had been treated with medications to adequate dosing and time standards.

Poor Mr. O'Malley. The diagnosis of psychotic depression was missed, and neither his inpatient nor his outpatient doctor read his story accurately. They did not offer appropriate treatments nor did they undertake the laboratory tests (such as the dexamethasone suppression test) that might have ensured Mr. O'Malley's diagnosis and adequate treatment.

---

*Dr. Fink is Professor of Psychiatry and Neurology Emeritus at State University of New York at Stony Brook and Professor of Psychiatry at Albert Einstein College of Medicine. Dr. Fink began his experience with ECT in January 1952. After extensive studies of ECT mechanisms and changes in the electroencephalogram, he was sidetracked into psychopharmacology—as an investigator in the Early Clinical Drug Evaluation Program. Popular recognition of the limitation of psychoactive drugs brought him back to ECT in the mid-1970s. He published his textbook, Convulsive Therapy: Theory and Practice, in 1979; launched the quarterly scientific journal Convulsive Therapy in 1985; produced the video Informed ECT for Patients and Their Families in 1986; and produced the trade book Electroshock: Restoring the Mind in 1999. In 2003, he published Catatonia: A Clinician's Guide to Diagnosis and Treatment (Fink and Taylor 2003), a joint effort with M.A. Taylor.

The diagnosis of psychotic depression was described in 1977 by Glassman and his associates. Before 1977, all psychotic patients in the United States were believed to have Schizophrenia, even when depression or mania was in the foreground. The researchers had treated a cohort of severely depressed patients with adequate trials of Tofranil (imipramine) monitored by serum blood levels (Kantor and Glassman 1977). The treatment had failed to be useful in 13 patients who were then treated until remission with ECT. In examining the records of these patients, the authors noted that each had been psychotic as well as severely depressed. The researchers offered a diagnosis of psychotic depression separate from that of Schizophrenia. Within a few years, this observation was confirmed, and a subtype of Major Depressive Disorder for those patients with psychotic features was included in DSM-III.

Psychotic depressed patients did not respond to antipsychotic medicines alone. They did improve, however, when antipsychotic and antidepressant medicines were combined using large doses of both medicines, equivalent to 200–300 mg of amitriptyline (Elavil) and 16–64 mg of perphenazine (Trilafon). By 1985, it was clear that the efficacy of antidepressants alone was 30%, antipsychotic agents alone was 50%, and combined antidepressant and antipsychotic agents was 70% (Kroessler 1985). These observations have been repeatedly confirmed (Kho et al. 2003; Parker et al. 1992; Vega et al. 2000).

Not one of the modern antidepressant drugs (SSRIs, selective norepinephrine reuptake inhibitors, etc.) has been adequately tested for its efficacy in psychotic depression. I cannot distinguish these agents for efficacy, but, given the weak evidence for efficacy of the latest antidepressants in hospitalized depressed patients, I do not feel justified in offering the newer compounds for psychotic depression. We lack evidence of the efficacy of SSRIs and antipsychotic drugs, and it would be hazardous to assume that they are either "adequate" or "inadequate." The evidence for the older medicines, by contrast, is quite strong. Nor has any atypical antipsychotic drug been shown to be effective in treating psychotic depression, either alone or in combination with an antidepressant.

What treatments are effective in psychotic depression? ECT offered remission in 80% of those treated (Kho et al. 2003; Kroessler 1985; Parker et al. 1992; Vega et al. 2000). In the past decade, however, we have learned how to administer ECT with increasing efficacy and even greater safety, so that the present remission rate (i.e., full remission from illness, not just a 50% improvement in rating scale scores!) is 95% with bitemporal ECT (Petrides et al. 2001). A similar conclusion is presented in the independent Belgian study by Birkenhäger et al. (2003).

ECT is not only effective in relieving psychotic depression, but it also does so very rapidly. Within 12 days (six ECT treatments), 45% remitted; within 3 weeks (nine ECT treatments), 80% remitted; and all had remitted by 4 weeks (12 ECT treatments) (Husain et al., in press).

Had Mr. O'Malley been offered ECT at the outset, he probably would have been home rather quickly and recovered after 6 weeks. Continuation ECT on a biweekly or monthly schedule for 4–6 months would have sustained improvement without additional medications (Fink et al. 1996).

What of laboratory testing? Surely the inpatient physicians should have examined Mr. O'Malley's neuroendocrine status. In patients with psychotic depression, serum cortisol levels are elevated, diurnal rhythm is lost, and exogenous steroids do not suppress the elevated levels. The dexamethasone suppression test uses 1 mg or 2 mg of oral dexamethasone as the test steroid. When severe depressive illness is relieved, the dexamethasone suppression test normalizes. A return to an abnormal dexamethasone suppression test (elevated cortisol levels that do not suppress with dexamethasone) heralds an impending relapse (Rush et al. 1996).

Poor Mr. O'Malley. Why was he treated so poorly, and why was ECT not offered? The failure to properly diagnose psychotic depression is one factor. Even if his depression was properly diagnosed, ECT is rarely used. The faculties of the major universities do not recommend it, because many universities have no facility for ECT. ECT is widely seen as difficult, expensive, and brain damaging. Expert treatment algorithms offer ECT, if they offer it at all, as the last resort. In a detailed review of the treatment of psychotic depression, the national expert Alan Schatzberg (2003, p. 21) writes, "While ECT is a remarkably effective treatment for psychotic depression, requirements for its use are stringent, and public perception about the overall appropriateness of shock treatment is negative." In the summary, Schatzberg concludes, "While there are sufficient data to recommend ECT for the treatment of psychotic depression, there are both real and perceived drawbacks to ECT; therefore it may be best considered after other options have failed" (p. 22). The shadow of *One Flew over the Cuckoo's Nest* still plagues this treatment option, which is unfortunate and unjustified because the film depicted the use of ECT without anesthesia, a practice that has not occurred in the United States for decades. Had Mr. O'Malley been the chief executive officer of a local company, the spouse of the hospital director, or some other VIP, however, he or his spouse would have demanded, and he would have received, the most effective treatment—ECT.

Mr. O'Malley, treated as the retiree that he was, seen as having infinite time to remain ill, is offered the conventional wisdom that the latest pills with lesser efficacy but greater presumed safety will eventually be useful. Sometimes, however, such a plan goes awry, as the patient sees no end to his pain, and suicide becomes the only option. That is particularly shameful because ECT is very effective at reducing suicidal thoughts (Kellner et al., submitted).

How are we to appreciate the choice of treatments for psychotic depression? Imagine a patient arriving at the hospital with high fever, chills, cough, and chest pain, and the physical examination is positive for a bacterial pneumonia. Would the physician consider palliative treatment, aspirin, or the least effective antibiotic? Unlikely. He or she would probably prescribe the most effective antibiotic for the condition, at the same time sampling the sputum to assess the sensitivity of the infectious agent to that antibiotic. Similarly, for psychotic depression, ECT is the primary treatment and should be prescribed without delay. It is effective and safe.

Psychotic depression is as severe an illness as psychiatrists have to treat. The mortality rate is significantly greater for psychotic depression than for nonpsychotic depression, with 41% versus 20% of patients, respectively, dying within 15 years of hospital admission (Vythilingham et al. 2003).

Mr. O'Malley was badly served by his therapists. His condition was not promptly recognized. The primary treatment, ECT, was not discussed or considered. Palliative medications were offered, but, even at best, these medicines are effective only half of the time and only after many months. The failure to prescribe ECT is indefensible.

References

Birkenhäger TK, Pluijms EM, Lucius SAP: ECT response in delusional versus non-delusional depressed inpatients. J Affect Dis 74:191–195, 2003

Fink M: Electroshock: Restoring the Mind. New York, Oxford University Press, 1999

Fink M, Taylor MA: Catatonia: A Clinician's Guide to Diagnosis and Treatment. Cambridge, UK, Cambridge University Press, 2003

Fink M, Abrams R, Bailine S, et al: Ambulatory electroconvulsive therapy. Task Force Report of the Association for Convulsive Therapy. Convulsive Ther 12:42–55, 1996

Husain M, Rush AJ, Fink M, et al: Speed of response and remission in major depressive disorder with acute ECT: a Consortium for Research in ECT (CORE) report. J Clin Psychiatry (in press)

Kantor SJ, Glassman AH: Delusional depressions: natural history and response to treatment. Br J Psychiatry 131:351–360, 1977

Kellner C, Fink M, Knapp R, et al: Bilateral ECT rapidly relieves suicidality. Am J Psychiatry (submitted)

Kho KH, van Vreeswijk MF, Simpson S, et al: A meta-analysis of electroconvulsive therapy efficacy in depression. J ECT 19:139–147, 2003

Kroessler D: Relative efficacy rates for therapies of delusional depression. Convulsive Ther 1:173–182, 1985

Mulsant BH, Haskett RF, Prudic J, et al: Low use of neuroleptic drugs in the treatment of psychotic major depression. Am J Psychiatry 154:559–561, 1997

Parker G, Roy K, Hadzi-Pavlovic D, et al: Psychotic (delusional) depression: a meta-analysis of physical treatments. J Affect Dis 24:17–24, 1992

Petrides G, Fink M, Husain MM, et al: ECT remission rates in psychotic versus non-psychotic depressed patients: a report from CORE. J ECT 17:244–253, 2001

Rush AJ, Giles DE, Schlesser MA, et al: The dexamethasone suppression test in patients with mood disorders. J Clin Psychiatry 57:470–484, 1996

Schatzberg AF: New approaches to managing psychotic depression. J Clin Psychiatry 64 (suppl 1):19–23, 2003

Vega JAW, Mortimer AM, Tyson PJ: Somatic treatment of psychotic depression: review and recommendations for practice. J Clin Psychopharmacol 20:504–519, 2000

Vythilingham M, Chen J, Bremner JD, et al: Psychotic depression and mortality. Am J Psychiatry 160:574–576, 2003

Junior Executive

Joan Demarest is a 38-year-old junior executive with a master's degree in business administration who, for the last year and a half, has worked on a marketing team in a large pharmaceutical firm. She is referred by a colleague for "supportive" treatment. She complains of being tired, uninterested in life, and "depressed" about everything: her job, her husband, and her prospects for the future.

She has had two previous extensive courses of psychotherapy for persistent feelings of depressed mood, inferiority, and pessimism, which she claims to have had since she was 16 or 17. These symptoms have waxed and waned. During her senior college year, she describes a 3-month period when, in addition to her chronic symptoms, she was not sleeping, was not eating, and probably had sufficient symptoms to meet the criteria for a Major Depressive Episode. She saw a therapist twice weekly for 3 years while in college and a psychoanalyst 2–3 times weekly for 2.5 years overlapping graduate school.

Although she did reasonably well in college, she often ruminated about students who were "genuinely intelligent." She rarely dated during college and graduate school and would never go after a guy she thought was "special," always feeling inferior and intimidated. Whenever she met such a man, she acted stiff and aloof or walked away as quickly as possible, only to berate herself afterward and then fantasize about him for months. She claimed that her previous therapies had helped her to better understand herself but had little, if any, effect on her depressive symptoms.

Just after graduation, she married her husband, whom she had dated for a year. She thought of him as reasonably desirable, although not "special," and married him primarily because she felt she "needed a husband" for companionship. Shortly after their wedding, the couple started to bicker. She rarely complains directly to him but disapproves of his clothes, his job, and his parents; he, in turn, accuses her of being rejecting and moody. Her social life with her husband involves several other couples. The man in these couples is usually a friend of her husband's. She is sure that the women find her uninteresting and unimpressive and that the people who seem to like her are probably as boring as she is. She now wonders whether her marriage was a mistake and sometimes thinks that she would leave her husband were she not afraid to be alone. They have had no children, in part because she felt inadequate to be a mother.

Recently, she has also been having difficulties at work. She is assigned the most menial tasks and is never given an assignment of importance or responsibility. She has trouble concentrating, and rarely demonstrates assertiveness or initiative to her supervisors. She views her boss as self-centered, unconcerned, and unfair, but nevertheless admires his success. She thinks that she will never go far in her profession because she does not have the right "connections," and neither does her husband.

DSM-IV-TR Casebook Diagnosis of "Junior Executive"

Ms. Demarest has had a chronically depressed mood since adolescence. Because her depression is currently not severe enough to meet the criteria for a Major Depressive Episode, and the mood disturbance and associated symptoms have persisted for more than 2 years, the diagnosis is most likely either Dysthymic Disorder or Major Depressive Disorder in Partial Remission. Because her depression did not begin with a Major Depressive Episode and there is no evidence of either specific etiological factors such as a general medical condition or chronic substance use, or of a Manic or Hypomanic episode in her lifetime, the diagnosis is Dysthymic Disorder (DSM-IV-TR, p. 380).

Discussion of "Junior Executive" by John C. Markowitz, M.D.*

The diagnosis of Dysthymic Disorder is frequently missed (Markowitz et al. 1992). Clinicians may focus on recent depressive symptoms and diagnose Major Depressive Disorder, but in fact the symptoms more likely represent a worsening of Dysthymic Disorder. About a third of all depressions are chronic: These can be categorized as either Dysthymic Disorder; Major Depression, chronic (in which the individual chronically has the full depressive syndrome); or recurrent Major Depressive Disorder without full interepisode recovery. The course of chronic depressions has been shown to be worse than that of episodic Major Depressive Disorder. As in Ms. Demarest's case, Dysthymic Disorder typically leads sooner or later to a Major Depressive Episode. Such cases are referred to as *double depression* (Keller and Shapiro 1982)—that is, Major Depressive Disorder superimposed on Dysthymic Disorder. It is unlikely that this actually represents two separate disorders but, rather, the addition of a couple of acute symptoms to persistent dysthymia. Patients with Dysthymic Disorder often present for treatment when their depressive symptoms become severe enough to warrant a diagnosis of Major Depressive Disorder, although such was not the story in Ms. Demarest's case.

A second diagnostic confusion is whether the patient has a Depressive Personality Disorder or a chronic mood disorder: Are the symptoms a trait or a (chronic) state? Patients tend to experience a chronic simmering depression *as* their personality. Such confusion is understandable considering that, as far back as they can recall, they may have always felt that way. Historically, such patients were believed to have a personality disorder and typically received long-term psychotherapy, whereas pharmacological treatment was not considered. Since 1980, the *Diagnostic and Statistical Manual of Mental Disorders* has classified chronic milder depressive symptoms as a Mood Disorder (Dysthymic

*Dr. Markowitz is Associate Professor of Psychiatry at Weill Medical College of Cornell University and Research Psychiatrist at the New York State Psychiatric Institute in New York City. Dr. Markowitz was trained in interpersonal psychotherapy (IPT) by the late Gerald L. Klerman, M.D., who, with Dr. Myrna Weissman, developed IPT in the 1970s. Dr. Markowitz is the author of Interpersonal Psychotherapy for Dysthymic Disorder (Markowitz 1998) and coauthored Comprehensive Guide to Interpersonal Psychotherapy (Basic Books, 2000) with Drs. Weissman and Klerman.

Disorder) rather than a personality disorder, a nosological change that has encouraged the often successful use of pharmacotherapy.

Ms. Demarest is unusual in that she is married. Because of their interpersonal difficulties, most patients with Dysthymic Disorder either have never married or have separated or divorced. Like Ms. Demarest, patients with dysthymia believe that they are boring and inadequate and feel uncomfortable in social situations. Emotional intimacy would require them to expose their self-perceived inner deficits. Interpersonal difficulties are indeed a hallmark of chronic depression. The patient's cognitive and emotional sense of inadequacy—feeling guilty, helpless, hopeless, worthless, like a fraud—is often more prominent than are neurovegetative depressive symptoms, such as problems with sleep and appetite. (That is, the DSM-IV Appendix B alternative symptom criteria for Dysthymic Disorder, which are based on research findings, are more germane than the standard criteria.) Dysthymic individuals tend to function better at work—where a job description provides role definition—than in the less structured social domain.

Ms. Demarest is 38 and seeks treatment for the third time. This is consistent with the findings of studies of chronically depressed outpatients who typically are in their 30s, have had unsuccessful treatment with psychotherapy, and yet rarely have had an adequate trial of antidepressant medication. These patients present with infectious discouragement, and often demoralize their therapists as well. It is important that the clinician not share the patient's discouragement, because effective treatments exist.

Antidepressant pharmacotherapy is the best proven treatment and should be considered the first-line intervention. All classes of antidepressant medications tested to date have worked about equally well, but selective serotonin reuptake inhibitors are most commonly used. The specific choice of medication depends on several factors, including response to previous medications, the match of the medication's effects with prominent symptoms (e.g., a sedating drug for a patient with insomnia), the medication's common side effects (e.g., increased activation, sexual dysfunction, weight gain), and interactions with other medications. With this patient, as with most patients, I would probably start with a selective serotonin reuptake inhibitor, first carefully informing her of its likely benefits, side effects, and course of action.

Medication may relieve decades-long symptoms in a matter of a few weeks (Kocsis et al. 1988) and improve social and vocational functioning as well (Markowitz 1994). To some patients, the sudden discovery of normal mood (euthymia) can feel like a personality change. Treatment should proceed as it would for Major Depressive Disorder: adequate doses of medication for an adequate acute duration—at least 8 weeks. Response rates are slightly lower (closer to 50%) than for Major Depressive Disorder (60%–70%) but are still substantial. If patients do not respond to a therapeutic dosage after 6–8 weeks, augmentation with or switching to another medication may well work. Because dysthymic patients are easily discouraged, therapists should take pains to ensure that patients do not blame themselves for treatment nonresponse and persevere with another treatment trial that might work. Once patients respond to medication, they tend to need years of maintenance pharmacotherapy to protect against relapse.

Psychotherapy has been less well studied but is likely helpful (Markowitz 1998), perhaps optimally in conjunction with medication (Keller et al. 2000), both to relieve symptoms and to help develop needed interpersonal skills. Time-limited psychotherapies such as cognitive-behavioral therapy (CBT), interpersonal psychotherapy (IPT), and the cognitive-behavioral analysis system of psychotherapy (CBASP) were designed to treat mood disorders. Given the risk of relapse, a successful acute course of such psychotherapies would need to be followed by continuation and maintenance psychotherapy. This approach is analogous to ongoing pharmacotherapy for this chronic disorder.

CBT is a diagnosis-targeted treatment based on the observation that depressed patients have characteristically distorted thoughts (e.g., "I'm a loser," "People don't find me interesting," "My life situation is overwhelming," "Nothing will ever get any better"), which seem to arise "automatically." Ideas such as "My work is slipshod" both are painful and inhibit normal functioning. CBT therapists encourage patients to examine and test these mood-congruent thoughts rather than simply believing them. Homework includes mutually agreed-on behavioral tasks—going out for a walk, for example, rather than sitting at home—and writing down and assessing the automatic thoughts. In research studies of CBT, the therapy is time limited (12–20 sessions). CBT has been better tested for acute Major Depressive Disorder than for chronic Mood Disorders.

IPT, also time-limited (12–16 acute sessions) and diagnosis-focused, addresses the relationship between a patient's mood and his or her life situation. It is based on the observation that depressive episodes tend to occur not in a vacuum but in the context of a difficult life situation: the death of a significant other, a problematic relationship, or some other life change. Working on interpersonal functioning and solving the life crisis also relieves mood. For Ms. Demarest, IPT might focus on her marital dispute or her work role, particularly on her inability to express her needs to her husband and at work. The model of IPT was developed to treat acute depression and requires some adaptation for patients with chronic mood syndromes (Markowitz 1998). IPT has demonstrated efficacy in the treatment of acute Major Depressive Disorder; ongoing research is assessing its benefits for chronic Mood Disorders (Browne et al. 2002; Markowitz 2003).

CBASP (McCullough 2000), which combines aspects of CBT, IPT, and psychodynamic psychotherapy, was compared to pharmacotherapy in one large trial for patients with chronic Major Depressive Disorder. (Chronic Major Depressive Disorder is related but not identical to Dysthymic Disorder.) CBASP is a highly structured treatment that focuses on how chronically depressed patients handle or mishandle interpersonal situations. CBASP worked as well as medication, and the combination of medication plus CBASP worked better than either treatment alone (Keller et al. 2000). The combination of time-limited psychotherapy and antidepressant medication may be the optimal treatment for many chronically depressed patients.

Psychoanalytically oriented therapy or psychodynamic psychotherapy, although in widespread clinical use, has not been systematically tested as a treatment for dysthymic patients. Its focus on the past may be less helpful than one of the previously discussed therapies, which help patients to solve current problems (Markowitz 1994).

In treating Ms. Demarest, I would present her with her diagnosis of Dysthymic Disorder and explain the range of treatment options. Inasmuch as she has never had an antidepressant medication trial despite years of having the disorder, I would recommend that she seriously consider one, explaining the strong research evidence for the efficacy of pharmacological treatment. She might respond rapidly to this medication and possibly need no additional treatment. On the other hand, it is unlikely that pharmacological treatment—even if largely successful in treating her mood symptoms—would solve her problems with her husband. For that reason, I would also suggest she consider focal, time-limited psychotherapy.

If Ms. Demarest refused medication after an extended discussion of its advantages and disadvantages, I would suggest treatment with IPT, CBT, or CBASP. Marital therapy might be another option. If, at the end of that time-limited treatment, the patient had not improved, she and I might by then have built enough of a treatment alliance to negotiate a pharmacotherapy trial. Regardless of which intervention ultimately worked, Ms.

Demarest would likely need ongoing treatment in order to maintain euthymia and to have the opportunity to develop new social skills.

As with treatment-resistant depression, an important aspect of treating chronic mood syndromes is that the therapist remain hopeful and optimistic. If one intervention does not work, the therapist should ensure that the patient does not give up or blame him- or herself. Hopelessness is a symptom of depression and particularly of chronic depression, but the prognosis is never hopeless.

References

Browne G, Steiner M, Roberts J, et al: Sertaline and/or interpersonal psychotherapy for patients with dysthymic disorder in primary care: 6-month comparison with longitudinal 2-year follow-up of effectiveness and costs. J Affect Disord 68:317–330, 2002

Keller MB, Shapiro RW: "Double depression": superimposition of acute depressive episodes on chronic depressive disorders. Am J Psychiatry 139:438–442, 1982

Keller MB, McCullough JP, Klein DN, et al: The acute treatment of chronic major depression: a comparison of nefazodone, cognitive behavioral analysis system of psychotherapy, and their combination. N Engl J Med 342:1462–1470, 2000

Kocsis J, Frances AJ, Voss C, et al: Imipramine and social-vocational adjustment in chronic depression. Am J Psychiatry 145:997–999, 1988

Markowitz JC: Psychotherapy of the post-dysthymic patient. J Psychother Pract Res 2:157–163, 1993

Markowitz JC: Psychotherapy of dysthymia. Am J Psychiatry 151:1114–1121, 1994

Markowitz JC: Interpersonal Psychotherapy for Dysthymic Disorder. Washington, DC, American Psychiatric Press, 1998

Markowitz JC: Interpersonal psychotherapy for chronic depression. J Clin Psychol 59:847–858, 2003

Markowitz JC, Moran ME, Kocsis JH, et al: Prevalence and comorbidity of dysthymic disorder among psychiatric outpatients. J Affect Disord 24:63–71, 1992

McCullough JP: Treatment for Chronic Depression: Cognitive Behavioral Analysis System of Psychotherapy. New York, Guilford, 2000

Dolls

Rocky is an 8-year-old boy for whom his parents seek treatment because "he wants to be a girl." The patient's major playmate is his younger sister. Although his parents are trying to foster friendships with other boys, Rocky prefers to play with girls or to be with his mother or a female babysitter. He refuses to participate in rough play with boys and physical fighting, although he is well built, above average in height for his age, and well coordinated. At home, he engages in much make-believe play, invariably assuming female roles. When playing house with his younger sister, he plays the "mother" or "big sister" role and leaves the male role to her. He likes to imitate female television figures, such as Brenda from *Beverly Hills 90210* or Bart Simpson's sister Lisa. Similarly, he likes to playact female characters from various children's books.

Rocky has never been interested in toy cars, trucks, or trains but is an avid player with dolls (baby dolls, Barbie, and family dolls) and enjoys playing with kitchen toys. He also likes to pretend he is a bride, a pregnant woman, a female teacher, or a lady doctor. He is good at drawing and is very interested in drawing female figures. Although his parents try to restrict the activity, he engages in a lot of cross-dressing. Sometimes, he uses a quilt or a towel around his middle for a skirt or a T-shirt or nightgown for a dress. He does not use any female underwear or bathing suits. He likes bows in his hair and may use an underskirt or a veil on his head to imitate long hair. He loves dancing, preferably in dresses. He is very interested in jewelry, has plastic necklaces, and pretends at times to wear earrings. Also, he pretends to apply lipstick (with Chapstick) and would use real lipstick and perfume if his mother would let him. He states, "I want to be a girl" often when he is unhappy (e.g., when he started kindergarten, when he felt in competition with his younger sister).

On physical examination, Rocky is found to have normal male genitalia. His intellectual development is apparently normal. Although he is somewhat reluctant, he is able to describe much of what his parents have related about his toy and game preferences. He says that he does

not want to be a boy because he is afraid he will have to play with soldiers or play army with other boys when he grows bigger. He wishes a
fairy could change him into a girl. What he likes about being a girl is
wearing dresses, long hair, and jewelry.

Family history, pregnancy, birth, and early development are all normal. The parents do not show any overt psychopathology. The patient's problems seem to have started with the birth of his younger
sister, when he was age 2. For the first 4 months of her life, his sister
had digestive problems and required a great deal of parental attention
and care. Rocky then began to display definite signs of regression—he
played the baby role again, wanting to drink from a bottle and be held
and carried. His mother gave in to some extent. Both parents and
babysitters think that cross-dressing and wanting to be a girl date back
to that time, although before the birth of his sister, there were already
some instances of Rocky's imitating long hair by wearing a towel on
his head. When the patient was 4, his sister got a baby doll, which he
took from her. Around this same time, he spent a vacation with his sister at their grandparents' house and complained that his sister got
more attention than he did, ending with the familiar, "Why can't I be a
girl? Why didn't God make me a girl? Girls get to dress up, get to wear
pretty things."

Rocky was enrolled in nursery school at age 3, and he initially displayed much separation anxiety. He appeared more sensitive than the
other children, always seemed to feel threatened by them, and did not
stand up for himself. His teacher noted from the beginning that he
dressed up very frequently, said that he wanted to be a mother when
he grew up, and refused to engage in rough-and-tumble activities. In
the third grade, his classroom teacher closed off the doll corner because of his preoccupation with doll play.

DSM-IV-TR Casebook Diagnosis of "Dolls"

There should be little question about the diagnosis in this case.
Rocky has a strong and persistent identification of himself as a female. He frequently states his desire to be a girl—not just play a

female role. He is preoccupied with female stereotypical activity, preferring to play with girls and pretending that he is a girl, and frequently cross-dresses. He plays exclusively with stereotypically female toys such as dolls. When imitating characters from books and television, he always chooses female characters. There is also evidence of a persistent discomfort with being a boy. He rejects stereotypical male toys and activities and shows an aversion toward rough-and-tumble play.

These are the characteristic features of Gender Identity Disorder (GID) as seen in a male (DSM-IV-TR, p. 581). When this disorder is diagnosed in a female, the desire to be male because of a profound discontent with being a female needs to be distinguished from the desire merely to have the perceived cultural advantages associated with being a male.

Discussion of "Dolls"
by Kenneth J. Zucker, Ph.D.*

Rocky presents with a very typical constellation of indicators that characterize boys who meet the DSM-IV-TR criteria for GID. He shows a strong cross-gender identification and a rejection of, or discomfort with, stereotypical masculine behaviors that are commonly displayed by boys in Western cultures. Rocky not only manifests a great deal of cross-gender behavior but also verbalizes unhappiness about being a boy, which is perhaps best captured by the term *gender dysphoria*. Apart from his cross-gender identification, Rocky has a history of separation anxiety, and he appears to be a temperamentally sensitive youngster. These characteristics are also common among boys with GID, who often show *internalizing* as opposed to *externalizing* behavior problems.

Dr. Zucker is Head of the Gender Identity Service in the Child, Youth, and Family Program at the Centre for Addiction and Mental Health–Clarke Division in Toronto, Ontario. The Gender Identity Service has assessed approximately 700 children and adolescents with gender identity issues since the late 1970s. Dr. Zucker has published more than 100 articles and book chapters on gender identity differentiation and its disorders. He has served on the DSM-III-R, DSM-IV, and DSM-IV-TR Subcommittees on Gender Identity Disorder. Since 2002, he has been Editor of Archives of Sexual Behavior, *a peer-reviewed scientific journal.*

The initial evaluation would profit by obtaining additional information about his relationships with both his mother and his father, particularly during the years that the signs of GID first emerged. It is possible that with the health difficulties experienced by his younger sister, he experienced his mother as less accessible and available to him, and it is unclear what role his father played in his earlier years. When the examiner provides feedback to the parents, they could be informed that Rocky does appear to be unhappy about being a boy and that the goal of treatment would be to try and help him to feel more comfortable as a boy. Along similar lines, Rocky should be asked whether he would like to meet with a "talking doctor" to see if there are ways to help him feel happier about being a boy.

My approach to treatment would be a combination of individual therapy with Rocky, counseling with the parents, and specific recommendations for the parents to carry out in his naturalistic day-to-day environment. Individual therapy would be used with Rocky to explore his fantasies that being a girl would make his life better (e.g., that being a girl would allow him to have a closer relationship with his mother [as he appears to have experienced her attention to his sister as a kind of abandonment], which would help him work through his feelings of jealousy toward his younger sister; and that being a girl would solve his problem of "having" to be aggressive and boisterous [as he perceives other boys to be], which would help him work on his idealization of girls and devaluation of boys).

Parent counseling would explore some of the individual and systemic factors that might have been involved in the genesis and/or perpetuation of his problem and to support them in helping Rocky feel better about himself as a boy. In Rocky's day-to-day environment, the parents would be encouraged to set limits on his pervasive cross-gender behavior (e.g., his cross-dressing and emulation of females in fantasy play) because the continuation of such behaviors only serves to self-reinforce his fantasies about being a girl. They would also be encouraged to let Rocky know that they understand his confusion about being a boy and that they were going to try and help him to feel happier about himself as a boy.

A key aspect of intervention in the naturalistic environment is for the parents to work hard on finding boys with whom Rocky can establish enduring friendships. This might involve, with the help of a teacher, the identification of potential boy playmates whom Rocky would not perceive as too threatening and with whom he might be able to develop friendships. Regular "play dates" with other boys would be one way Rocky could come to feel more comfortable as a boy via engagement in shared activities. Counseling sessions with the parents would provide a forum to discuss the changes instituted in Rocky's naturalistic environment and to evaluate what is working and what is not working.

Many parents of boys with GID want to know about the long-term outcome (e.g., whether it is prognostic of a later homosexual orientation or whether it is prognostic of a later desire to have sex-reassignment surgery). In my experience, parents vary considerably in their attitudes toward homosexuality: Some parents are uncomfortable about such an outcome (e.g., for reasons related to stigma and prejudice and religious values). Other parents are very accepting and will typically indicate that their main goal is in helping their son feel comfortable about his gender identity.

Some critics of the treatment of boys with GID argue that it is instituted as a kind of "backdoor" maneuver to prevent later homosexuality by both homophobic parents and therapists. Other critics argue that treatment of boys with GID is doomed to failure because it is the child's "essential" nature. Both lines of criticism locate the problem not in the child but in the attitudes of the family and society at large. Such critics typically do not accept the possibility that family factors might be involved in the genesis and/or perpetuation of GID, that the child may be experiencing internalized distress about his status as a boy, or that there is any developmental flexibility vis-à-vis gender identity differentiation (i.e., that the natural history does not inevitably lead to a persistence of GID in adolescence and adulthood).

In my experience, there are several factors that contribute to the difficulty of treating boys with GID: the age of the child (older); presence of severe comorbid psychiatric problems in the child; presence of severe psychopathology in the parents, as well as chronic marital discord; and marked ambivalence on the parents' part in valuing their child as a boy. With age and the persistence of GID, the child can become more rigid and "locked in" to the fantasy of sex change; comorbid psychiatric difficulties in the child often require attention in their own right and are a large factor in the child's concomitant social difficulties with other children. Psychiatric difficulties in the parents often make it harder for them to be available to their child and to initiate changes in the naturalistic environment. Ambivalence toward the child's gender identity often makes it harder for the parents to separate their own issues from the child's. As one mother commented, "Well, if he wants to have a sex change, then I guess I will get the daughter I always wanted."

If Rocky's parents are able to commit to a therapeutic change process, I would expect that he will be able to resolve his unhappiness about being a boy. He will be successful in developing friendships with other boys, and this will contribute to a same-gender identification. There will be a fading of his cross-gender identification, and he will be able to identify positive attributes about being a boy.

If Rocky does not respond to treatment, it is likely that he will become increasingly withdrawn. By late childhood, many boys with GID are rejected by both boys and girls. The increased sense of gender dysphoria would result in Rocky becoming increasingly preoccupied with wanting to change his sex, which would interfere with regular activities, including school performance. If Rocky's gender dysphoria persisted into adolescence, he might require placement in an alternative school milieu in which there is greater tolerance for youngsters who do not "fit in"—for whatever reason. By adolescence, Rocky might be struggling to decide whether he is gay or transsexual. In some youngsters, an increasing awareness of homoerotic feelings can intensify the desire to change sex (e.g., "If I were a girl, then my sexual attraction to boys would be 'normal'"). Thus, "internalized homophobia" can be a further factor in accelerating the idea of a sex change. Some clinicians advocate puberty-blocking hormonal treatment, as the development of secondary sex characteristics (e.g., facial and body hair) are experienced as severely aversive. The "real-life" test of living in the social role of the opposite sex would be required before initiating contrasex hormonal treatment and, much later, surgical genital reassignment.

In my experience, the most common diagnostic error committed by clinicians is that they do not take parental concerns seriously during the preschool years, when the GID is in its phase of *in statu nascendi*. Clinicians might take the position that the behavior "is only a phase" that the child will grow out of or might state that "all children do this," and there is nothing atypical about the child's cross-gender behavior. The most common treatment error made by clinicians is to make no effort to develop a case formulation that takes into account predisposing biological/temperamental factors, intrapsychic issues, and systemic factors in the child. An authoritarian approach to treatment ("just tell him he can't cross-dress") is likely to be unsuccessful because of its failure to take a multifactorial approach to intervention and to understand the subjectivity that underlies the fantasy solution of wanting to become a member of the opposite sex.

Since the late 1970s, I have assessed about 430 preadolescent children who have been referred for gender identity problems. My experience in treatment of these youngsters suggests that the majority can be helped so that the desire to change sex does not persist into adolescence and adulthood. This contrasts with my experience in treatment of adolescents with GID, for whom the prognosis for psychological change is much poorer, and, for these youngsters, it is often the case that contrasex hormonal and surgical sex change may well be the best methods of treatment to resolve the underlying gender dysphoria. Thus, my perspective is strongly developmental: There is more plasticity and malleability in gender identity during childhood than in adolescence.

Based on current data on long-term follow-up for boys with GID, the most likely outcome for Rocky is a homosexual sexual orientation without co-occurring gender dysphoria. One should, however, keep in mind that a minority of boys with GID persist with their desire to change sex in adolescence (with a co-occurring sexual attraction to biological males) and a minority of boys with GID desist in their desire to change sex as well (with a co-occurring sexual attraction to biological females). It is still difficult to predict long-term outcome in individual cases.

Suggested Reading

Coates S, Wolfe S: Gender identity disorder in boys: the interface of constitution and early experience. Psychoanalytic Inquiry 15:6–38, 1995

Cohen-Kettenis PT, Owen A, Kaijser VG, et al: Demographic characteristics, social competence, and behavior problems in children with gender identity disorder: a cross-national, cross-clinic comparative analysis. J Abnorm Child Psychol 31:41–53, 2003

Green R: The "Sissy-Boy Syndrome" and the Development of Homosexuality. New Haven, CT, Yale University Press, 1987

Meyer-Bahlburg HFL: Gender identity disorder in young boys: a parent- and peer-based treatment protocol. Clinical Child Psychology and Psychiatry 7:360–377, 2002

Newman LE: Treatment for the parents of feminine boys. Am J Psychiatry 133:683–687, 1976

Rosenberg M: Children with gender identity issues and their parents in individual and group treatment. J Am Acad Child Adolesc Psychiatry 41:619–621, 2002

Smith YLS, van Goozen SHM, Cohen-Kettenis PT: Adolescents with gender identity disorder who were accepted or rejected for sex reassignment surgery: a prospective follow-up study. J Am Acad Child Adolesc Psychiatry 40:472–481, 2001

Zucker KJ: Gender identity disorder in children and adolescents, in Treatments of Psychiatric Disorders, 3rd Edition, Vol 2. Edited by Gabbard GO. Washington, DC, American Psychiatric Press, 2001, pp 2069–2094

Zucker KJ, Bradley SJ: Gender Identity Disorder and Psychosexual Problems in Children and Adolescents. New York, Guilford Press, 1995

Zucker KJ, Bradley SJ: Gender identity disorder, in Handbook of Infant Mental Health, 2nd Edition. Edited by Zeanah CH. New York, Guilford Press, 2000, pp 412–424

Edgy Electrician

A 27-year-old married electrician complains of dizziness, sweating palms, heart palpitations, and ringing of the ears of more than 18 months' duration. He has also experienced dry mouth and throat, periods of extreme muscle tension, and a constant "edgy" and watchful feeling that has often interfered with his ability to concentrate. These feelings have been present most of the time over the previous 2 years; they have not been limited to discrete periods. Although these symptoms sometimes make him feel "discouraged," he denies feeling depressed and continues to enjoy activities with his family.

Because of these symptoms, the patient had seen a family practitioner, a neurologist, a neurosurgeon, a chiropractor, and an ear-nose-throat specialist. He had been placed on a hypoglycemic diet, received physiotherapy for a pinched nerve, and been told he might have "an inner ear problem."

He also has many worries. He constantly worries about the health of his parents. His father, in fact, had a myocardial infarction 2 years previously but is now feeling well. He also worries about whether he is "a good father," whether his wife will ever leave him (there is no indication that she is dissatisfied with the marriage), and whether co-workers on the job like him. Although he recognizes that his worries are often unfounded, he cannot stop worrying.

For the past 2 years, the patient has had few social contacts because of his nervous symptoms. Although he has sometimes had to leave work when the symptoms became intolerable, he continues to work for the same company he joined for his apprenticeship after high school graduation. He tends to hide his symptoms from his wife and children, to whom he wants to appear "perfect," and reports few problems with them as a result of his nervousness.

DSM-IV-TR Casebook Diagnosis of "Edgy Electrician"

This man has consulted numerous physicians for his symptoms, but the absence of preoccupation with fears of having a specific physical disease precludes a diagnosis of Hypochondriasis. He recognizes that his worries are often excessive, but they do not have the intrusive and inappropriate quality that characterizes the obsessions of Obsessive-Compulsive Disorder.

His predominant symptom is excessive and uncontrollable anxiety and worry for most of the time over the past 2 years. This suggests the diagnosis of Generalized Anxiety Disorder (GAD). He also has the characteristic associated symptoms of feeling on edge, difficulty concentrating, and muscle tension. His worries cause him significant distress and impair his social functioning. The diagnosis of GAD (DSM-IV-TR, p. 476) is made in this case because the worries are not confined to the features of another Axis I disorder (e.g., worrying about having a panic attack, as in Panic Disorder, or being embarrassed in public, as in Social Phobia), the symptoms do not occur only during the course of a Mood or Psychotic Disorder, they are not the direct effects of a substance (e.g., drugs of abuse or medication) or a general medical condition (e.g., hyperthyroidism), and the disturbance has persisted for more than 6 months.

Discussion of "Edgy Electrician" by Laszlo A. Papp, M.D.*

The electrician's description of himself as simply "edgy" may reflect his wish to minimize the severity of his condition and understate the anguish most patients with GAD experience. In truth, his debilitating symptoms, both somatic and psychological, clearly interfere with most areas of his life. Our patient, not surprisingly, seems reluctant to label himself "mentally" ill and potentially could go undiagnosed and untreated for many years. Depending on his health insurance plan and the most prominent physical symptom at the time, he will most likely continue to undergo extensive cardiovascular, gastrointestinal, and neurological workups, and after experimenting on his own with various alternative and herbal remedies, he may finally accept a psychiatric referral.

Unfortunately, his problems will not be over then. Even when properly diagnosed and treated, GAD tends to run a chronic course with periodic exacerbations, and it is frequently comorbid with depression and other Anxiety Disorders. Although progress has been made, GAD remains one of the most treatment-resistant conditions. Often, "treatment responders" continue to have residual symptoms with persisting functional impairment and associated high relapse rates (Ballenger et al. 2001).

The diagnosis of GAD, although highly reliable, can be difficult to make. Compared to other Anxiety Disorders, the symptoms are most similar to normal anxiety. But our electrician will have to understand that his type of anxiety—chronic, pervasive, excessive, and uncontrollable, involving routine daily activities and resulting in functional impairment—is far from normal. Nonpathological anxiety is usually facilitating (e.g., anxiety about failing an examination motivates one to study), does not manifest as disabling physical symptoms, and is not characterized by a preoccupation with worries about catastrophic future events.

---

*Dr. Papp is Associate Professor of Psychiatry at the College of Physicians and Surgeons of Columbia University, Director of the Biological Studies Unit at the New York State Psychiatric Institute, and Director of Anxiety Disorders Research at Hillside Hospital in New York City. Dr. Papp is the recipient of several Federal and private research grants, among them an Independent Scientist Award from National Institutes of Health and an Independent Investigator Award from National Alliance for Research on Schizophrenia and Depression. He has published extensively on the diagnosis, treatment, and psychobiology of Anxiety Disorders.

Pathological worry has been identified as one of the pathognomonic features of GAD. We can safely bet on his affirmative answer to the assessment question, "Do you worry excessively about minor matters?" whereas a negative response would effectively rule out the diagnosis of GAD. Patients with GAD consistently report a greater number of worry areas compared to patients with other Anxiety Disorders and nonanxious controls, but the particular pattern of worry content is highly variable and does not consistently identify patients with GAD. Some have argued that the symptom of worry in GAD is simply a distraction that serves to protect the patient from dealing with his or her "real" problems (e.g., low self-esteem). This hypothesis, akin to the "unconscious conflict" paradigm of psychodynamic thinking, has yet to be empirically tested, and, in any case, is unlikely to sit well with our electrician.

Whereas Anxiety Disorders, including GAD, are common in alcoholics, patients with GAD are much less likely to self-medicate their anxiety with alcohol and other substances than patients with Panic Disorder and Social Phobia. If it is confirmed that our electrician's anxiety is not limited to another Axis I disorder or due to substance use or a medical condition, the diagnosis of GAD would be justified.

In selecting the type of treatment, his clinician will have to take into consideration comorbidity (both psychiatric and medical); course of illness; prior response to treatments, if any; family history of psychiatric disorders; Personality Disorders/traits; and patient's choice/preference and sense of control. Because specific symptoms of an Anxiety Disorder, such as fear or worry, frequently cut across a number of DSM categories and certain features of GAD, such as duration of symptoms and the definition of "excessive" worry, are somewhat arbitrary, his treatment will have to accommodate a dimensional diagnostic approach as well (e.g., treatment for a symptomatic period lasting less than 6 months or prominent social avoidance or depression, even if he did not meet the criteria for Social Anxiety Disorder or Dysthymia).

The course of GAD is chronic with fluctuating severity and symptom patterns. The onset of symptoms in the electrician's mid-20s is fairly typical but, owing to the unreliability of retrospective self-report, his family should be asked about evidence suggesting an earlier onset of Anxiety Disorder, such as childhood fears, school problems, and behavioral inhibition. Patients with GAD with an onset prior to age 10 may have a more malignant type of the disorder that is more difficult to treat successfully. Early-onset GAD is more likely to have gradual onset, comorbid depression, and other Axis I and Axis II disorders and run a more chronic course (Papp and Kleber 2001). The clinician is advised to find out if our electrician's social isolation and perfectionism are related to a Personality Disorder or trait (e.g., avoidant or obsessive-compulsive personality features). Treatment resistance in GAD may be associated with an 80% rate of comorbid Personality Disorder. Although no specific Personality Disorder has been identified to be typically comorbid with GAD, Avoidant, Dependent, and Obsessive-Compulsive Personality Disorders and traits are most common.

Our patient is fairly typical in that he has more than adequate documentation of the absence of any "organic" abnormalities, but the evaluation of the rare anxious patient without prior medical workup should always include a thorough physical examination; blood tests for chemistry, hematology, and thyroid function; urinalysis; and an electrocardiogram. If neurological abnormalities are suspected, a neurological examination may need to be supplemented with appropriate brain-imaging studies. Prominent nocturnal pathology (e.g., middle of the night awakenings, excessively loud snoring) should be investigated in a sleep laboratory.

So, what is the current state-of-the-art treatment for our electrician?

We hope that he will be spared from the perennial debate over the supremacy of biological versus psychological approaches that only confuses patients. As the artificiality of this dichotomy is increasingly recognized, a pragmatic, unbiased approach in treatment research has begun to examine the merits of combined somatic and psychological treatments of anxiety. Although medication management of Anxiety Disorders with or without psychotherapy has been demonstrated to be very efficacious, because of its much lower incidence of side effects and lack of medical contraindications, a nonpharmacological treatment is almost always preferable if comparable efficacy can be established.

Assuming that this case represents a "pure" form of GAD (i.e., no apparent medical or psychiatric comorbidity), the recommendation should minimally include cognitive-behavioral therapy (CBT) using a modular approach (Gorenstein et al. 1999). A CBT package for GAD generally includes didactic information on the nature of anxiety, self-monitoring of anxiety, relaxation training, cognitive therapy, and exposure to anxiety-provoking stimuli. The principal methods used in a cognitive-behavioral approach include progressive muscle relaxation and diaphragmatic breathing training (i.e., slow abdominal breathing to replace superficial chest breathing exhibited by many anxious patients), cognitive restructuring (i.e., countering unrealistic, catastrophic

thoughts), worry behavior prevention (analogous to "response prevention" for Obsessive-Compulsive Disorder), problem solving, interoceptive exposure (controlled exposure to sensations of autonomic arousal
such as voluntary hyperventilation), cognitive-behavioral strategies
for coping with medication use and physical symptoms (routinized,
regularly scheduled medical checkups, realistic assessment of new
physical symptoms, anticipated side effects and dangers of medications, etc.), daily activity structuring, in vivo exposure (gradual exposure to feared and avoided situations or activities), and sleep hygiene
(stimulus control, regular bedtime and wake-up time).

CBT could be augmented with as-needed benzodiazepines such as
Ativan (lorazepam), Xanax (alprazolam), Klonopin (clonazepam),
and/or beta-blockers such as Inderal (propranolol) to facilitate exposure and to tone down autonomic arousal, but antidepressants may be
preferable (see later). Significant leeway should be given to the patient
to decide the sequence and timing of these interventions (e.g., medication can be introduced before, during, or after CBT, and frequency and
content of CBT sessions can vary). Because learning and retention may
be affected directly, and because the use of benzodiazepines may serve
as an avoidance strategy, some psychotherapists advocate anxiolytics
other than benzodiazepines, such as once-a-day antidepressants if
used in combination with CBT.

Given his apparent inclination to "medicalize" his condition, we
should accept his likely preference for medications alone. As the therapeutic alliance develops, CBT techniques will naturally complement
medication management even without formal psychotherapy. The
choice among the many efficacious pharmacological agents is usually
made based on side effects and individual patient characteristics (Papp
1999). Benzodiazepines, the traditional pharmacological option for
GAD, have been gradually replaced by antidepressants as first-line
anxiolytics. Long-term use of benzodiazepines can be problematic, and
the relapse rate after discontinuation is high. Nevertheless, benzodiazepines can be useful when the need for immediate benefits outweighs
their risks (e.g., development of tolerance, emergence of withdrawal
symptoms when lowering the dose, cognitive impairment) and the
side effects of the alternatives are unacceptable (e.g., weight gain, sexual dysfunction). Data do not support the advantage of any one benzodiazepine over the others, and correlation has not been established
between clinical response and dose or plasma level. A daily equivalent
of 15–25 mg of Valium (diazepam) is usually sufficient to relieve most
of the symptoms in the majority of patients with GAD. Both somatic

and, to a lesser extent, psychic anxiety symptoms respond within the first week of treatment. Tolerance to the sedative effects of benzodiazepines develops quickly, but the antianxiety effect of a given dose is usually well maintained over time.

The 5-HT$_{1A}$ agonist BuSpar (buspirone) was also promoted as an alternative to benzodiazepines, but clinical experience has been disappointing. Although BuSpar is safe and well tolerated and is less likely to induce drowsiness compared to benzodiazepines, the initial side effects of nausea, dizziness, and gastrointestinal irritation may be problematic, and the onset of action is delayed for an average of 4–5 weeks. Because BuSpar and the benzodiazepines do not have antidepressant effects, comorbid or emergent depressive symptoms should further justify the use of antidepressants. Although controversial, the theory that GAD may represent a prodromal state toward Major Depressive Disorder (or, alternatively, that GAD and Major Depressive Disorder may represent different symptomatic expressions of the same underlying pathophysiological condition) would also argue for antidepressants as preventive treatment.

In the absence of contraindications, the currently recommended first-line medication is one of the selective serotonin reuptake inhibitors (SSRIs) or Effexor (venlafaxine), with or without as-needed benzodiazepines or beta-blockers, to provide immediate benefits during the 4–5 weeks it takes for the antidepressant to kick in. A substantial body of evidence supports the acute benefits of Effexor and Paxil (paroxetine) in GAD and the long-term effectiveness of Effexor in maintaining improvement in GAD, and promising trials are ongoing with several other SSRIs and other "novel" antidepressants (Salzman et al. 2001).

Tricyclic antidepressants are also effective in treating patients with GAD. Doses and response patterns are similar to those observed in Panic Disorder. Increased initial physiological symptoms and anxiety may be related to side effects such as dry mouth, constipation, sedation, and positional hypotension rather than to the hypersensitivity syndrome (increased anxiety and panic attacks on initiating antidepressants) described in Panic Disorder. Because of significant comorbidity in these trials, the efficacy of tricyclic antidepressants in GAD may not be independent of their antipanic and antidepressant properties.

Insomnia, a symptom that is not reported in this case, is a frequent symptom of GAD and should be addressed specifically by selecting a sedating antidepressant given at bedtime, or a hypnotic, like Ambien (zolpidem), and/or adding the "sleep hygiene" module of the CBT package.

Because GAD is a chronic, frequently lifelong condition, treatment should probably be continued indefinitely but perhaps intermittently. Intermittent brief treatments may prove to be the best long-term strategy (Rickels and Schweitzer 1998). In general, the lowest dosage of medication that controls the patient's symptoms should be prescribed. A slow, gradual taper of medication may be attempted after 1 year in symptom-free patients. Recurrence should be retreated promptly. Longer duration treatments seem to confer the benefits of improved functioning, fewer residual symptoms, and lower relapse rates, but it is unknown whether the type of treatment (i.e., pharmacological, psychological, or the combination of the two) matters in conferring the long-term benefits. Patients with predominantly somatic symptoms and/or early-onset GAD may require ongoing pharmacotherapy, whereas those with primarily excessive worry and/or late-onset GAD may be better controlled by regularly practiced CBT techniques. Because it is not known what is required for the proper long-term clinical management of patients with GAD who responded to either CBT or medication, the most prudent approach is to schedule follow-up appointments at increasing intervals in order to continually monitor the course of illness. Although, for the time being, a cure may be elusive for patients who have GAD, with proper management, our electrician should enjoy long intervals of no or only minimal symptoms.

References

Ballenger JC, Davidson JRT, Lecrubier Y, et al: Consensus statement on generalized anxiety disorder from the International Consensus Group on Depression and Anxiety. J Clin Psychiatry 62 (suppl 11):53–58, 2001

Gorenstein EE, Papp LA, Kleber MS: Cognitive-behavioral treatment of anxiety in later life. Cognitive and Behavioral Practice 6(4):305–319, 1999

Papp LA: Anxiety disorders: somatic treatment, in Kaplan and Sadock's Comprehensive Textbook of Psychiatry, 7th Edition. Edited by Sadock BJ, Sadock VA. Baltimore, MD, Williams & Wilkins, 2000, pp 1490–1498

Papp LA, Kleber MS: Diagnosis and epidemiology of generalized anxiety disorder, in Textbook of Anxiety Disorders. Edited by Stein DJ, Hollander E. Washington, DC, American Psychiatric Press, 2001, pp 109–118

Rickels K, Schweitzer E: The spectrum of generalized anxiety in clinical practice: the role of short-term, intermittent treatment. Br J Psychiatry 173:49–54, 1998

Salzman C, Goldenberg I, Bruce SE, et al: Pharmacologic treatment of anxiety disorders in 1989 versus 1996: results from the Harvard/Brown Anxiety Disorders Research Program. J Clin Psychiatry 62:149–152, 2001

Cry Me a River

A **38-year-old** clerical worker described to a psychiatrist how she had been experiencing a disabling sleep problem for a year and a half. She usually goes to bed at 6:00 P.M. and sleeps straight through until 7:00 A.M. The reason that she presents for help now is that, last month, her driver's license was suspended after she fell asleep while driving her car out of a parking lot and hit a telephone pole. As a result, she now has to arise at 6:00 A.M. to use public transportation to arrive in time for work at 8:15 A.M. Upon arising, she typically feels groggy and "out of it." During the day she remains sleepy. She frequently falls asleep on buses, missing her stop. She recently took a sales job after work, from 6:00 P.M. until 10:00 P.M. two nights a week, in an attempt to remain on her feet at least some of the time that she is away from her office job. On weekends, she remains in bed asleep all day, arising only to go to the toilet or for meals, except on an occasional Saturday when she does her routine chores.

The patient does not believe that she snores during sleep (as would be likely in a Breathing-Related Sleep Disorder), and she denies nightmares (as in Nightmare Disorder), sleepwalking (as in Sleepwalking Disorder), or sudden loss of muscle tone (cataplexy) or feelings of paralysis upon awakening, both symptoms of Narcolepsy.

Before the onset of her sleep problem, the patient generally required only 6–7 hours of sleep a night. During the first year of her "sleepiness" she began to treat herself with caffeine, drinking up to 10 cups of coffee and 1–2 liters of cola daily.

In addition to the sleepiness, the patient has had severe, recurrent periods of depression since approximately age 13. For several months before the evaluation, she was having crying spells in her office. These sometimes would come on so suddenly that she had no time to run to the restroom to hide. She acknowledged trouble concentrating on her job and noted that she was getting little pleasure from her work, which she used to enjoy. She has been harboring angry and pessimistic feelings for the past several years and noted that these were more severe recently as she had allowed her diabetes and weight to get out of control. She felt guilty that she was physically damaging herself and slowly dying in this way. She sometimes thought that she deserved to be dead.

She had been treated from age 18 to age 33 with psychotherapy, during which time her depression gradually worsened. More recently, she had been given trials of antidepressants, including imipramine, desipramine, and fluoxetine, which had each made improvements in mood and wakefulness that lasted several months. She tended to fall asleep during evening group psychotherapy sessions.

The patient's diabetes was diagnosed at age 11. She first lost control of her weight and her blood sugar during her teenage years, then regained it, but she has frequently lost control since then. At this evaluation, she weighed about 30% above her ideal weight and was on 52 units of insulin daily, but she neither kept regular mealtimes nor tested her blood regularly. Results of recent random blood-sugar determinations were abnormally high. Significant diabetic retinopathy had developed, compelling her to use a magnifying glass for reading. She had mild hypertension without apparent diabetic kidney disease and took one diuretic tablet daily.

The patient had done poorly in high school and had gone to business school for 4 years but had failed to graduate. She had had some hope of a romantic relationship but never had a steady boyfriend. She lives at home with her mother and has no close friends outside her family. On close questioning, it became apparent that the onset of the sleep problems and the beginning of the most recent period of depression had coincided.

The patient's family history revealed that one of her five siblings took a nap each afternoon and slept 7 hours nightly. Otherwise, there was no history of Sleep Disorder, diabetes, or treatment for depression in the patient's family.

As the patient described her problem to the psychiatrist, she gazed continually downward and conversed in a low monotone. She answered questions dutifully but without elaboration. She shed copious tears.

The patient was admitted to the hospital for studies. Nursing observations documented that the patient slept 12–15 hours daily. She was much impaired in tests of vigilance, which involved her pushing a button whenever the letter *X* appeared in a series of letters visually presented at one per second; she averaged 4% correct responses during two trials, compared with a normal score of 66%–78%. She had an average multiple sleep latency (i.e., onset of sleep after lights out) of 8.5 minutes during four polygraphically recorded daytime naps, a result consistent with only mild sleepiness. Nocturnal sleep monitoring revealed an abnormally short REM latency of 2 minutes and an abnormal increase (42%) in the amount of REM sleep. The nocturnal sleep monitoring revealed no other abnormality. The patient had only 2% wakefulness, much less than expected in a prolonged recording; this was consistent with her daytime sleepiness. She continued to sleep for 9.5 hours, until she had to be awakened so the laboratory could be used for daytime purposes.

DSM-IV-TR Casebook Diagnosis of "Cry Me a River"

Although this patient experiences recurrent periods of depression, her predominant complaints are of excessive daytime sleepiness (falls asleep on buses, remains in bed all day on weekends) and prolonged transition to the fully awake state (feels groggy and "out of it" on awakening). The sleep laboratory findings (prolonged sleep, impaired vigilance, short rapid eye movement [REM] latency, increased REM activity) confirm her complaints of hypersomnia.

Because the onset of her sleep disturbance seems to have coincided with the most recent recurrence of her depression, it seems reasonable to conclude that the hypersomnia is related to the Mood Disorder. Therefore, the principal diagnosis is Hypersomnia Related to Major Depressive Disorder (DSM-IV-TR, p. 650). The recurrent episodes of depression warrant the additional Axis I diagnosis of Major Depressive Disorder, Recurrent (DSM-IV-TR, p. 376).

Discussion of "Cry Me a River" by Charles F. Reynolds III, M.D.*

The clerical worker described here has highly disabling daytime sleepiness in the context of an early-onset and recurrent depressive illness (apparently nonbipolar) and insulin-dependent diabetes mellitus (which is poorly controlled), with significant diabetic retinopathy and mild hypertension. The history of recurrent depression antedates the complaint of excessive sleepiness, and the onset of sleep problems coincided with the most recent siege of her depression.

It is important to realize that the patient's daytime sleepiness is truly a life-threatening condition because it occasioned a motor vehicle accident. (The case history gave no indication that the motor vehicle accident was a suicide attempt, although, clearly, this possibility cannot be excluded.) It is very unusual to have this degree of daytime sleepiness associated only with a Mood Disorder. Coexistent sleep-disordered breathing (i.e., the occurrence of frequent apneic episodes during sleep, associated with loud snoring, obesity, hypertension, cognitive impairment, and daytime sleepiness) and/or narcolepsy-cataplexy would be high in the differential diagnosis of this patient's symptoms, and periodic limb movement disorder (nocturnal myoclonus) would also be a possibility to be ruled out with polysomnographic evaluation. If the underlying problem were a periodic limb movement disorder, the polysomnograph would show frequent episodes of lower limb myoclonic activity associated with brief arousals on the electroencephalogram (producing a picture of shallow, fragmented sleep).

Patients with *any* of these sleep disorders frequently develop clinically significant depressive symptoms. However, sleep laboratory evaluation apparently failed to provide objective evidence of primary

---

*Dr. Reynolds is Professor of Psychiatry, Neurology and Neuroscience at the University of Pittsburgh School of Medicine, where he directs the National Institute of Mental Health–sponsored Intervention Research Center for Late Life Mood Disorders and serves as Senior Associate Dean. Dr. Reynolds chaired the 2001 Depression and Bipolar Support Alliance Consensus Conference on Unmet Needs in the Diagnosis and Treatment of Late Life Mood Disorders, the proceedings of which appeared in the Archives of General Psychiatry. In 2002–2003, he served on the Institute of Medicine's study of "Reducing Suicide: A National Imperative," published by the National Academy of Sciences press. He is a member of the National Mental Health Advisory Council and President of the American College of Psychiatrists.

sleep pathologies, such as apneic episodes, oxyhemoglobin desaturation, nocturnal myoclonus, or repetitive sleep-onset REM periods during the daytime nap test (necessary to confirm a diagnosis of narcolepsy). (We are not actually told in the case history about the absence of these polysomnographic findings but assume that they were checked and appropriately ruled out. If this is the case, the diagnostic possibilities mentioned were not supported.) The occurrence of a sleep-onset REM period at night has been noted in persons with narcolepsy and also in those with severe depression, including psychotic depression. Clinical evaluation failed to support a diagnosis of psychotic depression, however, and was also negative with respect to a history of cataplexy (i.e., loss of voluntary muscle control triggered by strong emotions, leading to falls).

The coexistence of insulin-dependent diabetes mellitus, depression, and daytime sleepiness is clinically important and key to further treatment planning. Depression is often an unwanted cotraveler with diabetes mellitus and significantly complicates the management of the diabetes. At the same time, some diabetic patients develop sleep-disordered breathing, which may mediate the occurrence of daytime sleepiness. The patient's excessive weight obviously complicates the management of her diabetes and places her at risk for worse hypertension and the subsequent development of sleep-disordered breathing. Another medical issue that arises with this clinical presentation is the differential diagnostic possibility of hypothyroidism, which could be associated with symptoms of depression and excessive sleepiness, as well as with sleep-disordered breathing. It was not clear that hypothyroidism had been ruled out. Two final diagnostic possibilities are drug (including alcohol or stimulant) abuse/dependence and idiopathic daytime hypersomnolence (or primary hypersomnolence in DSM-IV-TR terminology), a condition of chronic daytime sleepiness, with multiple sleep latency test findings similar to those presented here, not accounted for by narcolepsy-cataplexy or a sleep apnea syndrome. There was no reported history of alcohol, tobacco, stimulant, or other substance abuse or dependence, although the patient was self-medicating with excessive amounts of caffeine. Furthermore, the fact that her sleepiness apparently coincided with a major depressive episode rather than following a chronic course is evidence against a diagnosis of chronic idiopathic or primary hypersomnolence.

So, on balance, the most likely, and parsimonious, diagnostic formulation is hypersomnia related to Major Depressive Disorder, assuming that sleep-disordered breathing, narcolepsy, periodic limb movement disorder (nocturnal myoclonus), drug abuse/dependence, and hypothyroidism were truly ruled out in the course of her workup. The occurrence of depression may be associated with poor medical compliance with the patient's insulin regimen and other behavioral management, which may have been prescribed as part of chronic disease management for her diabetes. As well, both depression and its attendant sleep disturbance may lead to significant cognitive impairment, even in a young patient.

In my experience, the most common mistake that clinicians make in evaluating a patient who has both depression and hypersomnia is failure to evaluate and treat adequately for coexisting Mood Disorder and primary sleep disorders, such as sleep apnea or narcolepsy-cataplexy. To some extent, this failure reflects the fact that these disorders are traditionally the province of different medical specialists—psychiatry, pulmonology, and neurology. Adequate evaluation of a complaint of daytime sleepiness should include a diary of the patient's sleep-wake schedule and habits; attention to health habits, including substance use; collection of information from the patient's bed partner or significant other about sleep-related behaviors such as snoring, apnea, or leg jerks; attention to medical conditions that can cause daytime fatigue and sleepiness (especially diabetes and hypothyroidism); attention to the patient's safety while driving (often patients should be advised not to drive until their problem with excessive daytime sleepiness is diagnosed and corrected); and appropriate sleep laboratory evaluation to rule in or rule out primary sleep pathologies.

We are told that trials of antidepressant pharmacotherapy had helped the patient, including imipramine, desipramine, and fluoxetine, each of which was associated with improvement in mood and wakefulness "that lasted several months." This observation suggests that treatment of the primary Mood Disorder led to improvement in sleep symptoms, which was probably secondary to the Mood Disorder (rather than vice versa). On the other hand, the history is vague with respect to the actual antidepressant treatment received by this patient and why the effect did not last longer than several months. Did the patient discontinue treatment, or did it stop working? Why were several different medications used?

Treatment planning for this patient needs to address both her Mood Disorder (recurrent unipolar depression) and the coexisting chronic medical disorders of insulin-dependent diabetes, obesity, and hypertension. The goals of treatment should include getting the patient's symptoms of depression all the way to remission; keeping her in remission; and improving her adherence to the medical and behavioral management of her obesity, diabetes, and hypertension. Achieving these goals will depend on good coordination of her medical and psychiatric care. Given the fragmentation of our health care delivery system, this coordination is difficult to implement, even in the best of treatment settings.

Because of the severe and recurrent nature of the patient's depressive illness, I would use pharmacotherapy as a component of her treatment, using an antidepressant that is alerting rather than sedating and one that is unlikely to lead to further weight gain or exacerbate her hypertension. More alerting selective serotonin reuptake inhibitors (SSRIs) such as Celexa/Lexapro (citalopram/escitalopram) or Zoloft (sertraline) would be medically appropriate in my opinion. On the other hand, agents that cause sleepiness or lead to weight gain (e.g., Remeron [mirtazapine]) or may be associated with further elevation of systolic blood pressure or elevation of cholesterol (e.g., Effexor [venlafaxine]) would be relatively less helpful in this situation. If need be, I also would add a stimulant as a short-term augmenting strategy to the primary SSRI pharmacotherapy to help the patient with her incapacitating daytime sleepiness. Because of her hypertension, I would choose low-dose Provigil (modafinil) rather than Ritalin (methylphenidate) or Dexedrine (dextroamphetamine). Twenty years ago, I might have prescribed a monoamine oxidase inhibitor (MAOI) like Parnate (tranylcypromine) because of the clinical picture of atypical Major Depression (with hypersomnia). I would now consider the MAOI to be a second- or third-line agent for this patient.

Pharmacotherapy is unlikely to be enough, however, to get this patient to remission and keep her there. She needs to make some lifestyle changes and maximize her compliance with good diabetes care (which is already, in this case, associated with end-organ disease—retinopathy—and disability, in turn a risk factor for more recurrences of depression). In this context, the history suggests that the patient needs to stabilize her sleep-wake schedule and spend less time in bed. I would work with her to define a realistic sleep-wake schedule with no more than 8 hours of time in bed, based on her history of sleep need. At the same time, this patient needs a reason to get up in the morning—she is socially isolated and apparently has few vocational or social interests to engage her. These aspects of her functioning also need to be addressed, possibly via interpersonal psychotherapy or cognitive-behavioral therapy.

Given the chronic and recurrent nature of the patient's episodes of depression, she is at high risk for recurrences. Therefore, I would recommend that she consider maintenance antidepressant pharmacotherapy as a means for prolonging her recovery and remaining out of disabling episodes. A recent review has shown that continuing treatment with antidepressants reduces the odds of relapse by 70% (Geddes et al. 2003). Further counseling for good behavioral health practices, including weight management and sleep hygiene, would also be medically appropriate to achieve the goal of keeping her depression-free and diminishing the risks for further medical complications of either her diabetes or her depression.

Ultimately, this patient illustrates the inseparability of mental and physical health in diagnostic assessment and treatment planning to assure maximal quality of life.

Reference

Geddes JR, Carney SM, Davies C, et al: Relapse prevention with antidepressant drug treatment in depressive disorders: a systematic review. Lancet 361:653–661, 2003

My Fan Club

During the course of a routine physical examination, Nick, a 25-year-old single black man, suddenly started crying and blurted out that he was very depressed and was thinking about a suicide attempt he had made when he felt this way as a teenager. His doctor referred him for a psychiatric evaluation.

Nick is tall, bearded, muscular, and handsome. He is meticulously dressed in a white suit and has a rose in his lapel. He enters the psychiatrist's office, pauses dramatically, and exclaims, "Aren't roses wonderful this time of year?" When asked why he has come for an evaluation, he replies laughingly that he has done it to appease his family doctor, "who seemed worried about me." He has also read a book on psychotherapy and hopes that "maybe there is someone very special who can understand me. I'd make the most incredible patient." He then takes control of the interview and begins to talk about himself, after first remarking, half jokingly, "I was hoping you would be as attractive as my family doctor."

Nick pulls out of his attaché case a series of newspaper clippings; his resume; photographs of himself, including some of him with famous people; and a photocopied dollar bill with his face replacing George Washington's. Using these as cues, he begins to tell his story.

He explains that in the last few years he has "discovered" some now-famous actors, one of whom he describes as a "physically perfect teenage heartthrob." He volunteered to coordinate publicity for the actor, and as part of that, posed in a bathing suit in a scene that resembled a famous scene from the actor's hit movie. Nick, imitating the actor's voice, laughingly and then seriously, describes how he and the actor had similar pasts. Both were rejected by their parents and peers but overcame this to become popular. When the actor came to town, Nick rented a limousine and showed up at the gala "as a joke," as though he were the star himself. The actor's agent expressed annoyance at what he had done, causing Nick to fly into a rage. When Nick cooled down, he realized that he was "wasting my time promoting

151

others, and that it was time for me to start promoting myself." "Someday," he said, pointing to the picture of the actor, "he will want to be president of my fan club."

Nick has had little previous acting experience of a professional nature, but he is sure that success is "only a question of time." He pulls out some promotional material he has written for his actors and says, "I should write letters to God—He'd love them!" When the psychiatrist is surprised that some materials are signed by a different name than the one Nick has given the receptionist, Nick pulls out a legal document explaining the name change. He has dropped his family name and taken as his new second name his own middle name.

When asked about his love life, Nick says he has no lover, and this is because people are just "superficial." He then displays a newspaper clipping in which he had letterset his and his ex-lover's names in headlines that read: "The relationship is over." More recently he has dated and adored a man with the same first name as his own, but as he became disenchanted, he realized that the man was ugly and an embarrassment because he dressed so poorly. Nick then explains that he owns over 100 neckties and about 30 suits, and is proud of how much he spends on "putting myself together." He has no relationships with other homosexual men now, describing them as "only interested in sex." He considers heterosexual men as "mindless and without aesthetic sense." The only people who have understood him are older men who have suffered as much he has. "One day, the mindless, happy people who have ignored me will be lining up to see my movies."

Nick's father was very critical, was an alcoholic who was rarely around, and had many affairs. His mother was "like a friend." She was chronically depressed about her husband's affairs and turned to her son, often kissing him good night, until he was 18, when she started an affair of her own. Nick then felt abandoned and made his suicide gesture. He described a tortured childhood, being picked on by his peers for looking odd, until he began bodybuilding.

At the end of the interview, Nick is referred to an experienced clinician associated with the clinic, who charges a minimal fee ($10), which he can afford. However, Nick requests a referral to someone who would offer him free treatment, seeing no reason for paying anyone as the therapist "would be getting as much out of it as [he] would."

DSM-IV-TR Casebook Diagnosis of "My Fan Club"

What is remarkable about Nick is his unabashed grandiosity and preoccupation with unrealistic fantasies of success. His behavior and attitude are arrogant and haughty. He believes that he is so special that he is entitled to be treated gratis. He is preoccupied with envy of the stars that he emulates and presumes that others are envious of him. He seems to require constant attention and admiration, and we strongly suspect that he is unable to recognize and experience how others feel (lack of empathy). He can adore and flatter others if they are of use to him, but he quickly changes his mind if they are not, coldly devaluing them and pointing out their flaws. This pervasive pattern of grandiosity and need for admiration indicates Narcissistic Personality Disorder (DSM-IV-TR, p. 717).

Nick also has many of the features of Histrionic Personality Disorder (DSM-IV-TR, p. 714). He uses physical appearance to draw attention to himself, expresses emotions with inappropriate exaggeration and theatricality, is probably uncomfortable in situations in which he is not the center of attention, and undoubtedly displays rapidly shifting and shallow expressions of emotions. Therefore, we would note histrionic traits on Axis II.

In addition, there are many suggestions of the pervasive pattern of instability of interpersonal relationships, self-image, and affects that are characteristic of Borderline Personality Disorder (DSM-IV-TR, p. 710). Therefore, we would also note these traits on Axis II.

Discussion of "My Fan Club" by Otto Kernberg, M.D.*

This patient immediately raises a fundamental differential diagnostic question: Is it a case of a Narcissistic Personality Disorder, as suggested in the *DSM-IV-TR Casebook* diagnosis, or is it a hypomanic episode in a Bipolar Disorder? The patient's dramatic entry; his laughing, somewhat inappropriately, at the beginning of the session; the inappropriate degree of familiarity in his reaction to the examiner; his inordinate grandiosity; the jocular behavior; and his information that he owns over 100 neckties and about 30 suits and is proud of how much he spends on "putting myself together," all would fit with the diagnosis of a hypomanic episode. It is very important, therefore, to investigate whether Nick is presently experiencing a distinct period of persistently elevated or expansive mood that is clearly different from his usual affective condition. I would explore in great detail whether this is a particular episode, distinctively different from the patient's functioning at other times and if it turned out to be such an episode, whether it is related to substance abuse. Investigation of whether the patient presently has an unusual degree of energy and optimism that does not correspond to his usual experience and whether there is significant insomnia associated with such an episode would facilitate the differential diagnosis.

If it turns out that Nick's affect is not abnormally euphoric and his present behavior corresponds to a chronic or permanent characterological constellation rather than to an acute discontinuous episode, I would feel reassured that this is not a hypomanic episode.

---

*Dr. Kernberg is Professor of Psychiatry at the Joan and Sanford I. Weill Medical College of Cornell University and Director of the Personality Disorders Institute at The New York Presbyterian Hospital–The Weill Medical College of Cornell University, Westchester Division. He is also Training and Supervising Analyst at Columbia University Center for Psychoanalytic Training and Research.

Dr. Kernberg's major professional and research interests include the psychopathology and treatment of severe Personality Disorders and theory and technique of psychoanalytic modalities of treatment. He is the author of 10 books and coauthor of nine others, including Love Relations: Normality and Pathology (New Haven, Yale University Press, 1995); Ideology, Conflict, and Leadership in Groups and Organizations (New Haven, Yale University Press, 1998); Aggressivity, Narcissism, and Self-Destructiveness in the Psychotherapeutic Relationship (New Haven, Yale University Press, in press); and Object Relations, Affects, and Transference: Contemporary Developments and Controversies (New Haven, Yale University Press, in press).*

Let us assume that further inquiry permits us to discard the diagnosis of a hypomanic episode. Under these circumstances, the differential diagnosis would center on that of a severe Personality Disorder, and, indeed, as proposed in the *Casebook* discussion, the most likely diagnosis would be Narcissistic Personality Disorder. The histrionic elements described in the mental status examination may be consistent with a Narcissistic Personality Disorder and would not, by themselves, justify the diagnosis of a Histrionic Personality Disorder, nor do I believe that the information presented in this case justifies the diagnosis of Borderline Personality Disorder. The patient's severe pathology of object relations (the inappropriate familiarity with the examining psychiatrist, idealization and devaluation of his ex-lover, sexual instability, arrogant dismissal of other men) and his likely identity disturbance may correspond to the syndrome of identity diffusion that is common to all severe Personality Disorders.

Identity diffusion is characterized by a lack of integration of the concept of the self and the concept of significant others. It is reflected in an unrealistic assessment of the self and severe difficulties in assessing others in a realistic way, accompanied by the absence of appropriate empathy with others' emotional experiences. Patients with severe Narcissistic Personality Disorders typically present with identity diffusion, and they may present with generalized lack of impulse control, severely limited tolerance for anxiety, and chronic breakdown in their capacity for work or any intimacy, all of which would support the diagnosis of a Narcissistic Personality Disorder functioning on an overt borderline level. (The designation of *overt borderline level* refers to the presence of lack of anxiety tolerance, lack of impulse control, and lack of capacity for investment in work or creative pursuits beyond their survival level. These are nonspecific manifestations of severe personality disorders also called *borderline personality organization*, all of which are also characterized by severe identity disturbance—*identity diffusion*—and predominance of primitive defensive operations. In contrast, *neurotic personality organization* refers to less severe personality disorders that present with well-integrated identity and high-level defensive operations that are only diagnosable in intensive psychotherapeutic encounters.) This degree of severity of pathological narcissism should not be confused with a borderline personality proper. In clinical practice, unfortunately, this confusion is not infrequent and leads to unexpected complications in the psychotherapeutic treatment of patients who were diagnosed erroneously as having a Borderline Personality Disorder. These complications include negative therapeutic reactions, incapacity to establish a dependent relationship with the therapist, an extraordinary degree of arrogance and devaluation in the transference, and others.

Nick reports a homosexual identity, and the combination of homosexuality and a Narcissistic Personality Disorder often makes for a more difficult treatment course because of the use of the homosexual identity as a secondary defensive operation to protect the pathological grandiose self, which is characteristic of the Narcissistic Personality Disorder.

An important differential diagnosis in this case is the syndrome of malignant narcissism (not included in the DSM-IV-TR classification system) and Antisocial Personality Disorder. The syndrome of malignant narcissism includes, in the presence of a Narcissistic Personality Disorder, severe paranoid features, ego-syntonic aggression (directed against others or the self), and antisocial behavior. Nick does not present with significant paranoid traits, and, so far, there is no evidence for major aggression or antisocial behavior (except the inappropriate imitation of a famous actor "as a joke"). However, because all Antisocial Personality Disorders do present a narcissistic character structure, or rather, because the Antisocial Personality Disorder really is an extreme form of Narcissistic Personality Disorder with complete breakdown or absence of internalized ethical and moral value systems (absence of superego functions), it is very important to investigate antisocial behavior in all patients with Narcissistic Personality Disorder. Antisocial behavior may take the form of either aggressive or passive-exploitive behavior (such as lying, stealing, irresponsibility with money, and conning others), and, should this patient present such behaviors, they probably would be of the passive/exploitive type, given the lack of evidence of manifest aggression in the diagnostic interaction. His inappropriate familiarity with the diagnostician seems more of a childlike nature than a threatening, aggressive invasiveness.

Regarding the prognosis for Nick's treatment, the most important issues are the following: The first is the extent to which there is evidence of antisocial behavior—the more severe the antisocial features, the worse the prognosis, to the extent that an Antisocial Personality Disorder proper would practically present a zero prognosis for all psychotherapeutic modalities of treatment. A second prognostic feature is the presence or absence of secondary gain, a major problem in the treatment of severe Personality Disorders. So far, there is no evidence in the information provided of such secondary gain. Nick is not depending on chronic social support systems obtained on the basis of his personality disorder, and there is no indication of major exploitive or parasitic tendencies derived from his probable incapacity or unwillingness to work. Information regarding his work history and the nature of his intimate relationships would be crucial from a prognostic viewpoint: The more impoverished the capacity for object relations, the worse the prognosis. The features referred to before as indicating overt borderline functioning also would worsen the prognosis or, rather, move the treatment recommendation into a supportive—in contrast to a psychodynamic or exploratory—direction.

Regarding the treatment of Nick, he was already referred to an experienced clinician who was willing to see him at a minimal fee. The patient, however, requested a referral to somebody who would offer him free treatment, indicating, it seems to me, not only his narcissistic character (as the therapist would be "getting as much out of it as he would") but also his relatively poor motivation for treatment at this point.

The treatment of the patient with Narcissistic Personality Disorder is essentially psychotherapeutic. Patients who are functioning relatively well in social situations, in their work commitments or profession, and in their capacity to establish some degree of consistent, long-term relationships are candidates for psychoanalytic treatment. Given these patients' strong defenses against dependent relationships, standard psychoanalysis offers a specific technique for the treatment of their character structure that has been developed in recent years (Kernberg 1989) and offers an optimal treatment for the better-functioning patients with narcissism.

In the present case, however, because of the severity of the illness as reflected in the impression Nick conveys of severe disturbances in his social life, in his work, and probably also in his intimate relationships and in the gross manifestations of his lack of ordinary tact and sensitivity in social interactions, the optimal treatment would be a psychotherapy for severe Personality Disorders geared to modifying the personality structure proper—that is, a specific psychodynamic psychotherapy such as we have developed at Cornell—namely, transference-focused psychotherapy (TFP). This treatment, however, requires at least two sessions per week over many months and the patient's acceptance of a treatment contract that would include his commitment to work and to maintain a minimal adaptation to ordinary life situations, which would facilitate the analysis of his pathological character patterns.

The process itself would test the patient's capacity for tolerating self-exploration and in-depth analysis of his pathological character defenses that would be activated in the treatment situation.

I believe it would be worthwhile to attempt this psychodynamic psychotherapeutic treatment if Nick agreed to the treatment conditions and agreed only to shift the treatment to a supportive psychotherapeutic modality if it turned out that he was not able to tolerate, or if he revealed his incapacity to benefit from, such an exploratory modality of treatment. If further exploration of this patient revealed that he was not able to tolerate TFP, if a treatment trial with TFP evolved in a negative way, or if further negative prognostic indicators would weaken the advisability of TFP, supportive psychotherapy would become the treatment of choice, along the lines of specific supportive psychotherapy techniques for borderline patients. (Supportive psychotherapy implies tactful confrontation of the patient's pathological behavior patterns; cognitive and affective support; reeducative reduction of transference regression, clarifying and reducing through education the inappropriate aspects of transferential behavior and the use of transference patterns for clarification of similar patterns outside the transference; and direct environmental interventions.)

As an alternative to such a supportive psychotherapy based on psychodynamic principles, a cognitive-behavioral approach might be indicated, geared to modifying dominant inappropriate behavior patterns in the context of cognitive and affective validation. However, a cognitive-behavioral approach may be particularly difficult with Nick because of the prevalence of narcissistic resistances that would affect all psychotherapeutic treatment approaches. I am referring to such patients' characteristic narcissistic defenses against dependency on the therapist, who patients may believe wants to humiliate them or make them feel inferior, with a consequent reinforcement of patients' dismissive, grandiose, and possibly arrogant reactions. In addition, the profound suspicion that such patients have regarding the authenticity of the therapist's interest in them and their fears of being exploited and depreciated—all of it a consequence of the projection of their own pathological grandiose self onto the therapist—may bring about significant negative transferences and even negative psychotherapeutic reactions. These transferences might optimally be resolved in TFP and negotiated in a psychodynamically informed supportive psychotherapy but, in any case, will represent significant obstacles in the treatment that could possibly be reflected in a premature dropout.

One major problem in this case is Nick's lack of motivation for treatment, linked with his apparent lack of concern over his difficulties and his denial of his failure in the area of his supposed interest—acting. His depreciation of other homosexual men, probably part of his general dismissive attitude toward others, reflects a deep depreciation of himself projected onto others, and he may be unconsciously afraid of treatment being a confrontation with his own denied feelings of inferiority, failure, and loneliness. In explaining to Nick his need for treatment, a tactful confrontation of his failure in work, in intimacy, and presumably also in his social life in general must be matched with an empathic understanding of his reluctance to recognize these issues, his fear of depression, and his profound anxiety over his situation. The extent to which Nick would be able to come to understand, as part of the diagnostic interviews, his need for treatment and evince a thoughtful reaction to the therapist's comments—in contrast to jocular dismissal of them—may provide more information as to the extent to which the insight-oriented TFP may be indicated, in contrast to a supportive or cognitive-behavioral psychotherapeutic treatment. In any case, in the course of the evaluation, I would explain to Nick that he has a significant personality disorder, characterized by profound difficulties in assessing himself and others in depth and in committing himself to work or a profession in a way that would ensure realistic—in contrast to fantasized—success in life.

The essential characteristic of TFP for severe personality disorders is the consistent analysis of the transference developments in order to resolve identity diffusion and the primitive defensive operations linked to this syndrome. In the case of a patient with narcissism, manifestations of the pathological grandiose self as they are activated in the treatment situation and their gradual exploration and resolution would be analyzed. This analysis facilitates the emergence of the patient's underlying primitive conflicts around dependency and love, the resolution of which will facilitate the consolidation of a real self and the capacity for mature relationships with significant others. My personal experience in using TFP with patients presenting with Narcissistic Personality Disorder is very positive among those who do not present significant antisocial features or secondary gain of treatment and whose talents, capacities, and life situation provide them with realistic alternatives to the difficulties created by having the disorder. The prognosis is not good, as mentioned earlier, for those patients with severe antisocial features and secondary gain of illness, and when so much has been ruined in their lives and so much time has gone by that it is preferable to use a supportive approach.

Another negative prognostic element that becomes crucial for some patients is an intense degree of aggression against others and self that may evolve as the expression of an inordinate wish to destroy the treatment out of unconscious envy of the therapist. Unconscious envy is a major emotional difficulty dominant in the underlying dynamics of patients with narcissism. Insofar as Nick does not seem to present negative aggressive features, if he were able to accept TFP, his prognosis would be relatively good. The prognosis with a supportive psychotherapeutic approach is variable; it depends on the nature of the joint agreement between the patient and therapist that can be reached regarding what issues need to be examined and changed in the patient's behavior in the course of the treatment.

In any case, the amelioration of this severe personality disorder requires many months of treatment and faces the risk of premature termination.

Reference

Kernberg OF: Guest editor: narcissistic personality disorder. Psychiatr Clin North Am 12(3), 1989

Suggested Reading

Clarkin JF, Yeomans FE, Kernberg OF: Psychotherapy for Borderline Personality. New York, Wiley, 1999

Kernberg OF: Severe Personality Disorders: Psychotherapeutic Strategies. New Haven, CT, Yale University Press, 1984

Kernberg OF: Aggression in Personality Disorders and Perversion. New Haven, CT, Yale University Press, 1992

Lady Macbeth

Interviewer: Tell me about when things were the hardest for you. When was that?

Patient: It was around Christmas time last year.

Interviewer: And you were how old then?

Patient: 13.

Interviewer: You're 14 now, right?

Patient: Yes.

Interviewer: When things were really at their worst, can you tell me what it was that was disturbing to you at that time?

Patient: Well, the major part about it was that, like all these things that I did, they were really stupid, and they didn't make any sense; but I'm still gonna have to do it and, it was sort of like being scared of what would happen if I didn't do it.

Interviewer: What were the things that you were doing?

Patient: In the morning when I got dressed, I was real afraid that there'd be germs all over my clothes and things, so I'd stand there and I'd shake them for half an hour. I'd wash before I did anything—like if I was gonna wash my face, I'd wash my hands first; and if I was gonna get dressed, I'd wash my hands first; and then it got even beyond that point. Washing my hands wasn't enough, and I started to use rubbing alcohol. It was wintertime and cold weather, and this really made my hands bleed. Even if I just held them under water, they'd bleed all over the place, and they looked terrible, and everyone thought I had a disease or something.

Interviewer: And when you were doing that much washing, how much time every day did that take, if you added up all the different parts of it?

Patient: It took about 6 hours a day. In the morning I didn't have a whole lot of choice, because I had to get up at 6:00 A.M. and get ready for school. All I'd do was get dressed as best I could. I didn't even have time to brush my hair. At the time I never ate breakfast, so all these things…it was just so complex that I didn't have time to do anything.

Interviewer: You also told me about other things in addition to the washing and worrying about dirt: that you would have plans about how you would do other things.

Patient: Okay, well, they were like set plans in my mind that if I heard the word, like, something that had to do with germs or disease, it would be considered something bad and so I had things that would go through my mind that were sort of like "cross that out and it'll make it okay" to hear that word.

Interviewer: What sort of things?

Patient: Like numbers or words that seemed to be sort of like a protector.

Interviewer: What numbers and what words were they?

Patient: It started out to be the number 3 and multiples of 3 and then words like "soap and water," something like that; and then the multiples of 3 got really high, they'd end up to be 123 or something like that. It got real bad then.

Interviewer: At any time did you really believe that something bad would happen if you didn't do these things? Was it just a feeling, or were you really scared?

Patient: No! I was petrified that something would really happen. It was weird, because everyone would always say how sensible I was and intelligent. But it was weird because I tried to explain it in order to really make them understand what I was trying to say and they'd go, you know, like, "Well, that's stupid," and I knew it; but when I was alone, things would be a lot worse than when I was with this group, because if I was around friends, that would make me forget about most of this. But when I was alone it…like, my mind would wander to all sorts of things and I'd get new plans and new rituals and new ideas, and I'd start worrying more and more about people that could get hurt that I cared about and things that could really go bad if I didn't.

Interviewer: Who were the people you'd worry most would get hurt?

Patient: My family, basically my family.

Interviewer: Any particular people in your family?

Patient: Well, like my grandmother—she's 83 and you know, I was just worried that…I know that she's old and she's not gonna be around much longer, but I was worried that maybe something I did could cause her to get really, really sick or something.

Interviewer: Had anything like this ever been on your mind before you were 13, when this started?

Patient: Well, let's see…my mother, her family has always been mostly real neat people and extremely clean and so that could have affected it, because I was growing up in that sort of background. But I always like to be clean and neat, and I was never really allowed to walk around the house with muddy shoes or anything like that, so…

Interviewer: But your concerns about cleanliness, about how many times you did things—have they ever gotten in the way of your doing things that you wanted to do?

Patient: Uh-huh. Many times. Like, I was supposed to go somewhere with a friend, and we were gonna leave at 11:00 A.M. and I wanted to take a shower before I left. So I had to get up about 6:00 A.M. in the morning, and sometimes I just won't even make it with 5 hours to do it.

Interviewer: And that was since you were 13. But what about any time in your life before that—had anything like this ever happened? Or as far as you know was this the first?

Patient: It was the first time.

Interviewer: Have you at any time felt that you had some other special idea about forces beyond you…about your being able to control things magically or be in control?

Patient: I'm really scared of supernatural things. I don't like to say that I believe in superstitions and things, but I guess I really do because they frighten me. When I was little they weren't really bothering me or anything, but now I avoid it as much as I can. Like, the number 13 now, if it came up, you know, it wouldn't bother me, but I'd rather have the number 7 instead.

Interviewer: So you are superstitious, but you've never heard any special voice talking to you or…

Patient: Yeah, I have. It's like…if I tried to describe it, people would think that I saw little people dancing around or something, and that was wrong because all it was, it wasn't like a voice, it was just like a thought.

Interviewer: More like being able to hear yourself think?

Patient: Right.

Interviewer: Have you ever seen things that other people couldn't see?

Patient: No.

Interviewer: I know you are doing very well here in school and on the ward here at the hospital. Do you have any signs left of the problems that you used to have with your rituals and compulsions?

Patient: Well, everyone is compulsive to a point. I can see little things that I still do. Like I will go over something twice, or three times, because that's a special number. Like, if I read something and I really don't understand it, maybe I would go over it one more time and then, say, one more time will make it three. But nothing really big. It's been really good, because now I am able to take a shower, and get dressed, and wash my face and brush my teeth, and all that stuff in like half an hour! That's really good for me because I wasn't able to do that before I came into the hospital.

Interviewer: So, in general it's fair to say it's things that just you would notice now, and probably someone sharing the room with you wouldn't be able to tell the other things you are still doing even though you know these little things are there. Good....Well, thank you very much.

DSM-IV-TR Casebook Diagnosis of "Lady Macbeth"

This adolescent girl articulately and vividly describes what it is like to have a severe form of Obsessive-Compulsive Disorder (OCD) (DSM-IV-TR, p. 462). She has both obsessions and compulsions, and both are a significant source of distress to her and interfere with her functioning.

The obsessions consist of ideas that (at least at some time during the course of the illness) intrude themselves into her consciousness and are experienced as inappropriate. For example, she has the idea that maybe she did something that could cause her grandmother to become sick. Another example is the thought that there are germs on her clothes. The need to neutralize such distressing thoughts has led to various compulsions that are repetitive, and she feels driven to perform according to rules that must be applied rigidly. For example, if she heard a word that suggested germs or disease, she had to undo it ("cross that out") by saying the number 3 and multiples of 3, or words like "soap and water." Although these behaviors were designed to prevent discomfort or some dreaded event, the activity was not connected in a realistic way to what it was designed to prevent and was clearly excessive. For example, she washed her hands for hours to prevent becoming infected by germs, to the point at which her hands would actually bleed. Although emotionally she reacted as if the dangers were real ("I was petrified that something would really happen"), intellectually she always knew that her fears were irrational and were not about real-life problems (her friends would say that it was stupid, and she knew that it was). In rare cases, during a severe episode of the illness, the person may no longer recognize that the obsessions or compulsions are excessive or unreasonable; in such instances, the diagnosis is specified as With Poor Insight.

Discussion of "Lady Macbeth" by Judith L. Rapoport, M.D.*

Lady Macbeth certainly has OCD. It is not surprising that she is only 13, because about one-half of patients with OCD have their onset by their 15th birthday. The discomfort she describes in connection with "having" to carry out washing rituals is the primary basis for classifying OCD as an Anxiety Disorder, but where OCD should really be placed remains a matter of debate. The patient's bleeding hands are also a frequent clinical sign, and in reticent children who, out of embarrassment or fear of being considered "weird," conceal their illness, the diagnosis of OCD may eventually be made by a consulting dermatologist (Rapoport 1987)! This family (and patient) was fortunate because she would

---

*Dr. Rapoport is Chief of the Child Psychiatry Branch at the National Institute of Mental Health in Bethesda, Maryland. She studied psychology as an undergraduate at Swarthmore College, where she wrote a paper on theoretical explanations of obsessions and compulsions. Her first patient as a psychiatric resident at the Massachusetts Mental Health Center was a patient with OCD who had been cured by an early (1950s) frontal lobotomy (a procedure that brought other severe impairments). She is the author of a best-selling book on OCD: The Boy Who Couldn't Stop Washing (Rapoport 1987) and carried out many of the earliest studies of drug treatment, brain imaging, and animal models of this disorder.

talk about her problem. Children so often suffer their OCD in silence that even those in treatment for depression or anxiety hold back from talking about obsessions or compulsions with their therapist (Berg et al. 1989). Unless the child is interviewed directly and specifically about OCD, the diagnosis will be missed in most cases (Rapoport et al. 2000). Lady Macbeth's openness with the interviewer is also encouraging.

This brief vignette raises several questions that need to be answered before this patient will be understood or appropriate treatment is chosen.

Does She Have Comorbid Conditions Such as Other Anxiety Disorders or Attention-Deficit/Hyperactivity Disorder or (Less Likely in a Female) Motor Tics?

Comorbidity affects treatment choices. When Attention-Deficit/Hyper-activity Disorder is severe, concurrent stimulant drug treatment can sometimes worsen OCD. Comorbid tics predict usefulness of augmentation with dopamine-blocking agents. Axis II disorders are associated with poor outcome for both drug and behavioral treatment.

The most frequent comorbid disorders are other Anxiety Disorders, Tourette's, or Attention-Deficit/Hyperactivity Disorder, but there is a broad range of increased comorbidity in childhood-onset cases, which includes developmental disorders, behavior disorders, and substance abuse (Swedo et al. 1989).

Is There a Family History of Obsessive-Compulsive Disorder or Related Disorders?

The allusion to her mother and her family being really neat and extremely clean is intriguing. The Leyton Obsessional Interview was developed in the United Kingdom for the study of "House-Proud Housewives"—a group of subjects with a blend of what we would now consider true OCD and Obsessive-Compulsive Personality Disorder. This is not unusual in the families of OCD "washers." Because Obsessive-Compulsive Personality Disorder is rarely comorbid with OCD, it may be that the "house-proud" relatives have mild cases of OCD. Only in-person interviews will make this distinction.

Family history is also important with respect to familial OCD, Tourette's Disorder, motor tics, and Bipolar Disorder and rheumatic fever–related Sydenham's chorea. Familial Tourette's Disorder and Chronic Motor Tic Disorder may be increased in male family members.

In adolescent-onset OCD cases, the OCD precedes the onset of bipolar illness by several years.

Was the Onset of Illness Sudden and in Response to an Infectious Illness?

In some pediatric cases, it appears that OCD is triggered by an infection. This is called *pediatric autoimmune neuropsychiatric disorders associated with* Streptococcus *infection* (or PANDAS) (Swedo et al. 1998), the only infection studied formally being group A beta-hemolytic *Streptococcus*. A strong case for the diagnosis of PANDAS can be made if there has been a sudden onset or dramatic worsening of the OCD symptoms in relation to clinical infection and a positive throat culture or laboratory test on two or more occasions (e.g., antistreptolysin-O titer) that parallels the course of the OCD symptoms. Research is being done to evaluate immunosuppressant treatment, as well as prophylactic treatment, with penicillin.

If Not Because of an Infection, Why Does Lady Macbeth Have Obsessive-Compulsive Disorder?

First of all, let's discuss the real Lady Macbeth. She had just committed murder and had several excellent reasons to be washing her hands so carefully! But Shakespeare's tragic villainess did not have OCD. Now, back to our case: Growing evidence implicates dysfunction of a particular neural circuitry—that between the basal ganglia and the frontal lobes—as causal in OCD. Both genetic and nongenetic influences appear important, but there is no clear candidate for either other than streptococcal infection noted earlier.

Treatment Choice

Things have changed dramatically for patients like Lady Macbeth. In the 1980s, she would have been offered exploratory psychotherapy. She now has several choices of drug and nondrug treatments for her OCD, each with demonstrated efficacy (Rapoport and Inoff-Germain 2000). Each has advantages, and treatment combinations are common. She may be a candidate for behavior therapy, which requires insight, motivation for change, and the ability to assess symptoms. Behavior therapy works particularly well for uncomplicated, highly motivated patients—

as seems to be the case here. The benefits of behavior therapy often carry over after the treatment sessions have stopped. The disadvantage is that this can be a long and stressful experience with intense exposure to the "trigger" stimulus (e.g., touching something "dirty" in Lady Macbeth's case) together with response prevention (e.g., not washing). Reported success stories in behavior therapy are of those who complete at least 12 hours of such exposures for each major symptom.

Medication is usually faster and helps many symptoms at once. There is a choice of at least six agents, all of which apparently work by blocking serotonin uptake. There are also two medications that can be used to augment a partial response. Although many, if not most, patients at some point try both approaches, based on this vignette at least, I think Lady Macbeth might start with behavior therapy alone. But, if after a few months (e.g., 3) there is not clear improvement, medication should be added.

One feels good about this case, as she presents; I give great odds on substantial and prompt improvement!

References

Berg CZ, Rapoport JL, Whitaker A, et al: Childhood obsessive-compulsive disorder: a two-year prospective follow-up of a community sample. J Am Acad Child Adolesc Psychiatry 28:528–533, 1989

Rapoport J: The Boy Who Couldn't Stop Washing. New York, EP Dutton, 1987

Rapoport J, Inoff-Germain G: Update on treatment of obsessive compulsive disorder. J Child Psychol Psychiatry 41:419–437, 2000

Rapoport JL, Inoff-Germain G, Weissman MM, et al: Childhood obsessive-compulsive disorder in the NIMH MECA study: parent versus child identification of cases. J Anxiety Disord 4:535–548, 2000

Swedo S, Rapoport JL, Leonard HL, et al: Obsessive compulsive disorders in children and adolescents: clinical phenomenology of 70 consecutive cases. Arch Gen Psychiatry 46:335–341, 1989

Swedo SE, Leonard HL, Garvey M, et al: Pediatric autoimmune neuropsychiatric disorders associated with streptococcal infections: clinical description of the first 50 cases. Am J Psychiatry 155:264–271, 1998

Toughing It Out

Mindy Markowitz is an attractive, stylishly dressed 25-year-old art director for a trade magazine who presents to an anxiety clinic after reading about the clinic program in the newspaper. She is seeking treatment for "panic attacks" that have occurred with increasing frequency over the past year, often 2 or 3 times a day. These attacks begin with a sudden intense wave of "horrible fear" that seems to come out of nowhere, sometimes during the day, sometimes waking her from sleep. She begins to tremble, is nauseated, sweats profusely, feels as though she is choking, and fears that she will lose control and do something crazy, like run screaming into the street.

Mindy remembers first having attacks like this when she was in high school. She was dating a boy her parents disapproved of and had to do a lot of "sneaking around" to avoid confrontations with them. At the same time, she was under a lot of pressure as the principal designer of her high school yearbook and was applying to Ivy League colleges. She remembers that her first panic attack occurred just after the yearbook went to press and she was accepted by Harvard, Yale, and Brown. The attacks lasted only a few minutes, and she would just "sit through them." She went to her family physician because she thought she might have something seriously wrong with her heart. After a complete physical examination and an electrocardiogram, he reassured her that it was "just anxiety."

Mindy has had panic attacks intermittently over the 8 years since her first attack, sometimes not for many months, but sometimes, as now, several times a day. There have been extreme variations in the intensity of the attacks, some being so severe and debilitating that she has had to take a day off from work.

Mindy has always functioned extremely well in school, at work, and in her social life, apart from her panic attacks and a brief period of depression at age 19 when she broke up with a boyfriend. She is a lively, friendly person who is respected by her friends and colleagues both for her intelligence and creativity and for her ability to mediate disputes.

Mindy has tried to ignore the attacks and has rarely limited her activities because of them. There have been a few times, even during the brief periods that she was having frequent, severe attacks, when she stayed at home from work for a day because she was exhausted from multiple attacks. She has never associated the attacks with particular places. She says, for example, that she is as likely to have an attack at home in her own bed as on the subway, so there is no point in avoiding the subway. Whether she has an attack on the subway, in a supermarket, or at home by herself, she says, "I just tough it out."

DSM-IV-TR Casebook Diagnosis of "Toughing It Out"

Mindy describes classic, unexpected panic attacks. They hit her unpredictably with a sudden burst of fear and the characteristic symptoms of autonomic arousal: sweating, trembling, nausea, and choking, all severe enough to make her fear she will lose control. Unlike most patients who have such severe panic attacks, she has never associated particular situations, such as crowded places or public transportation, with having the attacks. Therefore, she does not show any symptoms of agoraphobic avoidance. Thus, the diagnosis is Panic Disorder Without Agoraphobia (DSM-IV-TR, p. 440).

Note: This case is discussed first by Dr. Martin M. Antony and then by Dr. Donald Klein.

Discussion of "Toughing It Out" by Martin M. Antony, Ph.D.*

In many ways, Mindy's condition is an example of a typical case of Panic Disorder Without Agoraphobia. She is experiencing unexpected panic attacks and worries about the consequences of the attacks (e.g., that she might lose control). There doesn't appear to be any significant comorbidity other than a brief period of depression experienced 6 years earlier that was triggered by the breakup of a relationship.

In the treatment of Panic Disorder, there are three empirically supported approaches—cognitive-behavioral therapy (CBT), pharmacotherapy (e.g., imipramine, selective serotonin reuptake inhibitors [SSRIs], alprazolam, clonazepam), and a combination of CBT and pharmacotherapy. Studies on the relative efficacy of these approaches have been somewhat inconsistent, but generally, there is little evidence to suggest that any of these three approaches is more effective than the others, at least for the acute treatment phase (Antony and Swinson 2000; van Balkom et al. 1997).

In the long term, however, after treatment has been discontinued, there is evidence that patients who receive CBT fare better than patients who receive either medication or combined treatments (Barlow et al. 2000; Marks et al. 1993). Therefore, my preference for a case such as Mindy's would be to start with a course of CBT, assuming that she is interested in that option. If treatment with CBT is not effective after 8–10 sessions, or if it leads to only a partial response after 10–15 sessions, my recommendation would be to augment treatment with medication (probably an SSRI).

There are a number of effective cognitive-behavioral protocols for treating panic disorder (e.g., Clark et al. 1994; Craske and Barlow 2001). My own approach is adapted from David Barlow and Michelle Craske's panic control treatment, which includes psychoeducation, breathing retraining, cognitive restructuring, and exposure. However,

---

*Dr. Antony is Associate Professor in the Department of Psychiatry and Behavioural Neurosciences at McMaster University. He is also Chief Psychologist and Director of the Anxiety Treatment and Research Centre at St. Joseph's Healthcare in Hamilton, Ontario. Dr. Antony has published 11 books, including the Handbook of Assessment and Treatment Planning for Psychological Disorders (2002), Practitioner's Guide to Empirically Based Measures of Anxiety (2001), and Phobic Disorders and Panic in Adults: A Guide to Assessment and Treatment (2000).

in light of recent evidence showing that breathing retraining does not contribute significantly to outcome (Schmidt et al. 2000), I typically don't include it (unless a patient is bothered by hyperventilation).

CBT for panic disorder typically has 10–15 weekly sessions, each one lasting about 1 hour. The final few sessions often occur less frequently (e.g., every 2 weeks). The initial few sessions are focused on assessment and on providing education about the nature and treatment of panic. These sessions are followed by several sessions focusing almost exclusively on cognitive therapy strategies. Although the cognitive strategies are used throughout treatment, exposure techniques are introduced at around the fifth session. The final sessions are spent discussing termination of treatment and strategies for maintaining gains.

To start, I would begin with a thorough assessment. In addition to the features measured during a typical psychiatric assessment (e.g., diagnostic symptoms, family history, course of illness), there are other aspects of the problem that are of particular interest in a CBT-focused assessment for panic disorder. These include a detailed assessment of the patient's panic attacks, including their frequency, intensity, triggers, symptoms, associated cognitions, coping strategies, and other features.

In preparation for using cognitive strategies, it is important to understand the beliefs, predictions, and assumptions underlying the attacks. In Mindy's case, these seem to be thoughts about losing control or doing something crazy in public. In preparation for using exposure-based strategies, it is important to understand the triggers for Mindy's attacks. Although she doesn't have agoraphobia and her attacks are not triggered by particular places, it is still likely that triggers can be identified. These may include particular symptoms that she fears (e.g., trembling, nausea, sweating) or activities that trigger symptoms of arousal (e.g., exercise, drinking caffeine, sex, scary movies).

The treatment rationale would also be presented during the early sessions. This part of treatment is designed to educate the patient about the nature of panic attacks and panic disorder, to provide the patient with a model for understanding the problem, and to provide an overview of the treatment procedures. From a cognitive-behavioral perspective, Panic Disorder is thought to be maintained by a tendency to be fearful of benign physical sensations. Although most people tend to ignore symptoms such as dizziness or heart rate changes, individuals with Panic Disorder tend to interpret these symptoms as signs of impending danger.

As Mindy's therapist, I would discuss with her the notion that anxiety and fear are normal emotions experienced by everyone. Normalizing the experience of fear helps patients to become more accepting of their panic symptoms, which is the first step to overcoming the intense fear of having panic attacks. Mindy would also be encouraged to recognize that panic attacks are time limited. Although they are uncomfortable and frightening, panic attacks always come to an end, and they are almost never dangerous. Any misconceptions about panic that Mindy holds (e.g., that panic attacks could cause her to lose control) would be discussed, and corrective information would be presented.

Mindy would also be encouraged to think of her fear and anxiety in terms of three components—physical, cognitive, and behavioral. The physical component of fear includes all of the physical arousal symptoms that she experiences during the attacks. The cognitive component includes her fearful misconceptions, predictions, and beliefs about the dangers of panic attacks and symptoms (e.g., "I will lose control"), as well as her tendency to attend to threat-related information (e.g., scanning her body for feared symptoms). The behavioral component includes any actions that Mindy takes to control her fear or prevent her panic attacks. For many individuals with Panic Disorder, these behaviors include avoidance of panic triggers (e.g., exercise, caffeine) and engaging in various safety behaviors (e.g., carrying a mobile phone in case of an "emergency," lying down whenever the slightest symptom is experienced, checking one's pulse repeatedly). Once Mindy understands her symptoms in terms of these three components, the treatment procedures would be introduced.

Cognitive therapy is designed to target the cognitive component of fear by changing fearful thoughts about panic attacks. Exposure targets fearful behaviors (e.g., avoidance, safety behaviors) by compelling patients not to use their typical avoidance strategies, thereby showing them that their symptoms are not dangerous. Other strategies (e.g., breathing retraining, medications) are designed to influence the physical component. Intervening at any of these levels is assumed to lead to changes in the other two components. To reinforce the material discussed in the initial sessions, Mindy would be encouraged to read a self-help manual that describes the nature and treatment of panic from a cognitive-behavioral perspective (Zuercher-White 1997).

Around the time of the third session, Mindy would be taught to use cognitive restructuring to challenge anxious thinking—in particular, her tendency to overestimate the likelihood of negative consequences occurring (probability overestimations) and her tendency to exaggerate the impact of such consequences if they were to occur (catastrophic thinking). She would be encouraged to record her anxious thoughts in diaries and to use a variety of techniques to examine the evidence for her thoughts. Mindy would also be encouraged to conduct behavioral experiments to test out the accuracy of her predictions. For example, if she is convinced that unless she escapes during a panic attack she will lose control and run screaming into the street, Mindy would be encouraged to stay where she is during her next attack to learn that she will not, in fact, lose control. Although cognitive strategies would be introduced over a period of two sessions, she would be encouraged to continue using the strategies throughout the remaining sessions (and between sessions, for homework), and some time at the start of each session would be spent reviewing her use of the cognitive therapy techniques.

Exposure would be introduced at around the fifth session. Because Mindy does not report any agoraphobic avoidance, her treatment would not include much situational exposure. However, if she does avoid any arousal-producing activities, such as exercise or sex, she would be encouraged to begin to incorporate these into her routine. In addition, Mindy would be taught to use interoceptive exposure, which essentially involves exposure to feared physical symptoms. Initially, Mindy would attempt a series of exercises designed to trigger panic-like sensations (e.g., hyperventilation, aerobic exercise, breathing through a straw, spinning in a chair), and her responses would be recorded. The exercises that most strongly triggered feelings similar to her panic attacks would be noted, and Mindy would be instructed to repeat these exercises until they no longer produced fear. Exposure practices would occur in the therapist's office and during homework, between sessions, both at her home and in situations in which she typically experiences panic-like feelings (if any such situations can be identified).

Over the next few sessions, Mindy would continue to practice both the cognitive therapy and exposure strategies. If she reports a tendency to hyperventilate, breathing retraining might be included to teach her to slow down her breathing. The last few sessions would focus on helping Mindy to plan for the future. She would be encouraged to continue to use the cognitive-behavioral strategies after treatment has ended and to call her therapist for a booster session if the need arises.

Although most patients respond well to CBT alone, some require other treatment approaches. If Mindy did not respond to CBT, I would recommend adding medication. In all likelihood, I would suggest starting with a low dosage of an SSRI and increasing the dose gradually (agitation and anxiety can be side effects of SSRI treatment in the first few weeks). While waiting for the SSRI to begin working, a low dosage of a benzodiazepine (e.g., clonazepam) would help to decrease her anxiety, although I would gradually discontinue the benzodiazepine after 4–6 weeks.

Mindy's prognosis is very good. Most of the predictors of negative outcome in the treatment of Panic Disorder (e.g., chronic life stress, severe agoraphobia, comorbid personality disorders) do not appear to be an issue for her. There is a good chance that Mindy could completely beat her panic attacks in a relatively short time. If this does not happen, chances are very good that her symptoms would at least be significantly improved by the end of treatment.

References

Antony MM, Swinson RP: Phobic Disorders and Panic in Adults: A Guide to Assessment and Treatment. Washington, DC, American Psychological Association, 2000

Barlow DH, Gorman JM, Shear MK, et al: Cognitive-behavioral therapy, imipramine, or their combination for panic disorder. JAMA 283:2529–2536, 2000

Clark DM, Salkovskis PM, Hackmann A, et al: A comparison of cognitive therapy, applied relaxation and imipramine in the treatment of panic disorder. Br J Psychiatry 164:759–769, 1994

Craske MG, Barlow DH: Panic disorder and agoraphobia, in Clinical Handbook of Psychological Disorders, 3rd Edition. Edited by Barlow DH. New York, Guilford Press, 2001, pp 1–59

Marks IM, Swinson RP, Basoglu M, et al: Alprazolam and exposure alone and combined in panic disorder with agoraphobia: a controlled study in London and Toronto. Br J Psychiatry 162:776–787, 1993

Schmidt NB, Woolaway-Bickel K, Trakowski J, et al: Dismantling cognitive-behavioral treatment for panic disorder: questioning the utility of breathing retraining. J Consult Clin Psychol 68:417–424, 2000

van Balkom AJLM, Bakker A, Spinhoven P, et al: A meta-analysis of the treatment of panic disorder with or without agoraphobia: a comparison of psychopharmacological, cognitive-behavioral, and combination treatments. J Nerv Ment Dis 185:510–516, 1997

Zuercher-White E: An End to Panic: Breakthrough Techniques for Overcoming Panic Disorder, 2nd Edition. Oakland, CA, New Harbinger Publications, 1997

Discussion of "Toughing It Out" by Donald Klein, M.D.*

Mindy may have been asked about, or is only telling, half of the story. Whoever provided this skimpy history apparently refrained from probing. The problem is the inconsistencies between the unbelievably stoical history, the hair-raising symptomatic description, and the intelligent, educated patient.

This Ivy League graduate has waves of "horrible fear" for 8 years, with distressing physical and mental symptoms and apprehensions about losing her mind, but she accepts her doctor's reassurance that it's "just anxiety" because she is otherwise perfectly healthy. What is worse is that this statement is the reason accepted by the mental health professional who evaluated her. In my experience, it is extremely unlikely that a patient who has been experiencing severe panic attacks for 8 years would be reassured by proclaiming that it is just anxiety. Obvious inconsistencies in a patient's history always require a more detailed evaluation, accompanied by gentle confrontation if necessary (e.g., "these panic attacks were so bad you felt like you were losing your mind…. I'm surprised that simple reassurance from your doctor would have been so effective.")

---

*Dr. Klein is Professor of Psychiatry at Columbia University, College of Physicians and Surgeons, as well as Director of Research at the New York State Psychiatric Institute. In 1962, Dr. Klein and Dr. Max Fink at Hillside Hospital found, in a placebo-controlled, randomized trial, that depressed patients benefited from the antipsychotic chlorpromazine, as did patients treated with the first tricyclic antidepressant, imipramine. This finding challenged the watertight distinction between antipsychotics and antidepressants.

Two years later, in 1964, on the basis of a double-blind, placebo-controlled trial, Dr. Klein suggested that "anxiety" was not a single affect. Spontaneous panic and anticipatory anxiety are distinguished by their distinct responses to medication. The first American textbook in clinical psychopharmacology, Diagnosis and Drug Treatment of Psychiatric Disorders (1969), was coauthored by Dr. Klein and Dr. John M. Davis.

Dr. Klein fostered innovative recategorizations of depressive and anxiety disorders, including atypical depression and social anxiety disorder, while demonstrating the unique benefits of the neglected monoamine oxidase inhibitors. His recent suffocation false-alarm theory of "spontaneous" panic has generated much controversy due to the claim that panic is not fear because of the lack of hypothalamic-pituitary-adrenal activation, the distinctive acute air hunger that does not occur in danger-engendered fear, and the lack of effect of tricyclic antidepressants on ordinary fear.

Mindy's panic attacks are called "classic," but they are not exactly classic. Sudden dyspnea, experienced as air hunger, is the common salient somatic feature of recurrent spontaneous panics. This is not apparent in the case description, although "choking" may actually be the label for dyspnea used by the patient. It should not be assumed that the terms the patient uses to describe her experience of her symptoms are identical to those used by the evaluator. Spontaneous panic attacks without dyspnea do occur, but they are usually sporadic rather than recurrent, less severe, and more frequent in males. (They also respond best to high-potency benzodiazepines.) The reason given for the absence of phobic avoidance is not a counterexample of agoraphobic reasoning. The travel restrictions of patients with agoraphobia are not due to having more panic attacks when away than when at home but rather to the feared lack of access to ready help if severe panic should strike (e.g., "going crazy," one of the patient's perceived possibilities).

Somehow, the attacks are perceived as not likely to be catastrophic by this patient despite the described symptoms. What disorders should be considered besides Panic Disorder?

Number one is covert drug abuse—probably marijuana, possibly mixed with cocaine. This hypothesis is consonant with these features:

1. Onset during association with disreputable boyfriend
2. Marked irregularity of attack pattern
3. Apparent avoidance of medical attention, which may indicate covert knowledge of probable precipitant and fear of detection
4. Absence of phobia, indicating possible knowledge that the attacks are precipitated by drugs rather than indicative of some impending catastrophe
5. Unpersuasive rationalization for the absence of phobia
6. Marijuana and cocaine are frequent precipitants of recurrent panics

The diagnostic assessment apparently did not include queries about drug use and abuse or about smoking tobacco, which is now known to be a major risk factor for Panic Disorder (as is being female and having a history of depression).

Atypical depression (i.e., depression characterized by symptoms such as oversleeping and overeating) is occasionally associated with recurrent panic attacks that often do not incite phobic reactions. However, atypical depression is usually chronically problematic and not brief and infrequent, as described by this patient. Yet another problem with this assessment is that it is based entirely on the patient's narrative. Depressed patients, particularly those who aspire to "tough it out," often deny and minimize.

Temporal lobe epilepsy should also be considered in the differential diagnosis. In temporal lobe disorder, patients frequently have waves of fear. Surprisingly, temporal lobe disorder is often associated with creative activities. Exploring the possibility of temporal lobe epilepsy, I would want to know the following: Does the patient keep a journal or diary? Is she shy? Is she hypergraphic? Is she cosmically or mystically inclined? Does she have olfactory hallucinations? Just what is her social and sex life like? We know nothing about Mindy's family history, premenstrual exacerbations, or nocturnal attacks.

In my practice, patients are asked to come to the first interview with the person who knows them best, usually a spouse but maybe a parent, child, or friend. Patients are also sent forms before their appointment and are asked to provide a narrative summary of their illness, a detailed record of past treatments and medications, general medical and psychiatric symptomatology, and doctor and hospital records. After reviewing this material, I initially see the patient and informant together, pointing out that it is valuable to obtain another person's perspective. Both minimization and dramatization, which would only be guesswork if the patient was seen alone, become apparent in a joint interview. After 15–20 minutes I thank the informant and continue with the patient for the next hour. On rare occasions, review of the written material prompts seeing the patient alone at first.

The initial review takes 1.5 hours. This amount of time usually suffices for a working diagnosis and treatment plan but not always. (Expressions of shocked indignation may now be heard from managed-care aficionados!) Is this economical?

I believe that the major difference between good and bad care is the thoroughness of evaluation and close monitoring of treatment. Many so-called refractory cases benefit from quite simple interventions for which indications had been missed. Others benefit from discontinuing toxic medication regimens.

Critical attention to the level of evidence that justifies the use of particular diagnostic and therapeutic techniques is crucial. However, my emphasis on thoroughness should not be used as a rationalization for indefinitely prolonged, goal-less explorations. Comparative treatment outcome data is, unfortunately, rare and heavily influenced by the allegiance of the treatment providers to particular forms of treatment.

Suggested Reading

Fyer AJ, Mannuzza S, Chapman TF, et al: Effects of specific phobia comorbidity on the familial transmission of panic disorder. Am J Med Genetics (submitted)

Goetz RR, Klein DF, Papp LA, et al: Acute panic inventory symptoms during CO_2 inhalation and room-air hyperventilation among panic disorder patients and normal controls. Depress Anxiety 14(2):123–136, 2001

Klein DF: Evidence for the validity of the concept of panic disorder. Eur Neuropsychopharmacol 8 (suppl 2):S57–S60, 1998

Klein DF: Panic and phobic anxiety: phenotypes, endophenotypes, and genotypes. Am J Psychiatry 155(9):1147–1149, 1998

Klein DF, Preter M: Panic, suffocation false alarms, separation anxiety and endorphins. Behav Brain Sci (submitted)

Marshall R, Blanco C, Printz D, et al: A pilot study of noradrenergic and HPA axis functioning in PTSD vs. panic disorder. Psychiatry Res 110(3):219–230, 2002

Martinez JM, Coplan JD, Browne ST, et al: Respiratory variability in panic disorder. Depress Anxiety 14:232–237, 2001

Sheikh JI, Leskin GA, Klein DF: Gender differences in panic disorder: findings from the National Comorbidity Survey. Am J Psychiatry 159:55–58, 2002

Sinha SS, Coplan JD, Pine DS, et al: Panic induced by carbon dioxide inhalation and lack of hypothalamic-pituitary-adrenal axis activation. Psychiatry Res 86:93–98, 1999

Slattery MJ, Klein DF, Mannuzza S, et al: Relationship between separation anxiety disorder, parental panic disorder, and atopic disorders in children: a controlled high-risk study. J Am Acad Child Adolesc Psychiatry 41(8):947–954, 2002

Child Psychiatrist

Dr. Crone, a single, 35-year-old child psychiatrist, has been arrested and convicted of fondling several neighborhood boys, ages 6–12. Friends and colleagues were shocked and dismayed, as he had been considered by all to be particularly caring and supportive of children. Not only had he chosen a profession involving their care, but he had also been a Cub Scout leader for many years and also a member of the local Big Brothers.

Dr. Crone is from a stable family. His father, who had also been a physician, was described as a workaholic, spending little time with his three children. Dr. Crone never married and, when interviewed by a psychiatrist as part of his presentence investigation, admitted that he experienced little, if any, sexual attraction toward females, either adults or children. He also denied sexual attraction toward adult men. In presenting the history of his psychosexual development, he reported that he had become somewhat dismayed as a child when his boy friends began expressing rudimentary awareness of an attraction toward girls. His "secret" at the time was that he was attracted more to other boys and, in fact, during childhood often played "doctor" with other boys, eventually progressing to mutual masturbation with some of his friends.

His first sexual experience was at age 6, when a 15-year-old male camp counselor performed fellatio on him several times over the course of the summer—an experience that he had always kept to himself. As he reached his teenage years, he began to suspect that he was homosexual. As he grew older, he was surprised to notice that the age range of males who attracted him sexually did not change, and he continued to have recurrent erotic urges and fantasies about boys between the ages of 6 and 12. Whenever he masturbated, he would fantasize about a boy in that age range, and on a couple of occasions over the years had felt himself to be in love with such a youngster.

Intellectually, Dr. Crone knew that others would disapprove of his many sexual involvements with young boys. He never believed, however, that he had caused any of these youngsters harm, feeling instead that they were simply sharing pleasurable feelings together. He yearned to be able to experience the same sort of feelings toward women, but he never was able to do so. He frequently prayed for help and that his actions would go undetected. He kept promising himself that he would stop, but the temptations were such that he could not. He was so fearful of destroying his reputation, his friendships, and his career that he had never been able to bring himself to tell anyone about his problem.

DSM-IV-TR Casebook Diagnosis of "Child Psychiatrist"

Dr. Crone experiences recurrent intense sexual urges and sexually arousing fantasies involving sexual activity with prepubescent boys. He has acted on these fantasies and urges on many occasions. This alone is sufficient to make the diagnosis of Pedophilia (DSM-IV-TR, p. 572). The diagnosis would also be made if Dr. Crone had never acted on these fantasies and urges but was markedly distressed by them or if they caused interpersonal difficulties.

Discussion of "Child Psychiatrist" by Fred S. Berlin, M.D., Ph.D.*

A psychiatric diagnosis is simply a shorthand way of conveying useful information. The term *pedophilia* denotes that an individual's sexual ori-

Dr. Berlin is an Associate Professor of Psychiatry at The Johns Hopkins University School of Medicine and an attending physician at The Johns Hopkins Hospital. He is also the founder of The Johns Hopkins Sexual Disorders Clinic and the Director of the National Institute for the Study, Prevention and Treatment of Sexual Trauma. He has been an invited participant at a White House Conference on Child Sexual Abuse, and he has been invited to address the Juvenile Justice Subcommittee of the U.S. Senate, as well as Colleges of Judges in several states, on related matters. He has been the recipient of a contract from the National Institute of Mental Health to provide an annotated bibliography of sex offender treatment and of a grant from the Guggenheim Foundation to study the biology of sexual disorders. He has also provided consultation to the European Parliament. The program that he directs has been designated a National Resource Site by the U.S. Department of Justice. The published recidivism rate for men treated for pedophilia at that program has been less than 8%.

entation (usually a male's) is directed either in whole or in part toward prepubescent children. Thus, although Dr. Crone has been diagnosed with Pedophilia, contrary to what some might believe, the term conveys no information whatsoever about his character, temperament, honesty, integrity, attitudes, or intellectual level, nor does it convey any information about either the presence or absence of additional Axis I or Axis II comorbid conditions. The fundamental treatment focus in working with him must be directed toward his disordered sexuality, rather than toward more peripheral concerns (Berlin and Krout 1986). In the course of treating Dr. Crone, it will also be important to determine whether any comorbid conditions, such as depression, personality disorder, or alcoholism, are present, and, if so, to treat them as well.

The public often uses the term *pedophilia* as a stigmatizing pejorative label, and persons with the condition are frequently portrayed as subhuman predators. In point of fact, persons with pedophilia can differ from one another in the expression of their sexuality, just as individuals whose sexual orientation is directed toward adults do. Whereas some persons with pedophilia may simply feel a sense of lust, many, as seems likely in Dr. Crone's case, enjoy the companionship of children and have a genuine affection for them (Money 1980). Usually, the issue is not a lack of concern for them but a sexual attraction to them, which, if enacted, can damage what, in other ways, may have been a caring relationship. In therapy, I would reassure Dr. Crone that I had an appreciation of that fact. At the same time, he must appreciate why such behavior is criminal.

In treating a patient such as Dr. Crone, it is important to recognize that he has not simply chosen to experience sexual attraction to young boys. As youngsters, none of us paused to weigh our options, deciding whether to grow up to be attracted either to women, men, girls, or boys. Likely, no one would choose to develop a sexual orientation that is directed toward prepubescent youngsters—and neither did Dr. Crone. One known etiological risk factor for the development of pedophilia is having been sexually abused during childhood, and Dr. Crone, like many men with the disorder, is indeed a former victim (Freund and Kuban 1994). This too, will likely need to be addressed in his treatment.

Historically, there have been a number of misconceptions about pedophilia that have sometimes led to misdirected treatments—treatments that should be avoided in this instance. For example, some have speculated that pedophilic behavior is more about power and control than about sexuality. Others have suggested that persons with the disorder turn to children because they lack the maturity, confidence, and social skills necessary to attract other adults. However, neither of these formulations can explain why it is that Dr. Crone can ordinarily get an erection only in response to fantasies about prepubescent boys. Teaching him social skills might only serve to enhance his capacity to interact more successfully with children, and therefore I would not consider that to be either a necessary or an appropriate component of his care.

Early psychodynamic theories postulated that pedophilia develops when something has gone wrong during the formative childhood maturation process (Freud 1985). Through subsequent therapy, one could develop insight regarding the etiology of the problem, thereby leading to a cure. Were a therapist to consider an individual such as Dr. Crone to have been cured, presumably it would then be safe for him to be around children. Sadly, in the past, many therapists have endorsed such an option. On the other hand, if part of Dr. Crone's treatment requires that he make every effort to avoid situations of temptation that he may not be capable of handling, then he should refrain from any unnecessary contacts with youngsters. Pedophilia is a chronic disorder that cannot be cured, and successful treatment, with a primary goal of abstinence from any and all sexual contacts with children, requires that the individual being treated not place himself in circumstances in which he is vulnerable or "tempted" (Fagan et al. 2002). Insight-oriented psychotherapy is not the treatment of choice for pedophilia, and Dr. Crone should be informed that maintaining proper behavioral control, rather than insight about the etiology of his condition, is the primary goal of his treatment.

Some behavior therapists have tried to recondition sexual orientation, the intent being to extinguish pedophilic arousal, replacing it instead with a newly developed erotic attraction to adults (Kelly 1982; Marks 1981). In the laboratory, using the penile plethysmograph as a monitor, erotic arousal patterns can be transiently changed. However, it is not clear that such changes will carry over outside of the laboratory in such a fashion that sexual orientation will have been permanently reconditioned. How many men could be reconditioned to permanently lose their attraction toward adult women, while at the same time learning to acquire a sustained sexual interest in prepubescent boys? The answer is "probably none." For that reason, I would not attempt to recondition Dr. Crone's erotic arousal pattern.

Bolstering my decision not to try to decondition Dr. Crone's pedophilic sexual makeup would be the knowledge that although some previously learned physiological responses (e.g., salivating in response to the sound of a bell) can be unlearned via a process known as *classical conditioning*, certain other psychobiological responses, even if learned originally, cannot be unlearned. *Imprinting* is a type of learning that, once acquired, becomes in effect "stamped in" in such a fashion that deconditioning does not subsequently occur (Hess 1966). Sexual orientation, if learned (and that is uncertain), may be acquired via imprinting, or being "stamped in" in such a way that deconditioning becomes extremely difficult if not impossible. Because of my belief that any attempt to decondition pedophilic cravings is unlikely to be successful, my treatment of Dr. Crone would be geared toward helping him develop the ability to consistently resist succumbing to unacceptable cravings—cravings that are still likely to remain episodically present. An analogous approach is ordinarily used to treat both drug addiction and alcoholism.

The presence of strong pedophilic cravings can color perceptions, leading to distorted thinking (e.g., self-deception, denial, and rationalization). Dr. Crone's statement that he and the boys with whom he has been involved were simply sharing pleasurable feelings likely represents such a cognitive distortion. I would use group therapy treatment to confront in a firm, yet supportive, fashion any such distortions in an effort to help him better appreciate the true ramifications of his behavior (Hall 1995; Marshall and Barbaree 1990). Dr. Crone has intimated, probably correctly, that he had not ever intended to cause harm to a child. What he may have failed to appreciate is that behaviors can sometimes be wrong even when no harm was intended and even when no harm has occurred. Adult sexual interactions with a prepubescent child involve a multitude of both potential harms and violations of trust, facts that can be better appreciated by Dr. Crone via the group therapy process. The group therapy process should also help him to become more aware of situations that can heighten the risk of relapse, while discussing and reinforcing various relapse prevention strategies (Fuller 1989). Group therapy can also encourage the development of a positive social support network, while serving as a reminder of the need to maintain daily self-vigilance.

Patients such as Dr. Crone often require a great deal of emotional support—a kind of support that group therapy can also provide. One patient whom I have treated for pedophilia characterized himself as having a collateral disorder that he referred to as "posttraumatic pedophilia–related syndrome." He was calling attention to his intense awareness that pedophilia was viewed by society as evil and unforgivable.

The "syndrome" was characterized by a constant fear that others might find out about his "shameful secret attractions," chronic stress, low self-esteem, and a disturbing sense of isolation and estrangement. Even though he had not been engaging in any pedophilic behavior, he had continually felt bad about himself. It is very likely that Dr. Crone is experiencing similar feelings. However, in time, the esprit de corps of the group therapy setting may very well prove to be useful in ameliorating such distress. On the other hand, brief intervals of inpatient hospitalization might be required as a precaution were Dr. Crone to experience either a sense of heightened stress or an impending loss of control.

In some instances, psychotherapy alone, whether group or individual, may not be sufficient to treat pedophilia. Behaviors energized by powerful biological drives, whether involving a hunger for alcohol, heroin, sex, or even just food, can often stress, and sometimes ultimately overcome, volitional resolve. However, a person such as Dr. Crone, who is, in a sense, hungering sexually for children, can often be helped by biological interventions that can decrease the intensity of his hunger (Berlin 1983). Although, in the past, the only method for biological intervention had involved the surgical removal of the testes (castration) to lower testosterone levels, today a variety of prescription drugs can accomplish that same end (Berlin et al. 1995; Bradford 2000; Freund 1980).

Dr. Crone could be administered 7.5 mg of Lupron Depot (leuprolide) intramuscularly once per month as an effective long-term sexual appetite suppressant. He should also be prescribed flutamide (a testosterone-receptor blocking agent), 250 mg po tid, during the first 2 weeks of Lupron therapy to protect against the transient increase in testosterone level that may occur before its subsequent sustained suppression. A complete blood cell count, comprehensive metabolic panel, follicle-stimulating hormone, luteinizing hormone, testosterone levels, and bone density monitoring (as osteoporosis is a potential side effect) should be repeated periodically (Rosler and Witzturn 1998). Weight and blood pressure readings should be closely observed. Dr. Crone has the exclusive form of pedophilia, and therefore he may feel little interest in developing a sexualized relationship with an adult. However, for a patient with the nonexclusive form of the disorder, it might be possible to prescribe sildenafil (Viagra) to enhance his capacity to sustain an erection with a consenting adult partner, without affecting the overall suppression of sexual drive induced by Lupron.

Because of his criminal conviction, Dr. Crone may be either on parole or on probation. If so, he may be required to undergo periodic polygraph testing or periodic testing involving penile plethysmography. He may even be wearing an ankle bracelet as part of ongoing electronic surveillance. Likely, he will be distressed about the fact that his name and address (which may include the address of his family) is on a "sex offender registry." In addition, his neighbors may have been publicly notified about his background. Under these circumstances, as his therapist, I would maintain a close working relationship with his probation officer (Gilligan and Talbot 2000). I would not tolerate noncompliance with treatment, but I would try to maintain Dr. Crone's confidentiality within the context of any relevant statutory requirements. Both Dr. Crone and I would need to understand our responsibilities to the community, and I would discuss his moral obligations with him. At the same time, as his therapist, I would work hard to establish and maintain a trusting doctor-patient relationship and to make clear that his well-being was of genuine concern to me. When treatment is successful, there is no conflict of interest between the patient and the community, as both constituencies are well served.

Both as a physician and as a patient, in conjunction with his therapy, Dr. Crone would likely want to learn more about pedophilia, including information about any relevant research, especially research that may better inform and guide future treatments. Therefore I would make him aware of investigations that have suggested that there may be a familial transmission of pedophilia (Gaffney et al. 1984) and of preliminary neurobiological research that has suggested the possibility of an abnormal release of gonadotropins within the brains of individuals with the condition (Gaffney and Berlin 1984). I would also give him information about a study utilizing positron emission tomography that has documented the release of endogenously produced opiates in specific brain regions during erotic arousal, which may relate to the addictive quality often observed clinically in sexually disordered individuals, such as himself (Frost et al. 1986).

In treating Dr. Crone, I would make him aware of research evidence suggesting that a majority of persons with pedophilia who remain fully compliant with properly administered treatment can do well. For example, in one community-based study involving more than 400 men with the disorder, the 5-year-plus criminal sexual recidivism rate was less than 8% (Berlin et al. 1991). Patients who had been fully compliant with treatment had an even lower recidivism rate of less than 3%.

Often, it is the psychiatrist who can provide the necessary lifeline to patients like Dr. Crone through a combination of therapeutic confrontation, relapse prevention guidance, emotional support, and pharmacological treatment that can enable such success to occur. In working with Dr. Crone, I would be cognizant of the fact that, as a consequence of scientific/medical advances, many persons previously thought to be lazy are now more properly seen as biologically depressed; that morbid obesity, once considered the sin of gluttony, is now viewed as a medical matter; and that alcoholism is no longer seen simply as an example of moral weakness. Although expecting him to behave morally, I would nevertheless reassure Dr. Crone that his disorder did not develop because of moral corruption.

References

Berlin FS: Sex offenders: a biomedical perspective and a status report on biomedical treatment, in The Sexual Aggressor: Current Perspectives on Treatment. Edited by Greer JB, Stuart IR. New York, Van Nostrand Reinhold, 1983, pp 82–123

Berlin FS, Krout E: Pedophilia: diagnostic concepts, treatment and ethical considerations. Am J Forensic Psychiatry 7:13–30, 1986

Berlin FS, Hunt WP, Malin HM, et al: A five-year plus follow-up survey of criminal recidivism within a treated cohort of 406 pedophiles, 111 exhibitionists, and 109 sexual aggressives: issues and outcome. Am J Forensic Psychiatry 12:5–28, 1991

Berlin FS, Malin HM, Thomas K: Nonpedophilic and nontransvestitic paraphilias, in Treatment of Psychiatric Disorders. Edited by Gabbard GO. Washington, DC, American Psychiatric Press, 1995, pp 1941–1958

Bradford JM: The treatment of sexual deviation using a pharmacological approach. J Sex Res 37:248–257, 2000

Fagan PJ, Wise TN, Schmidt CW, et al: Pedophilia. JAMA 288:2458–2465, 2002

Freud S: The sexual aberrations, in Three Essays on the Theory of Sexuality. Edited by Steiner BW. New York, Plenum, 1985, pp 259–324

Freund K: Therapeutic sex-drive reduction. Acta Psychiatr Scand 287 (suppl):5–38, 1980

Freund K, Kuban M: The basis of the abused abuser theory of pedophilia: a further elaboration of an earlier study. Arch Sex Behav 23:553–563, 1994

Frost JJ, Mayberg HS, Berlin FS, et al: Alteration in brain opiate receptor binding in man following sexual arousal using C-11 carfentanil and positron emission tomography, Proceedings of the 33rd annual meeting of the Society of Nuclear Medicine. J Nucl Med 27:1027, 1986

Fuller AK: Child molestation and pedophilia. JAMA 261:602–606, 1989

Gaffney GR, Berlin FS: Is there a hypothalamic-pituitary-gonadal dysfunction in pedophilia? Br J Psychiatry 145:657–660, 1984

Gaffney GR, Lurie SF, Berlin FS: Is there familial transmission of pedophilia? J Nerv Ment Dis 172:546–548, 1984

Gilligan L, Talbot T: Community Supervision of the Sex Offender: An Overview of Current Promising Practices. Silver Spring, MD, Center for Sex Offender Management, 2000, pp 1–16

Hall GC: Sexual offender recidivism revisited: a meta-analysis of recent treatment studies. J Consult Clin Psychol 63:802–809, 1995

Hess EH: Imprinting in animals, in The Biological Basis of Behavior. Edited by McGaugh JL, Weinberger NM, Whalen RE. San Francisco, CA, San Francisco Press, 1966, pp 107–111

Kelly RJ: Behavioral reorientation of pedophiliacs: can it be done? Clin Psychol Rev 2:387–408, 1982

Marks IM: Review of behavioral psychotherapy, II: sexual disorders. Am J Psychiatry 138:750–756, 1981

Marshall WL, Barbaree HE: Outcomes of comprehensive cognitive-behavioral programs, in Handbook of Sexual Assault: Issues, Theories and Treatment of the Offender. Edited by Marshall WL, Laws DR, Barbaree HE. New York, Plenum, 1990, pp 363–385

Money J: Love and Love Sickness. Baltimore, MD, The Johns Hopkins University Press, 1980

Rosler A, Witzturn E: Treatment of men with paraphilia with a long-acting analogue of gonadotropin-releasing hormone. New Engl J Med 338:416–422, 1998

Suggested Reading

Berlin FS: Pedophilia: when is a difference a disorder? Arch Sex Behav 31:1–2, 2002

Flashbacks

A 23-year-old Vietnam veteran was admitted to the hospital 1 year after the end of the Vietnam War, at the request of his wife, after he began to experience depression, insomnia, and "flashbacks" of his wartime experiences. He had been honorably discharged 2 years previously, having spent nearly a year in combat. He had only minimal difficulties in returning to civilian life, resuming his college studies, and then marrying within 6 months after his return. His wife had noticed that he was reluctant to talk about his military experience, but she wrote it off as a natural reaction to unpleasant memories.

The patient's current symptoms began, however, at about the time of the fall of Saigon. He became preoccupied with watching television news stories about this event. He then began to have difficulty sleeping and at times would awaken at night in the midst of a nightmare in which he was reliving his past war experiences. His wife became particularly concerned one day when he had a flashback while out in the backyard: As a plane flew overhead, flying somewhat lower than usual, the patient threw himself to the ground, seeking cover, thinking it was an attacking helicopter. The more he watched the news on television, the more agitated and morose he became. Stories began to spill out of him about horrifying atrocities like those he had seen and experienced, and he began to feel guilty that he had survived while many of his friends had not. At times he also seemed angry and bitter, feeling that the sacrifices he and others had made were all wasted.

The veteran's wife expressed concern that his preoccupation with Vietnam had become so intense that he seemed uninterested in anything else and was emotionally distant from her. When she suggested that they try to plan their future, including having a family, he responded as if his life currently consisted completely of the world of events experienced 2 years earlier, as if he had no future.

DSM-IV-TR Casebook Diagnosis of "Flashbacks"

This veteran has become totally preoccupied with his painful year in Vietnam. His combat experience obviously involved traumatic events in which he and others were threatened with death and that evoked feelings of fear and horror. He reexperienced this trauma through dreams and flashbacks. His responsiveness to his current environment became diminished (he was uninterested in things, was emotionally distant from his wife, and had a sense of a foreshortened future). In addition, he had symptoms of increased arousal (disturbed sleep, outbursts of anger, and exaggerated startle response). This is the full picture of Posttraumatic Stress Disorder (DSM-IV-TR, p. 467). The disorder is further subclassified as Chronic because the symptoms have been present for longer than 3 months, and Delayed to indicate that the onset of the symptoms occurred at least 6 months after the trauma.

Discussion of "Flashbacks" by Jonathan R. T. Davidson, M.D.*

This patient displayed a common symptom seen in people who experience a life-threatening trauma shared with others: a sense of guilt that they survived when others did not.

---

*Dr. Davidson is Professor in the Department of Psychiatry and Behavioral Sciences and Director of the Anxiety and Traumatic Stress Program at Duke University Health Systems in Durham, North Carolina. Dr. Davidson's work in the area of psychological trauma began while he was employed in the Veterans Administration (VA) in 1982 and has continued ever since. His work encompasses survivors from all kinds of trauma and includes biology, treatment, measurement, and epidemiology. During the past two decades, he has published extensively in these areas; he has served as Cochair of the DSM-IV Workgroup for Posttraumatic Stress Disorder (PTSD); has chaired, cochaired, or served as a member of numerous PTSD Advisory Boards; has reviewed the National Institute of Mental Health and VA merit review proposals; and has received funding from the National Institute of Mental Health to study PTSD. He has also coedited three books on PTSD: Posttraumatic Stress Disorder: DSM-IV and Beyond (American Psychiatric Press, 1993); Posttraumatic Stress Disorder: Diagnosis, Management and Treatment (Martin Dunitz Publishers, 2000); and Clinicians' Manual on Post-Traumatic Stress Disorder (Science Press Ltd., 2001).

A 23-year-old Vietnam veteran was admitted to the hospital 2 years after he had returned home from military service, which involved 1 year in combat. His symptoms are representative of chronic PTSD, and they were seemingly triggered by his watching television coverage of the fall of Saigon, which resulted in severe nightmares and flashbacks. It is not unusual for a patient's spouse or partner to be sufficiently concerned by manifestations of PTSD to seek treatment. Given the circumstance, it would be particularly important to establish that the patient had the same desire for treatment.

Before addressing issues of management, a number of points call for comment. First, it is noted that news media coverage may be connected to the intensity of symptoms. It is perhaps relevant to recall that, after the September 11 terrorist attacks, the amount of time spent watching television coverage correlated with severity of symptoms (Marshall and Galea 2004). We should be mindful of the extent to which trauma survivors engage in watching television or reading news material that could provoke further rumination and reintensification of trauma-related experiences.

Second, comorbid psychiatric disorders, such as depression and alcohol and substance abuse, are among the risk factors for developing PTSD, as well as complications in its management. Fortunately, these seem to be absent in this particular instance, thereby simplifying the management. Moreover, an additional factor—positive family history of psychiatric disorder—is also absent.

A third factor is the significant level of survivor guilt. Despite having been dropped from the list of diagnostic criteria in DSM-III-R, it remains a salient aspect of the disorder, commanding special attention. We learn that the patient was involved in perpetrating atrocities. One is reminded of Pitman and colleagues (1991), who found that prolonged exposure, which is often used effectively to treat PTSD, may have the capacity for unmasking anger or thoughts of suicide in subjects who have been involved in atrocities. The presence of guilt would not necessarily contraindicate prolonged exposure but would need to be considered in the patient's management.

A fourth consideration is the comparatively short duration of PTSD. Even though the correct diagnosis is chronic PTSD in this case, it is far less chronic than the mean 20 years of active symptoms that can characterize patients with PTSD (Kessler 2000). As a general rule, it is held that response to treatment may be better if the illness is of shorter duration. Counterbalancing this principle, however, is the need to establish that the patient is committed to treatment and that he is willing to tolerate the predictable bumps in the road that he will encounter, no matter what treatment approach is adopted.

Last, it is not clear whether the patient is employed. If he were employed, then one would need to inquire about the level of employer support he receives and the security of his job. If he is unemployed, then the possibility of vocational training might need to be discussed.

Treatment of this patient can be accomplished in a number of ways. Evidence is well established for the success of prolonged exposure, cognitive therapy, and anxiety management techniques. Generally, it appears preferable to follow one approach, as the combination is perhaps less effective (Foa 2000), but, even acknowledging this, combination approaches that use different psychotherapeutic techniques are still more effective than control treatments. Typically, prolonged exposure is administered over a course of 12–16 sessions; requires active participation by the patient, who is assigned homework between sessions; and requires in vivo exposure, as he describes in vivid detail, in the present tense, the events and his reactions to them. Particular themes may need to be explored in further detail. The issue of loss is likely to be important here, because the patient lost a number of good friends. As Foa (2000) has written, where there are issues of guilt, it may be necessary to use cognitive approaches before initiating prolonged exposure to the fear-bound parts of trauma. The patient's sense of meaninglessness of all the sacrifices that he and others made will need to be addressed and hopefully replaced with a greater sense of the significance and meaning in his present-day life.

Would this patient be suitable for psychotherapeutic treatments along the lines described above? Almost certainly the answer is yes. Whether he accepts and/or receives the method of treatment, however, is a matter to be discussed and negotiated at the beginning. We presume that he will have access to a qualified therapist, rather than one who offers generic psychotherapy. We also would have to assume that the patient is interested in traveling along this road and is willing to tolerate some intensification of symptoms (albeit in a supportive and structured environment) before he sees improvement. The support of his wife would also be important, and this seems to be a strength in his life.

Pharmacological treatment would be a second option. Data now show that most of the selective serotonin reuptake inhibitor (SSRI) drugs are effective in PTSD, including fluoxetine, sertraline, and paroxetine, all in double-blind studies, and fluvoxamine and citalopram in open-label studies. Choice of an SSRI will be determined by a number of factors. For instance, if cost were a major concern, then generic fluoxetine would be a reasonable choice. If sleep disturbance were profound, as it appears to be in this case, a drug such as paroxetine, which improves sleep, would be a consideration. Paroxetine is the only SSRI drug to have proven itself, relative to placebo, in combat veterans with PTSD. In favor of sertraline is the existence of long-term, relapse-prevention data that demonstrate that continuing with the drug beyond 9 months carries with it a five-times-greater likelihood of preventing relapse than discontinuation to placebo (Davidson et al. 2001). The availability of these data is an important consideration, because relapse-prevention effects for paroxetine or fluoxetine have not been demonstrated at the present time.

Drug interactions need to be kept in mind. In this patient's case, he is not taking any other medication, and therefore this simplifies the task. However, were he to be taking beta-blockers, for example, then there would be a greater case for choosing an SSRI that is less likely to inhibit the cytochrome P450 2D6 isoenzymes. Were he to be on a drug that was metabolized by the 3A4 isoenzyme system, as many are (including calcium-channel blockers, statins, and some benzodiazepines), it would be necessary to monitor for potentiation by drugs, such as fluvoxamine and nefazodone.

All of the SSRI drugs are broad spectrum in their effect—that is, they reduce the four main symptom groups in PTSD (reexperiencing, avoidance, numbing, and hyperarousal). They also improve quality of life, disability, and comorbidity. One drug, fluoxetine, has also been shown to strengthen resilience (Connor et al. 1999), an important aspect in the management of PTSD. Should SSRIs fail to work, then alternative effective drugs that can be used include mirtazapine, a dual-acting serotonergic and noradrenergic drug, as well as dual-acting tricyclics, such as amitriptyline and imipramine. Of relevance in the case of the tricyclics is their demonstrated efficacy in combat veterans who have PTSD (Davidson et al. 1990).

When we use an SSRI, the earliest symptoms to improve, often in the first week, are irritability and anger, which can therefore be a useful prognostic sign (Davidson et al. 2002). Failure to respond at all after the patient has been taking an SSRI for 4 weeks at an adequate dose may be a signal to consider switching drugs, although somebody who has shown minimal improvement even after 12 weeks is still capable of converting to a full responder after 4–5 months of treatment. The important study by Londborg and colleagues (2001) shows that full remission is attainable through pharmacotherapy, as is also the case with psychotherapy (Foa 2000). A further benefit of medication is its ability to relieve symptom burden and to restore a greater sense of control, such that it becomes possible for the patient to participate more effectively in psychotherapy.

Persisting nightmares in spite of otherwise effective pharmacotherapy could be treated with specific drugs, such as prazosin, clonidine, or antidepressants, with a marked hypnotic effect (e.g., trazodone, mirtazapine, and nefazodone).

A selection of self-rating scales is available to monitor treatment in patients with PTSD, and this can be a useful element in therapy. It allows the therapist and the patient to more accurately gauge what he or she is responding or not responding to.

As a combat veteran, this patient might find it helpful to participate in a local support group for colleagues who have gone through similar experiences. This could be arranged either through the local VA Medical Center or through his Veterans Center. Consideration of possible service-connected eligibility for VA benefits would be important to pursue.

The role of this patient's wife is critical. She is clearly invested in seeing him improve, as well as in making their marriage work. At this point in time, she is perhaps his strongest ally, and efforts need to be made during the course of treatment to keep this alliance strong. Failure to do so, coupled with poor motivation or poor compliance on the part of this patient, can eventually set up a high level of negative affect on the part of his wife. She may become resigned to failure, may pull back from the marriage, or may ultimately decide to separate, or they may reach a stalemate relationship in which hostility or passive-aggressive styles are all too evident. A spousal support group at the local Veterans Center would be helpful to her, as well as educational material regarding PTSD, available either from appropriate Web sites or printed brochures, books, etc.

Under the most favorable circumstances, we know that chronic PTSD can respond well to treatment, even after very many years. It is to be hoped that this patient, his wife, and his therapist sustain a high degree of commitment, enthusiasm, and positive expectations for this veteran to achieve an optimal outcome.

References

Connor KM, Sutherland SM, Tupler LA, et al: Fluoxetine in post-traumatic stress disorder. Br J Psychiatry 175:17–22, 1999

Davidson JRT, Kudler HS, Smith RD, et al: Treatment of PTSD with amitriptyline and placebo. Arch Gen Psychiatry 47:259–266, 1990

Davidson JRT, Pearlstein T, Londborg PD, et al: Efficacy of sertraline in preventing relapse of post-traumatic stress disorder: results of a 28-week double-blind, placebo-controlled study. Am J Psychiatry 158:1974–1981, 2001

Davidson JRT, Landerman LR, Farfel GM, et al: Characterizing the effect of sertraline in posttraumatic stress disorder. Psychol Med 32:661–670, 2002

Foa EB: Psychosocial treatment of posttraumatic stress disorder. J Clin Psychiatry 61 (suppl 5):43–51, 2000

Kessler RC: Posttraumatic stress disorder: the burden to the individual and society. J Clin Psychiatry 61 (suppl 5):4–12, 2000

Londborg PD, Hegel MT, Goldstein S, et al: Sertraline treatment of posttraumatic stress disorder: results of 24 weeks of open-label continuation treatment. J Clin Psychiatry 62:325–331, 2001

Marshall RD, Galea S: Science for the community: assessing mental health after 9/11. J Clin Psychiatry 65 (suppl 1):37–43, 2004

Pitman RK, Altman B, Greenwald E, et al: Psychiatric complications during flooding therapy for posttraumatic stress disorder. J Clin Psychiatry 52:17–20, 1991

Paranoid and Dangerous

Tracy Shaw, age 32, overweight, and wild looking, was brought to the psychiatric emergency room by the police after she had furiously shattered a full-length mirror in the principal's office of her child's school. The psychiatrist who examined her described her as "paranoid and dangerous to others" and recommended immediate hospitalization by two-physician certification if she refused to admit herself voluntarily.

Ms. Shaw refused voluntary admission. She stated that her suspicions concerning her child's unfair treatment in school were well founded and that she would harm no one. She acknowledged that she was particularly irritable and angry because she was premenstrual. Her husband supported her decision and assumed responsibility for her and for bringing her back to see the psychiatrist the next day. That evening her menses began.

When Ms. Shaw saw the psychiatrist the next day, she appeared to be a "different" person. She was relaxed, her anger and irritability had dissipated, and she displayed a sense of humor. However, she retained her conviction that the school principal owed her an explanation for his unfair treatment of her child.

Ms. Shaw gave a history of monthly premenstrual symptoms beginning at menarche but worsening since her 20s. The symptoms were not the same every month. Some months she would become depressed, with thoughts of suicide; other months she would crave chocolate and gain 5–10 pounds in 1 week; some months she would break out in hives; and there were months when she was free of symptoms. The symptoms were always predictable in their timing, occurring the week before her menses and remitting with its onset.

Ms. Shaw was the oldest daughter of a chronically depressed and fearful mother and an alcoholic businessman father. Before marriage, she was the caretaker of her family. Her mother recovered significantly during Ms. Shaw's adolescence, only to fail rapidly and die when her daughter left home and married after high school.

Currently, Ms. Shaw is the mother of four grade-school children; in addition, she has primary responsibility for a sibling with alcoholism who is dying of cancer, as well as for her disabled husband, who has been severely depressed and vocationally incapacitated since surgery 1.5 years ago. She lives with her in-laws. Both her husband and his parents have significant alcohol problems.

Ms. Shaw is still the family caretaker. "I can't live with myself unless I do it all. I feel guilty if I do something for myself." She can cope with the demands of her life and is not usually depressed, except during her premenstruum, when "the whole world closes in" and she feels "pulled down."

DSM-IV-TR Casebook Diagnosis of "Paranoid and Dangerous"

The uncontrolled behavior that led to Ms. Shaw's psychiatric evaluation suggested to the psychiatrist that she was psychotic and potentially dangerous to others and therefore in need of involuntary hospitalization. Fortunately, Ms. Shaw was able to convince the psychiatrist that she was not psychotic, but that she experienced episodic difficulties that always occurred in the few days before her menses and remitted when her menses began. Her symptoms vary from cycle to cycle and include depression, anger, irritability, and overeating. Between episodes she is apparently completely free of such symptoms.

This pattern of recurrent dysphoric episodes beginning in the premenstrual phase and remitting with the onset of menses suggests the Axis I diagnosis of premenstrual dysphoric disorder (DSM-IV-TR, p. 774), a diagnosis that is not in the official classification but is included in an appendix to DSM-IV-TR and is given as an example of Depressive Disorder Not Otherwise Specified in the DSM-IV-TR text. In order to confirm this diagnosis, it would be necessary to have Ms. Shaw make daily ratings of her mood and behavior for at least two cycles to document her impression that the changes are always associated with the menstrual cycle. In addition, it would be necessary to establish that at least five associated symptoms (e.g., decreased interest in usual activities, marked lack of energy, sleep disturbance, and other physical symptoms) have been present for most of the time during each symptomatic premenstrual phase.

Discussion of "Paranoid and Dangerous" by Teri Pearlstein, M.D.*

The description of Ms. Shaw by the psychiatrist as "paranoid and dangerous to others" when she was premenstrual but as a "different person" the day after menses illustrates the potentially markedly different presentations of the same woman in the luteal (premenstrual) and follicular (postmenstrual) phases of the menstrual cycle. "Manic-depressive" was an early clinical description of this phenomenon. The contrasting "Dr. Jekyll–Mr. Hyde" dichotomy has been captured by would-be humorists in newspaper cartoons, calendars, greeting cards, and coffee mugs. Buttons are sold with phrases like "Beware: I Am Armed and Have PMS," and the luteal phase has been likened to the "spin cycle of a washing machine." Such humor demeans women suffering from premenstrual symptoms by promoting the already ingrained view that such women are not to be taken seriously because of their unprovoked tears, intense anger, and mood lability. Although these women may later report that their premenstrual irritable and angry reaction seemed exaggerated, they often state that the issue that provoked the sudden reaction remains troublesome to them. In the case of Ms. Shaw, although in retrospect she may have agreed that her reaction was over the top, she continued to insist that the school principal did in fact treat her child unfairly and that he owed her an explanation for his unfair treatment. The goal of treatment for Ms. Shaw is not to eliminate disagreements with significant others in her life; the goal is to have her reactions to the events of daily life be in the same "proportion" in the luteal phase as during the follicular phase.

Ms. Shaw would initially receive a provisional diagnosis of Depressive Disorder Not Otherwise Specified based on her presenting symptoms, and she would then be asked to rate her symptoms daily for two complete menstrual cycles. Her clinician should provide her with a rating form that lists common premenstrual symptoms to be rated daily with anchor points ranging from "not present" to "severe," and her cli-

---

Dr. Pearlstein is Director of the Women's Behavioral Health Program at Women and Infants Hospital in Providence, Rhode Island, and Associate Professor of Psychiatry and Human Behavior at Brown Medical School. Dr. Pearlstein has authored several manuscripts on the diagnosis and treatment of premenstrual dysphoric disorder and has conducted numerous antidepressant and oral contraceptive trials for premenstrual dysphoric disorder.

nician should review these ratings to see how well her ratings correspond with her menstrual cycle. To meet the diagnostic criteria for premenstrual dysphoric disorder (PMDD) as specified in the Appendix of DSM-IV-TR, at least 5 out of 11 possible symptoms must be present in the premenstrual phase; these symptoms should be absent shortly after the onset of menses; and at least 1 of the 5 symptoms must be depressed mood, anxiety, lability, or irritability. The criteria for PMDD require some degree of functional impairment as a result of the premenstrual symptoms. If premenstrual symptoms are evident but they do not include the requisite type or number of symptoms, or if they are not severe enough to cause functional impairment, a woman would be said to have premenstrual syndrome (PMS), not PMDD. If mood or anxiety symptoms are present during the follicular phase and they are increased during the luteal phase, instead of having a diagnosis of PMDD, the woman would be described as having the premenstrual exacerbation of an underlying mood or anxiety disorder. Although most women with severe PMS or PMDD have similar symptoms each cycle, two cycles of ratings are recommended because there can be some variability in symptom severity. Ms. Shaw's presentation is unusual in that her symptoms vary considerably from cycle to cycle, including some symptom-free cycles.

Many women with premenstrual symptoms recognize the cyclic nature of their symptoms, conclude that their symptoms are "caused by hormones," and then describe their symptoms to their gynecologist or primary care clinician. Even though PMDD is clearly related to mood disorders, few women with premenstrual complaints present to a mental health clinician. Thus, Ms. Shaw is unusual in that the cyclic and dramatic nature of her symptoms led to her presentation in a psychiatric emergency setting, followed by an outpatient psychiatric evaluation. However, a small proportion of women may act on severe premenstrual suicidal impulses or have intermittent displays of violent behavior that will lead to psychiatric evaluation.

After the diagnosis of PMDD is established, Ms. Shaw's clinician should discuss the many treatment options that are available. Regardless of whether one presents to a medical or mental health clinician, selective serotonin reuptake inhibitors (SSRIs) are considered the first line of treatment by both psychiatric (Altshuler et al. 2001) and gynecologic (American College of Obstetrics and Gynecology 2000) expert consensus guidelines because of their efficacy and ease of administration. In the past, gynecologists and primary care clinicians were likely to prescribe oral contraceptives and other nonpsychotropic medications, but since the U.S. Food and Drug Administration approval of Sarafem (fluoxetine) in 2000, Zoloft (sertraline) in 2002, and Paxil CR (paroxetine CR) in 2003 for PMDD, medical clinicians are becoming more likely to administer an SSRI. Almost all double-blind, placebo-controlled studies of SSRIs have reported efficacy (Pearlstein 2002), with an average response rate of 60%–70% for the SSRI and approximately 30% for placebo. A meta-analysis of 15 randomized, double-blind, placebo-controlled SSRI trials in severe PMS and PMDD reported an almost seven-times-greater odds ratio in favor of response to SSRIs over placebo (Dimmock et al. 2000).

The effective doses in PMDD are equivalent to the doses that are effective in Major Depressive Disorder (MDD). However, several features of antidepressant use in PMDD are different than in MDD. Unlike with MDD, in which all antidepressants appear to be equally effective, serotonergic antidepressants are much more effective in treating PMDD, as compared to nonserotonergic antidepressants, such as bupropion or some tricyclic antidepressants. SSRIs also appear to have a rapid onset of action for relief of premenstrual symptoms, perhaps through modulation of hormonal or neurosteroid pathways. In contrast, SSRIs typically take 2–6 weeks to be effective in treating depression and anxiety disorders. Several studies have reported efficacy with dosing during the luteal phase of the cycle only (from ovulation to menses), with both luteal phase daily dosing of SSRIs and weekly fluoxetine (Pearlstein 2002). The efficacy of SSRI use on symptomatic luteal days only (symptom-onset dosing)—for example, a woman who takes an SSRI on only the 3 luteal days that she has premenstrual symptoms—has not yet been systematically demonstrated.

Another differentiation between the treatment of PMDD and MDD is the report by many women with PMDD of the return of premenstrual symptoms after the discontinuation of an SSRI. Although there are few systematic studies of the return of symptoms after discontinuation of an SSRI, many clinicians and women with PMS report that the premenstrual symptoms usually recur and may do so as quickly as the first cycle in which the patient is off of medication. Ms. Shaw is probably looking at years of SSRI use, perhaps until menopause. Luteal-phase dosing and daily dosing of SSRIs are approximately equivalent in efficacy, but Ms. Shaw might choose luteal-phase dosing of an SSRI to decrease possible side effects that may occur with long-term daily use, such as weight gain or sexual dysfunction.

Women with PMDD who plan to conceive often discontinue the SSRI medication before conception. However, some women choose to take the SSRI until conception. These women may choose an SSRI with a shorter half-life or luteal-phase dosing to minimize the fetal exposure to SSRI once conception occurs and they discontinue the SSRI. Because PMDD symptoms usually abate during pregnancy, pregnant women with previous PMDD generally do not need medication, but premenstrual symptoms usually recur once menses resume after giving birth. Women with PMDD are at increased risk for the future development of MDD (noted by the appearance of mood and anxiety symptoms during the follicular phase), and a switch to another class of antidepressant may be necessary to treat an episode of MDD.

A simplified view of the etiology of PMDD is that the hormonal changes at ovulation interact with "dysregulated" neurotransmitter or neurosteroid systems (Schmidt et al. 1998). The theory behind the treatment of PMDD is to "correct" the "dysregulation" with psychotropic medications or to induce an anovulatory state to avoid the hormonal "trigger" at ovulation each cycle. Thus, the second-line treatment for severe PMS and PMDD is the induction of anovulation with gonadotropin-releasing agonists, Danocrine (danazol), or other gonadal hormones (Pearlstein and Steiner 2000). Studies of gonadotropin-releasing agonists generally report efficacy, but adding back replacement estrogen and progesterone to decrease the medical risks associated with a prolonged hypoestrogenic state have led to the induction of mood and anxiety symptoms. Almost all studies of the luteal-phase administration of progesterone have not demonstrated superiority over placebo, and, to date, the few published reports of use of oral contraceptives have not suggested efficacy compared to placebo (Epperson et al. 1999; Kahn and Halbreich 2001). Most women with PMDD will respond to SSRIs, but a gonadotropin-releasing agonist would be a reasonable second option for Ms. Shaw if she did not respond.

Positive studies have been reported for at least some premenstrual symptoms treated with other serotonergic medications, such as Effexor (venlafaxine), Anafranil (clomipramine), L-tryptophan, and BuSpar (buspirone), with Xanax (alprazolam) during the luteal phase with a taper during menses; light therapy; bromocriptine; spironolactone; and other medications (Pearlstein 2002; Pearlstein and Steiner 2000). A recent comprehensive review of herbal medications and other alternative treatments suggested that no specific complementary treatment can be clearly recommended, but there is some research support for calcium and magnesium (Stevinson and Ernst 2001). Anecdotally, dietary changes, such as frequent feedings and increased complex carbohydrates, exercise, and relaxation, have been reported to be helpful for relieving premenstrual symptoms. Cognitive therapy has been reported to be beneficial for treating patients with PMDD in a few studies (Pearlstein and Steiner 2000). Ms. Shaw might particularly benefit from psychotherapy that incorporated cognitive techniques as well as addressing some of her considerable stressors. It is common for women with severe PMS or PMDD to have increased negative cognitions and to be more "pulled down" by stressors when they are in the premenstrual phase. Ms. Shaw states that she can cope with being a caretaker and with the "demands of her life" when she is not premenstrual. Individual psychotherapy could address Ms. Shaw's caretaking roles and emphasize her need to elicit support from others and decrease her expectations of herself when she is premenstrual.

References

Altshuler LL, Cohen LS, Moline ML, et al: The Expert Consensus Guideline Series. Treatment of depression in women. Postgrad Med (Spec No):1–107, 2001

American College of Obstetrics and Gynecology: Premenstrual syndrome, in ACOG Practice Bulletin. Washington, DC, American College of Obstetrics and Gynecology, 2000

Dimmock PW, Wyatt KM, Jones PW, et al: Efficacy of selective serotonin reuptake inhibitors in premenstrual syndrome: a systematic review. Lancet 356(9236):1131–1136, 2000

Epperson CN, Wisner KL, Yamamoto B: Gonadal steroids in the treatment of mood disorders. Psychosom Med 61(5):676–697, 1999

Kahn LS, Halbreich U: Oral contraceptives and mood. Expert Opin Pharmacother 2(9):1367–1382, 2001

Pearlstein T: Selective serotonin reuptake inhibitors for premenstrual dysphoric disorder: the emerging gold standard? Drugs 62(13):1869–1885, 2002

Pearlstein T, Steiner M: Nonantidepressant treatment of premenstrual syndrome. J Clin Psychiatry 61 (suppl 12):22–27, 2000

Schmidt PJ, Nieman LK, Danaceau MA, et al: Differential behavioral effects of gonadal steroids in women with and in those without premenstrual syndrome. N Engl J Med 338:209–216, 1998

Stevinson C, Ernst E: Complementary/alternative therapies for premenstrual syndrome: a systematic review of randomized controlled trials. Am J Obstet Gynecol 185(1):227–235, 2001

Toxic Neighborhood

Robert Cortland is a 38-year-old man who presents to a community mental health center for follow-up outpatient treatment after his third psychiatric hospitalization in 3 years. Despite holding degrees in pharmacy and dentistry, he has been unable to work for the past 3.5 years, receives disability insurance, and lives with his mother. He was prescribed lithium and Trilafon (perphenazine) on hospital discharge and complains of feeling tired, feeling angry at having been hospitalized, and having difficulty feeling any emotions ("Try-a-laughing on Tril-a-fon"). He claims not to feel depressed, irritable, or euphoric; denies changes in appetite or libido; and says he is sleeping about 9 hours a night. He denies hallucinations and problems with concentration, although he has difficulty responding clearly to many questions. He wants to move out of his mother's house because he is suspicious of the neighbors but feels guilty about abandoning his mother.

Dr. Cortland reluctantly recounts his psychiatric history. Fortunately, hospital records have also been forwarded to the evaluating psychiatrist. He initially presented for treatment 3 years ago. At that time, the police brought him to the psychiatric emergency service after neighbors reported that he was outside screaming at them through their windows to "turn the radiation off!" Police found him shirtless in 30°F weather and wearing a "samurai headband." Dr. Cortland was admitted and treated with Haldol (haloperidol) and Cogentin (benztropine). He is embarrassed about describing any other symptoms leading up to this first hospitalization but remembers being unable to sleep for days because he felt like his mind was "buzzing," his eyes were "bulging," and his bedroom was overheated. About 1 month before this episode, he decided that he no longer wanted to practice dentistry because it did not allow him to be creative enough with his hands, so he began painting "impressionistic" art on discarded window glass.

Dr. Cortland never returned to work after this first hospitalization, despite working briefly with an occupational therapist. Although he was referred to a psychiatrist for follow-up treatment, he missed "at least half" of his appointments and took Haldol only sporadically for 3 months before discontinuing it because it made him feel "dead." He spent most of his time over the next year painting in his basement and occasionally grocery shopping for his mother but otherwise was reclusive. He remained suspicious of his neighbors and glared at them in chance encounters. He described feeling down and discouraged during this time, unsure of what to do with his life, and afraid to interact with people because they might recognize that he was "crazy."

Dr. Cortland was admitted for his second psychiatric hospitalization approximately 1 year ago, after his mother called 911 because he again believed his neighbors were beaming microwaves at his bedroom from their satellite dish to keep him awake. In the hospital discharge summary, he was described as extremely agitated, threatening, and irritable, with pressured speech on admission. He was also suspected of hearing voices because of his extreme distractibility, although he denied it. In addition, he was reported to have had a fixed, persecutory delusion about his neighbors in the year before admission. He was discharged on Depakote (divalproex), Zyprexa (olanzapine), and Ativan (lorazepam).

Dr. Cortland was again "too proud" to follow up with outpatient treatment and discontinued his medication when his prescriptions ran out 1 month after discharge. He felt well for approximately 3 months but then resumed being reclusive, slept for more than 16 hours a day, stopped shaving, and bathed infrequently and only at his mother's insistence. He was admitted for the third time 2 months ago after appearing at the psychiatric emergency service because he "couldn't take it anymore." He had been driving aimlessly for hours on the interstate, often at high speeds, hoping he would be stopped and shot by police. He was agitated and irritable, believed that the Holy Spirit was sending messages through his painting, and believed that his neighbors were still aiming microwaves at his brain. He reported that he "could hear them scheming through the walls." He refused to resume Depakote and Zyprexa but gradually improved on lithium and Trilafon. Dr. Cortland appeared physically healthy on examination in the hospital, and there were no significant laboratory abnormalities, including normal thyroid function tests and brain magnetic resonance imaging.

Dr. Cortland is an only child and had always been somewhat of a "loner" growing up. He received a Registered Pharmacist degree in a 5-year college program, worked for several years as a pharmacist, and then successfully applied for admission to dental school. He operated a solo dentistry practice for 12 years. He lived at home with his mother all his life, feeling obligated to take care of her (although she is in good health) when his father died 15 years ago. He had several protracted periods of feeling down during college and dental school, usually because of rejection by women he was dating. He could not provide any more elaborate history of depressive symptoms. Dr. Cortland's father was "a strange man" but never received psychiatric care. His paternal uncle had "nervous breakdowns," and a paternal first cousin spent years in a state psychiatric facility.

DSM-IV-TR Diagnosis of "Toxic Neighborhood"

Dr. Cortland was hospitalized three times with symptoms that met diagnostic criteria for a manic episode (irritable mood, decreased need for sleep, pressured speech, racing thoughts, psychomotor agitation). Although he was not hospitalized for the treatment of depressive episodes, Dr. Cortland appears to have had at least two post-manic periods during which he had symptoms consistent with major depressive episodes. Each manic episode was complicated by the presence of psychotic features, which included persecutory delusions during two admissions and grandiose delusions and auditory hallucinations during at least one admission. Thus, Bipolar Disorder, Manic, Severe With Psychotic Features is a diagnostic consideration. However, Dr. Cortland's persecutory delusions regarding his neighbors never fully remitted and were present during intervals when he was neither manic nor depressed. In addition, he experienced residual disorganized thinking and behavior that impaired his ability to return to his premorbid level of functioning as a dentist. In fact, he was disabled. Because of the persistence of his delusions beyond the duration of prominent mood symptoms and because his mood episodes (manic and depressive) were present for a substantial portion of the total duration of his illness, Dr. Cortland's disturbance meets criteria for Schizoaffective Disorder, Bipolar Type. His course of illness was also complicated by his lack of insight and difficulty accepting that he had a major psychiatric disorder in need of ongoing treatment. These factors, coupled with uncomfortable side effects, consistently led to his lack of adherence to treatment recommendations. Finally, he appeared to have difficulty separating from his mother before the onset of his illness and had even greater difficulty since he became ill.

Follow-Up

The initial goal of treatment with Dr. Cortland was to establish a therapeutic alliance and gain his trust. His outpatient psychiatrist discussed Dr. Cortland's concerns about the side effects of his medication and invited his input as a pharmacist. Treatment alternatives were discussed, and Trilafon was tapered and discontinued over the next 2 weeks while Seroquel (quetiapine) was gradually titrated to a therapeutic dose. His mood brightened and he brought a window glass painting to his next visit. This gesture led to discussions over the next several visits of Dr. Cortland's career interests and plans. He was assigned a case manager and enrolled in a vocational rehabilitation program. His mood remained stable, although he continued to harbor suspicions that his neighborhood was "toxic." Several months later, Dr. Cortland and his mother sold their house and moved to a duplex apartment. There were no problems with their new neighbors. He began working at a craft supply store stocking shelves and adhered to his treatment visits and medication regimen. He continues to maintain this level of functioning and activity at 2 years in follow-up.

Discussion of "Toxic Neighborhood" by Paul E. Keck Jr., M.D.*

In my experience, one of the most difficult things about treating patients with Schizoaffective Disorder is distinguishing this illness from Schizophrenia and psychotic Mood Disorders. Mood disturbances and

*Dr. Keck is Professor of Psychiatry, Pharmacology, and Neuroscience; Vice Chairman for Research in the Department of Psychiatry at University of Cincinnati College of Medicine; and Associate Director of the General Clinical Research Center at Cincinnati Veterans Affairs Medical Center in Cincinnati, Ohio. Dr. Keck has published a number of studies and reviews of the nosological issues and pharmacological treatment regarding Schizoaffective Disorder. He is the editor of Managing Depressive Symptoms in Schizophrenia and coauthor of The Neuroleptic Malignant Syndrome and Related Conditions (American Psychiatric Publishing, 2003). Dr. Keck served on the American Psychiatric Association's Workgroup to Develop Practice Guidelines for Treatment of Patients With Bipolar Disorders (1994 and 2001).

psychosis characterize Schizophrenia, Schizoaffective Disorder, and psychotic Mood Disorders on cross-sectional evaluation. Historically, the presence of Schneiderian first-rank symptoms (e.g., delusions of thought broadcasting, thought insertion, thought withdrawal, being controlled by an outside force, and hearing two or more voices conversing with each other) or mood-incongruent delusions were considered useful clues toward a diagnosis of Schizoaffective Disorder or Schizophrenia rather than a psychotic Mood Disorder. However, a number of studies have demonstrated a lack of pathognomonic specificity of these psychotic symptoms (Spitzer et al. 1978). Thus, the primary means of distinguishing between these disorders relies on examining the temporal relationship of psychotic and affective symptoms. As a general rule, psychotic Mood Disorders are diagnosed when psychotic symptoms occur only in tandem with mood disturbances or episodes. Schizophrenia is diagnosed when mood episodes account for a small proportion of the total duration of the illness. Schizoaffective Disorder is diagnosed when mood symptoms are a significant part of the illness but psychotic symptoms also occur in the absence of mood episodes.

Schizoaffective Disorder, Depressive Type, in particular can be difficult to distinguish from Schizophrenia accompanied by depressive or negative symptoms. The diagnosis of Schizoaffective Disorder, Depressive Type, becomes clearer when depression has occurred during a substantial portion of the course of a patient's illness. For practical purposes, however, the pharmacological treatment of the depressive type of Schizoaffective Disorder and of Schizophrenia complicated by depressive or negative symptoms is likely to be the same (i.e., with an atypical antipsychotic medication with or without a concomitant antidepressant). Schizoaffective Disorder, Depressive Type, is also a consideration in the differential diagnosis of psychotic Major Depression or bipolar depression. This is especially difficult if a patient is presenting for treatment of psychotic and depressive symptoms for the first time. Again, for practical purposes, the acute pharmacological treatment of both the depressive type of Schizoaffective Disorder and psychotic depression would usually consist of an antipsychotic and antidepressant combination. The diagnosis of Schizoaffective Disorder, Depressive Type, would become a stronger consideration if psychotic symptoms recurred or persisted despite adequate treatment of the depressive episode.

Distinguishing between the bipolar type of Schizoaffective Disorder (in the manic phase) and Schizophrenia complicated by severe psychomotor agitation can also be challenging on cross-sectional evaluation.

The presence of euphoric mood, affective lability, diminished need for sleep, racing thoughts, pressured speech, and hypersexual behavior is more consistent with criteria for mania. More common scenarios include patients who present for treatment of a clear-cut manic episode who also have psychotic features and respond initially to combination treatment with a mood stabilizer and an antipsychotic but who then experience a recurrence of psychotic but not affective symptoms when antipsychotics are tapered or discontinued. Similarly, some patients with presumptive Bipolar Disorder are plagued by persistent residual thought disorder and/or persecutory or grandiose overvalued ideas, or frank delusions that persist in the absence of mood symptoms during maintenance treatment with a mood stabilizer. Such patients appear to require long-term maintenance treatment with an antipsychotic in combination with a mood stabilizer to treat these pernicious and persistent psychotic symptoms. In these scenarios, the diagnosis evolves from Bipolar Disorder to Schizoaffective Disorder, Bipolar Type.

Dr. Cortland's course of illness is representative of many patients with Schizoaffective Disorder, Bipolar Type. For the first 3 years after his initial psychiatric hospitalization, Dr. Cortland experienced a chronic, deteriorating pattern of illness. He experienced recurrent mood episodes, persistent residual delusions and disorganized thinking, very limited insight, poor treatment adherence, worsening social isolation, loss of his profession, and need to go on disability.

Formal diagnostic criteria for Schizoaffective Disorder were not operationalized until DSM-III-R (1987), drawing on criteria formulated by Spitzer et al. (1978) and Feighner et al. (1972). Two types of Schizoaffective Disorder are recognized in DSM-IV-TR: Bipolar and Depressive. Schizoaffective Disorder has been conceptualized as a form of Schizophrenia; a severe form of Mood Disorder; a transitional state between mood disorders and Schizophrenia; a combination of both syndromes; a distinct and homogeneous syndrome; and a heterogeneous syndrome encompassing variants of Schizophrenia, Mood Disorder, and combined forms of these disorders (Brockington et al. 1991; Maier et al. 1992; Maj 1984). Diagnostic boundaries between Schizophrenia complicated by depressive episodes and Schizoaffective Disorder, Depressive Type, are determined primarily by the relative duration of the depressive episode(s) in the context of the overall duration of the psychotic illness (Skodol 1987). To date, most studies suggest that Schizoaffective Disorder, Depressive Type, is more similar to Schizophrenia than Mood Disorder in family history, phenomenology, course of illness, and treatment response (Keck et al. 1994). In contrast, similar studies suggest that the Bipolar Type is more similar to Bipolar Disorder.

Despite ambiguity surrounding the nosological boundaries of Schizoaffective Disorder, the availability of diagnostic criteria has allowed significant improvement in the reliability of its diagnosis. For example, two studies, using test-retest reliability methods, found fair to good interrater reliability for Schizoaffective Disorder (Spitzer et al. 1978; Williams et al. 1992).

Although no national community-based epidemiological study of the prevalence of psychiatric disorders has included Schizoaffective Disorder, a number of studies have examined its prevalence in clinical settings. Pooled data from clinical studies indicated a mean prevalence of 16% of Schizoaffective Disorder among patients presenting for treatment in inpatient and outpatient settings (Keck et al. 1994). Thus, Schizoaffective Disorder is common in clinical settings.

Not surprisingly, because diagnostic criteria for this disorder are relatively new, little research has been conducted regarding the pharmacological treatment of Schizoaffective Disorder (Keck et al. 1994). Most studies of antipsychotics conducted over the past 40 years included patients with Schizophrenia and Schizoaffective Disorder together, without separately analyzing improvement in psychosis or assessing improvement in affective symptoms. Recently, with the advent of atypical antipsychotics, which appear to improve both manic and depressive symptoms, greater attention is being focused on the response of patients with Schizoaffective Disorder to these agents. However, many fundamental pharmacological treatment questions remain. For instance, as in Dr. Cortland's case, is combination treatment with a mood-stabilizing agent and an atypical antipsychotic drug superior to treatment with an atypical antipsychotic alone? Similarly, for patients with the Depressive Type of Schizoaffective Disorder, is treatment with an antidepressant and an atypical antipsychotic better than treatment with an atypical agent alone?

In Dr. Cortland's case, the psychological sequelae of Schizoaffective Disorder are similar to those that many patients with mood or psychotic disorders face—accepting the reality of having such an illness, redefining life goals, striving to regain functioning, coping with recurrent or residual symptoms and episodes, and adhering to medication regimens and minimizing side effects. Dr. Cortland attended psychotherapy meetings monthly. Initial goals were to help him identify signs and symptoms of his illness and to enlist the help of his mother in identifying them along with him. He spent considerable effort coping with the loss of his prior professional identity and adjusting to immediate-term, realistic goals, such as finding gainful employment and structuring his time productively. As he began working, attention shifted to discussions of his interactions with co-workers and customers, including taking constructive criticism and interacting with appropriate boundaries.

References

Brockington IF, Roper A, Copas J, et al: Schizophrenia, bipolar disorder and depression: a discriminant analysis, using "lifetime" psychopathology ratings. Br J Psychiatry 159:485–494, 1991

Feighner JP, Robins E, Guze SB, et al: Diagnostic criteria for use in psychiatric research. Arch Gen Psychiatry 26:57–63, 1972

Keck PE Jr, McElroy SL, Strakowski SM, et al: Pharmacologic treatment of schizoaffective disorder. Psychopharmacology 114:529–538, 1994

Maier W, Lichterman D, Minges J, et al: Schizoaffective disorder and affective disorders with mood-incongruent psychotic features: keep separate or combine? evidence from a family study. Am J Psychiatry 149:1666–1673, 1992

Maj M: Evolution of the American concept of schizoaffective psychosis. Neuropsychobiology 11:7–13, 1984

Skodol AE: Problems in Differential Diagnosis: From DSM-III to DSM-III-R in Clinical Practice. Washington, DC, American Psychiatric Press, 1987

Spitzer RL, Endicott J, Robins E: Research diagnostic criteria: rationale and reliability. Arch Gen Psychiatry 35:773–782, 1978

Williams JBW, Gibbon M, First MB, et al: The Structured Clinical Interview for DSM-III-R (SCID), II: multisite test-retest reliability. Arch Gen Psychiatry 49:630–636, 1992

Low Life Level

Louise Larkin is a pale, stooped woman of 39 years, whose child-like face is surrounded by scraggly blond braids tied with pink ribbons. She was referred for a psychiatric evaluation for possible hospitalization by her family doctor, who was concerned about her low level of functioning. Her only complaint to him was, "I have a decline in self-care and a low life level." Her mother reports that there has indeed been a decline, but that it has been over many years. In the last few months Louise has remained in her room, mute and still.

Twelve years ago, Louise was a supervisor in the occupational therapy department of a large hospital, living in her own apartment, and engaged to a young man. He broke the engagement, and she became increasingly disorganized, wandering aimlessly in the street, wearing mismatched clothing. She was fired from her job, and eventually the police were called to hospitalize her. They broke into her apartment, which was in shambles, filled with papers, food, and broken objects. No information is available from this hospitalization, which lasted 3 months, and from which she was discharged to her mother's house with a prescription for an unknown medication that she never had filled.

After her discharge, her family hoped that Louise would gather herself together and embark again on a real life, but over the years, she became more withdrawn and less functional. Most of her time was spent watching television and cooking. Her cooking consisted of mixing bizarre combinations of ingredients, such as broccoli and cake mix, cooking them, and then eating them alone because no one else in the family would eat her meals. She collected cookbooks and recipes, cluttering her room with stacks of them. Often when her mother entered her room, she would quickly grab a magazine and pretend to be reading, when in fact she had apparently just been sitting and staring into space. She stopped bathing and brushing her hair or teeth. She ate less and less, although she denied loss of appetite, and over a period of several years lost 20 pounds. She would sleep at odd hours. Eventually, she became enuretic, wetting her bed frequently and filling the room with the pungent odor of urine.

On admission to the psychiatric hospital, Louise sat with her hands tightly clasped in her lap and avoided looking at the doctor who interviewed her. She answered questions readily and did not appear suspicious or guarded, but her affect was shallow. She denied depressed mood, delusions, or hallucinations. However, her answers became increasingly idiosyncratic and irrelevant as the interview progressed. In response to a question about her strange cooking habits, she replied that she did not wish to discuss recent events in Russia. When discussing her decline in functioning, she said, "There's more of a take-off mechanism when you're younger." Asked about ideas of reference, she said, "I doubt it's true, but if one knows the writers involved, it could be an element that would be directed in a comical way." Her answers were interspersed with the mantra, "I'm safe. I'm safe."

DSM-IV-TR Casebook Diagnosis of "Low Life Level"

Several features of this case suggest the diagnosis of Schizophrenia. There are Louise's extreme decline in functioning over a period of several years and her many oddities of behavior and speech. In addition, there is no evidence of a mood disorder or of a general medical condition or substance that could account for this disturbance. What makes the diagnosis more problematic is the apparent absence of delusions or hallucinations, which are usually present during the active phase of Schizophrenia.

DSM-III and DSM-III-R did permit the diagnosis of Schizophrenia, even in the absence of delusions and hallucinations, if there were two of the following three symptoms: incoherence or marked loosening of association, catatonic behavior, or flat or grossly inappropriate affect. It would have been difficult to diagnose this as a case of Schizophrenia without stretching these criteria. Louise's speech is at times incoherent, but her affect, although described as shallow, is not flat or grossly inappropriate, and she has no catatonic symptoms. The criterion describing the characteristic symptoms of Schizophrenia in DSM-IV (and DSM-IV-TR) includes additional negative symptoms: alogia (poverty of amount or content of speech) and avolition (pervasive inability to persist in goal-directed activities). Because her speech is at times incoherent and she is unable to work or cope with more than minimal self-care (avolition), the DSM-IV-TR diagnosis would be Schizophrenia (DSM-IV-TR, p. 312).

Discussion of "Low Life Level" by Gerard E. Hogarty, M.S.W.*

I truly appreciate the opportunity to comment on an appropriate treatment plan for Louise. In spite of a gloomy presentation, I would not be pessimistic about her chance to recover a high quality of life.

Medical Diagnosis

A pale, "stooped," and likely malnourished 39-year-old woman, who is incontinent of urine and possibly experiencing a sleep reversal, first needs a thorough medical workup, including a visit to a gynecologist. Although no evidence of a contributing medical condition is believed to exist, half of patients with Schizophrenia harbor underlying medical disease (Goldman 1999). Although there is insufficient information for a definitive DSM-IV-TR diagnosis, Louise is clearly cognitively disorganized and thought disordered. Barring an underlying medical condition that has caused (or exacerbated) her cognitive decline, she is a candidate for a therapeutic dose of a first-line atypical antipsychotic medication, preferably one that will not raise her prolactin level if she has osteoporosis or osteopenia. In the absence of bone disease or other complicating factors (e.g., diabetes, hypercholesterolemia), an appetite-stimulating antipsychotic could be a good choice for this underweight woman. Louise might have had a negative experience with a conven-

Mr. Hogarty is Professor of Psychiatry at the University of Pittsburgh Medical Center. His grant support from the National Institute of Mental Health over the past 35 years has made the development and testing of many interventions possible, including Major Role Therapy (a clinical case management approach), Family Psychoeducation, Personal Therapy, and, more recently, Cognitive Enhancement Therapy.

tional neuroleptic when first hospitalized 12 years ago—one that could have accounted for her reluctance to fill a discharge prescription. A trusting relationship should lead to the assurance that the past need not be repeated, regarding the extrapyramidal side effects of conventional neuroleptics. But arm wrestling Louise over medication adherence would likely be as successful as pushing a rope. Outreach, patience, and an empathic, trusting relationship will be the key to successful treatment adherence. The point here is as follows: first things first. Psychosocial treatment does not presume to replace good medical diagnosis and management. If there is a Schizophrenia illness, psychosocial treatment will build on medication effects and then move well beyond the limitations of pharmacotherapy (Hogarty and Ulrich 1998).

Psychosocial Diagnosis

DSM-IV-TR is a necessary *classification* system. But diagnosis, which is needed for a thoughtful psychosocial treatment plan, represents *understanding*, including an understanding of the patient's past accomplishments, disappointments, hopes, skills, interests, temperament, learning capacity, psychosocial-biological needs, and personal narrative of "what went wrong." Unfortunately, Louise is typical of many acutely ill patients who, because of active psychotic symptoms, are poor informants of their personal history, thus making a DSM-IV-TR differential diagnosis quite difficult. I would begin the process of "understanding," which is needed for a correct diagnosis and relevant treatment plan, by vigorously pursuing the hospital records of the past 12 years and by immediately engaging her mother, who appears to be the only available informant (but others could be in the wings). Louise needs to be reassured that having all interested parties on board offers the best hope of eventual recovery. (The well-intended but misguided confidentiality laws of some states [e.g., New York] can often become the nemesis of appropriate treatment planning for adult psychotic patients.)

Louise's mother could likely profit from and appreciate a psychoeducation primer (Anderson et al. 1986), at least regarding basic information on the nature and treatment of severe mental illness. It should be offered with a message of hope that, going forward, life can indeed be better for her daughter. Having a family member aligned with the treatment plan offers an assurance of treatment adherence and, at the same time, can attenuate the guilt, self-blame, frustration, despair, and anxiety that are frequently associated with a loved one's decline

(Anderson et al. 1986). Louise's downward course is more of a testimonial to treatment neglect and a minimally responsive health care system than a confirmation of the myth that the inevitable course of Schizophrenia is one of irreversible deterioration.

What do we know at this point that might help to form a psychosocial diagnosis and treatment plan? First, Louise is apparently intelligent and probably well educated if, in fact, she functioned previously as an occupational therapy supervisor in a large hospital. At one time, she possessed the executive functions needed to manage her own affairs and to form an intimate relationship. Such premorbid competencies often indicate the potential for a very positive response to psychosocial treatment (Hogarty 2002; Hogarty et al. 2004). Louise's downward spiral is characteristic of the well-known process of "desocialization" (Cameron and Margaret 1951). Odd behavior, even in its mildest forms, can distance "normal" friends, co-workers, and family, depriving people such as Louise of meaningful interpersonal contact and bringing the lifelong process of "secondary socialization" to a halt (Brim 1966; Carter and Flesher 1995). Awareness of the basic rules of conduct results from "primary socialization" experiences learned early in life at the hand of one's parents (e.g., "Don't spill your milk"). But secondary socialization provides a person with continuous information throughout life regarding the implicit rules, vocabularies, and modes of conduct associated with acquired roles (such as becoming an occupational therapy supervisor, friend, or lover). Without a continuing opportunity for secondary socialization, these skills atrophy. The downward spiral of social withdrawal and isolation is also likely to have been facilitated by important neurobiological changes that accompany the onset and early course of Schizophrenia (Keshavan and Hogarty 1999). However, many of these anomalies might be reversed or compensated with treatment (e.g., Hogarty et al. 2004; Keshavan and Hogarty 1999; Penades et al. 2002).

There is no "quick fix" for Schizophrenia. Louise needs an immediate treatment plan appropriate to the *acute* phase, closely coupled with a *stabilization* phase intervention. Her cognitive disorganization provides a clue to potential long-term treatment needs in the *recovery* phase. Cognitively disorganized patients invariably have problems in information processing (e.g., selective attention) as well as with "working memory" and its related problem-solving difficulties. Being able to follow a cooking recipe (a less than successful passion for Louise) represents a formidable challenge to a person with attention and working memory problems. Similarly, Louise's incoherent account of her downward course speaks volumes about working memory difficulties as well. While waiting for more useful and valid information on psychiatric history, we can nevertheless proceed on the basis of what we do know.

Acute Phase Treatment

There are no psychosocial treatment "heroics" when a patient with Schizophrenia is acutely ill. Rather, the need to establish a therapeutic alliance (see Chapters 3 and 4 in Hogarty 2002) is, foremost, one that will provide the linchpin for a more accurate diagnosis, needs assessment, and treatment plan. Resistance might occur, but, with Louise's input into her own life plan, I believe that she would be responsive to an empathic, helping relationship. While waiting for the antipsychotic effects of medication to emerge, it is essential to create a "holding environment" (Winnicott 1965), including gaining control of destabilizing environmental events that can variably take the form of criticism, inappropriate expectations, losses, excessive stimuli, substance abuse, competing demands, and "insight-oriented" probing, to name a few. Louise also needs a case manager to smooth her community reentry and to secure supported and well-supervised housing. Medication adherence is a primary goal in the acute phase, together with dietary supervision in Louise's case. A skillful case manager should be able to access the needed resources, as well as monitor medication fidelity, nutritional intake, personal safety, and environmental sources of stress. Obtaining the life-sustaining benefits to which Louise is entitled (e.g., disability, housing, and health insurance benefits) is paramount. This is not the time to become conflicted about encouraging "dependency" (Hogarty 2002). Again keep in mind, first things first.

Stabilization Phase Treatment

On the assumption that Louise does have a Schizophrenia disorder, with time, she will likely be among the 85%–90% of compliant patients who achieve at least a partial response to a first- or second-line (clozapine) antipsychotic medication. Thus, a psychosocial treatment plan designed to facilitate and maintain *clinical stability* is the treatment of choice. Although I am admittedly biased, I would recommend our Personal Therapy (PT) approach (Hogarty 2002). (If positive symptoms of Schizophrenia persist in spite of adequate pharmacotherapy, a brief course of cognitive-behavioral therapy for Schizophrenia [Kingdon and Turkington 2002] could be tried before PT.)

PT is a three-phase, graduated approach to the control of external and internal sources of distress that might serve to destabilize a patient. Its phases are designed to accommodate the patient's stage of recovery and extend from simple exercises in stress avoidance during the Basic Phase to more sophisticated approaches at implementing acquired coping strategies in the community during the Advanced Phase. PT offers something of a smorgasbord of effective coping strategies within a phase that can be tailored to the individual patient's needs and preferences, thus avoiding the well-known "therapeutic stalemate." I would suggest the Basic and Intermediate Phases of PT for Louise that, if she were responsive, would make her an ideal candidate for a poststabilization, recovery phase intervention. (The Advanced Phase can be reserved for patients whose providers lack a recovery phase–cognitive rehabilitation intervention.) Louise is at least cognizant of her "decline in self-care and a low life level" and uses an autoprotective strategy to achieve self-control ("I'm safe"), not at all a bad foundation on which to build awareness and coping skills. (In all phases, PT attempts to capitalize on existing strengths.) The patient can be assured that PT is a method that has enabled many patients like her to reclaim their former level of functioning. At the least, the approach can help put Louise in control of her illness. The patient can be assured that her illness is not the result of personal failure and that she has an essential role in managing its course.

PT blends a number of established practice principles across three treatment phases, principles that change only in the degree of extension that accommodate the level of residual symptoms. Among these are 1) *psychoeducation* that moves from a basic understanding of the illness and how treatments work to a personalized knowledge of one's own vulnerabilities; 2) *role resumption* that begins with the graduated assumption of self-care activities and extends to (prevocational) community activities that provide the opportunity to test acquired skills under supervision; 3) *internal coping*, a centerpiece of PT that starts with the concept of "stress as a trigger" and extends through an appreciation of a potential march of symptoms (precursors, signs, symptoms, and eventual syndromes) to a personal understanding of one's own subjective cues of distress, including how and when to intervene; 4) *adaptive strategies* associated with internal coping that begin with basic social skills exercises in avoidance and prosocial responses and proceed to deep breathing, relaxation techniques, social perception training, reflective consideration, criticism management, and conflict resolution; and, finally, 5) *adjustment to disability*. An appreciation of the less apparent residuals of Schizophrenia, such as amotivation, mental fatigue, and abiding problems with attention and memory, can be identified *and* managed. Based on our long-term, randomized studies involving more than 150 patients (Hogarty 2002), I strongly believe that Louise would be among the vast majority of patients who can successfully complete the Basic and Intermediate Phases of PT over 12–15 months of individual, weekly (45-minute) sessions. If not, Louise might profit from a course of behavioral skills training (Heinssen et al. 2000) before resuming PT.

Recovery Phase Treatment

By now, Louise should have achieved a level of clinical stabilization such that the continuing services of a case manager might not be necessary, and, if indicated, she might well be able to resume independent living. Given Louise's premorbid competencies (including at least an average if not higher IQ), I would recommend our new Cognitive Enhancement Therapy (CET) approach (Hogarty and Flesher 1999a, 1999b). CET has recently demonstrated unprecedented effects on attention, executive functions, social cognition, and social adjustment among 121 (randomized) patients similar to Louise whose average illness duration exceeded 15 years (Hogarty et al. 2004). CET is a recovery phase intervention for patients with Schizophrenia who have achieved clinical stability but nonetheless remain socially and vocationally disabled. The "rate-limiting" factors of recovery have increasingly implicated residual deficits in neurocognition *and* social cognition (the ability to act wisely) (Hogarty and Flesher 1999a)—deficits that have both "state" characteristics (as are clearly apparent in Louise's acute condition) and "trait" or abiding characteristics that endure even when symptoms remit. CET integrates 75 hours of computer-assisted training in attention, memory, and problem solving with 1.5 hours per week (50 sessions) of social cognitive group exercises that encourage active mental processing, perspective taking, social context appraisal, negotiation, empathy, attention, and online working memory through a variety of secondary socialization experiences designed to increase the patient's interpersonal comfort and competencies. Simple "computer training" will likely not suffice because the residual neurocognitive deficits that are functionally disabling require active, in vivo, interpersonal negotiation. (The patient in supported employment who repeatedly "fails coffee break" and quits his or her job is not vocationally disabled simply because his or her reaction time is prolonged but also because of problems with perspective taking and with the appraisal of nonverbal cues and subtle rules of conduct that govern each and every social situation.) Fifteen to 18 months of CET, coupled with a course of preparatory, supported education, should leave Louise more than able to resume a rewarding life, be it a new vocation, a reentry into her earlier career, or a volunteer or supported job that would allow her to first "test the waters" of community reintegration. (The return to work or school should be gradual and accommodating of residual cognitive deficits *and* mental stamina.)

Postrecovery

As Louise resumes the roles that are meaningful to her, biweekly "booster" sessions will be indicated for at least 1 year. The patient with Schizophrenia who attempts a resumption of life goals is the one who most requires ongoing support. Tragically, treatment systems frequently reduce contact once a patient is symptomatically stable. Should Louise have a setback or even a temporary exacerbation of symptoms, she need not return to the "square one" of psychosocial treatment. Rather, after an appraisal of the circumstances and associated stressors that led to the temporary setback, a review and in vivo simulation of acquired skills appropriate to the relevant phase of PT or CET is often sufficient to reinstate the patient to the recent level of recovery. This cost-effective, psychosocial treatment algorithm is described elsewhere (Hogarty 2002).

Summary

I have briefly laid out an "evidence-based" treatment plan, but the sad reality of the current mental health environment is that Louise, and countless thousands like her, will be fortunate to receive even "warm medication" and a "friendly visitor" on occasion. Most severely mentally ill patients have been sacrificed on the altar of *managed cost*, whose pillars often extend deep into the soil of therapeutic nihilism. Even the consensus of psychosocial treatment experts has narrowly restricted available services to the most chronically impaired and nonfunctioning patients (McEvoy et al. 1999). In my lengthy experience, these patients are more often limited by reasons of mental insufficiency and/or organic brain disorder than by Schizophrenia! In my opinion, these comorbidities, when combined with the absence of an appropriate psychosocial treatment, have given Schizophrenia its fatalistic reputation. Patients who symptomatically recover and have greater rehabilitation potential are essentially ignored in consensus recommendations.

At the moment, we have an arsenal of effective but unused psychosocial treatments. For example, there are now more than 30 studies that demonstrate the efficacy of family psychoeducation, but the approach is rarely implemented. A commitment to establishing a *dedicated funding source* is required for the already-tested, efficacious psychosocial treatments that exist. Most costs of Schizophrenia are associated with preventable hospitalizations that follow the absence of outpatient psychosocial treatment. Problems with dissemination and implementation exist, but more often than not they can be traced to political and administrative issues involving insufficient funds. Although we lack the marketing resources of the pharmaceutical industry (that manages to get any number of expensive "me too" medications *quickly* implemented), collectively we *can* make the promise of effective psychosocial treatment a reality (as has been demonstrated in some European countries). Louise reminds us that there are substantial costs in *not* treating psychotic conditions *early* and *adequately* (Carr et al. 2003).

References

Anderson CM, Reiss DJ, Hogarty GE: Schizophrenia and the Family: A Practitioner's Guide to Psychoeducation and Management. New York, Guilford Press, 1986

Brim OG: Socialization through the life cycle, in Socialization After Childhood. Edited by Brim OG, Wheeler S. New York, Wiley, 1966, pp 3–49

Cameron N, Margaret H (eds): Desocialization, in Behavior Pathology. New York, Houghton Mifflin, 1951, pp 478–503

Carr VJ, Neil AL, Halpin SA, et al: Costs of schizophrenia and other psychoses in urban Australia: findings from the Low Prevalence (Psychotic) Disorders Study. Aust N Z J Psychiatry 37(1):31–40, 2003

Carter MJ, Flesher S: The neuro-sociology of schizophrenia: vulnerability and functional disability. Psychiatry 58:209–224, 1995

Goldman LS: Medical illness in patients with schizophrenia. J Clin Psychiatry 60 (suppl 21):5–10, 1999

Heinssen RK, Liberman RP, Kopelowicz A: Psychosocial skills training for schizophrenia: lessons from the laboratory. Schizophr Bull 26:21–46, 2000

Hogarty GE: Personal Therapy for Schizophrenia and Related Disorders: A Guide to Individualized Treatment. New York, Guilford Press, 2002

Hogarty GE, Flesher S: Developmental theory for a cognitive enhancement therapy of schizophrenia. Schizophr Bull 25:677–692, 1999a

Hogarty GE, Flesher S: Practice principles of cognitive enhancement therapy for schizophrenia. Schizophr Bull 25:693–708, 1999b

Hogarty GE, Ulrich R: The limitations of antipsychotic medication on schizophrenia relapse and adjustment and the contributions of psychosocial treatment. J Psychiatry Res 32:243–250, 1998

Hogarty GE, Flesher S, Ulrich R, et al: Cognitive enhancement therapy for schizophrenia: effects of a two-year randomized trial on neurocognition and behavior. Pre-publication report 2004

Keshavan MS, Hogarty GE: Brain maturational processes and delayed onset in schizophrenia. Dev Psychopathol 11:525–543, 1999

Kingdon DG, Turkington D: Cognitive-Behavioral Therapy of Schizophrenia. New York, Guilford Press, 2002

McEvoy JP, Scheifler PL, Frances A: The expert consensus guideline series: treatment of schizophrenia. J Clin Psychiatry 60 (suppl 11):1–80, 1999

Penades R, Boget T, Lomena F, et al: Could the hypofrontality pattern in schizophrenia be modified through neuropsychological rehabilitation? Acta Psychiatr Scand 105:202–208, 2002

Winnicott D: The Motivational Process and the Facilitating Environment. New York, International Universities Press, 1965

Under Surveillance

Mr. Simpson is a single, unemployed, 44-year-old white man brought to the emergency room by the police for striking an elderly woman in his apartment building. His chief complaint is, "That damn bitch. She and the rest of them deserved more than that for what they put me through."

The patient has been continuously ill since age 22. During his first year of law school, he gradually became more and more convinced that his classmates were making fun of him. He noticed that they would snort and sneeze whenever he entered the classroom. When a girl he was dating broke off the relationship with him, he believed that she had been "replaced" by a look-alike. He called the police and asked for their help to solve the "kidnapping." His academic performance in school declined dramatically, and he was asked to leave and seek psychiatric care.

Mr. Simpson got a job as an investment counselor at a bank, which he held for 7 months. However, he was receiving an increasing number of distracting "signals" from co-workers, and he became more and more suspicious and withdrawn. It was at this time that he first reported hearing voices. He was eventually fired and soon thereafter was hospitalized for the first time, at age 24. He has not worked since.

Mr. Simpson has been hospitalized 12 times, the longest stay being 8 months. However, in the last 5 years he has been hospitalized only once, for 3 weeks. During the hospitalizations he has received various antipsychotic drugs. Although outpatient medication has been prescribed, he usually stops taking it shortly after leaving the hospital. Aside from twice-yearly lunch meetings with his uncle and his contacts with mental health workers, he is totally isolated socially. He lives on his own and manages his own financial affairs, including a modest inheritance. He reads the *Wall Street Journal* daily. He cooks and cleans for himself.

Mr. Simpson maintains that his apartment is the center of a large communication system that involves all the major television networks, his neighbors, and apparently hundreds of "actors" in his neighborhood. There are secret cameras in his apartment that carefully monitor all his activities. When he is watching television, many of his minor actions (e.g., going to the bathroom) are soon directly commented on by the announcer. Whenever he goes outside, the "actors" have all been warned to keep him under surveillance. Everyone on the street watches him. His neighbors operate two different "machines"; one is responsible for all of his voices, except the "joker." He is not certain who controls this voice, which "visits" him only occasionally and is very funny. The other voices, which he hears many times each day, are generated by this machine, which he sometimes thinks is directly run by the neighbor whom he attacked. For example, when he is going over his investments, these "harassing" voices constantly tell him which stocks to buy. The other machine he calls "the dream machine." This machine puts erotic dreams into his head, usually of "black women."

Mr. Simpson described other unusual experiences. For example, he recently went to a shoe store 30 miles from his house in the hope of buying some shoes that wouldn't be "altered." However, he soon found out that, like the rest of the shoes he buys, special nails had been put into the bottom of the shoes to annoy him. He was amazed that his decision concerning which shoe store to go to must have been known to his "harassers" before he himself knew it, so that they had time to get the altered shoes made up especially for him. He realizes that great effort and "millions of dollars" are involved in keeping him under surveillance. He sometimes thinks this is all part of a large experiment to discover the secret of his "superior intelligence."

At the interview, Mr. Simpson is well groomed, and his speech is coherent and goal-directed. His affect is, at most, only mildly blunted. He was initially very angry at being brought in by the police. After several weeks of treatment with an antipsychotic drug that failed to control his psychotic symptoms, he was transferred to a long-stay facility with a plan to arrange a structured living situation for him.

DSM-IV-TR Casebook Diagnosis of "Under Surveillance"

Mr. Simpson's long illness apparently began with delusions of reference (his classmates making fun of him by snorting and sneezing when he entered the classroom). Over the years, his delusions have become increasingly complex and bizarre (his neighbors are actually actors, his thoughts are monitored, a machine puts erotic dreams in his head). In addition, he has prominent hallucinations of different voices that harass him.

Bizarre delusions and prominent hallucinations are the characteristic psychotic symptoms of Schizophrenia (DSM-IV-TR, p. 312). The diagnosis is confirmed by the marked disturbance in his work and social functioning and the absence of a sustained mood disturbance or a general medical condition or use of a substance that can account for the disturbance.

All of Mr. Simpson's delusions and hallucinations seem to involve the single theme of a conspiracy to harass him. This preoccupation with a delusion, in the absence of disorganized speech, flat or inappropriate affect, or catatonic or grossly disorganized behavior, indicates the Paranoid Type (DSM-IV-TR, p. 314), further specified as Continuous, as he has not been free of psychotic symptoms for many years.

Discussion of "Under Surveillance" by Thomas H. McGlashan, M.D.*

The common feature of paranoid patients is an overriding, watchful, suspicious interpretation of experience. These patients demand special consideration by virtue of being, without doubt, the most difficult pa-

---

*Dr. McGlashan is Professor of Psychiatry at the Yale University Department of Psychiatry. Schizophrenia has been a major focus of Dr. McGlashan's career, starting in residency at Massachusetts Mental Health Center with Elvin Semrad. He is a biological psychiatrist and psychoanalyst who has interdigitated research and treatment of psychiatric disorders, especially schizophrenia, since his training. This has included work on a first-episode schizophrenia unit at the National Institutes of Health with Will Carpenter and 15 years at Chestnut Lodge Hospital treating and tracking schizophrenic patients with many colleagues, notably Christopher Keats, with whom he wrote a book (McGlashan TH, Keats CJ: Schizophrenia: Treatment Process, and Outcome. Washington, DC, American Psychiatric Press, 1989), and Wayne Fenton, with whom he has written many papers on the course and therapy of schizophrenia. At Yale, he has articulated the reduced synaptic connectivity hypothesis of schizophrenia with Ralph Hoffman and initiated early identification and intervention research in schizophrenia both at home and abroad.

tients to treat psychotherapeutically. They invariably enter treatment under coercion and bristling with hostility. Convinced that people always misunderstand them, they trust no one.

Mr. Simpson represents the paranoid patient par excellence and, as such, is one of the most challenging persons any psychiatrist will ever treat. The patient's clinical history, symptoms, and severe functional deficits leave little doubt as to the diagnosis of Schizophrenia, Chronic Paranoid subtype, and there are no reasonable differential diagnostic entities to consider. The patient's symptoms are continuous, and his deficits in reality testing are particularly severe. He is totally disabled functionally with regard to work and social interactions. After 20 years of active psychosis and 12 hospitalizations, he presents any treater with a daunting challenge—any treater, that is, who is willing to try.

Mr. Simpson's overall prognostic potential is slim if the goal is symptomatic and functional recovery. His expected future course is likely to be an extension of his course over the last 20 years. Mr. Simpson assaulting an elderly female neighbor might signal further deterioration. If deterioration continues, his prospects for living outside of a long-stay asylum or jail will diminish drastically. On the other hand, the past 5 years have seen only one hospitalization, suggesting that his disorder could be mellowing.

Two additional elements bode ominously with respect to prognosis. The first is that his psychotic world of delusions and hallucinations literally fills his apartment and his life. His disorder is not just persecutory, it is also interesting, exciting, and, at times, amusing and gratifying. In short, his investment in psychosis is substantial compared to his investment in "real" life and people. The second ominous prognostic element is his obviously negative attitude toward any and all efforts at treatment—an attitude that has translated into noncompliant behavior with virtually every therapeutic encounter.

On the other hand, two positive prognostic elements stand out. One is his degree of organization. His affect is intact. He has few negative symptoms (e.g., lack of motivation, poverty of speech), and most of the time he displays little disorganization, all of which is consistent with the paranoid subtype. Most strikingly, he is self-sufficient and takes care of himself. He is almost certainly unable to work, but his modest inheritance keeps him off of disability and provides an illusion of instrumental self-sufficiency. The other positive prognostic development, paradoxically, is that he has broken the law and gotten himself into treatment as a consequence. He probably denies responsibility for the precipitating assault, but, nevertheless, his behavior has added a real problem to his delusional ones, and it could be the key to "locking" him into an adequate trial of treatment for the first time in his life. Mr. Simpson may not see his delusions and hallucinations as a problem, but no matter how intensely paranoid he may be about the police, unlike his other persecutors, they are real.

Two bodies of information would be especially desirable to have in evaluating his case. The first are records of his prior treatments, supplemented with whatever observations the patient is willing to share about his career as a "patient." The history indicates that a recent several-week trial of an antipsychotic drug failed to control his psychotic symptoms. Information regarding his compliance with this medication is crucial because it determines the direction of pharmacotherapeutic treatment planning. If he did not take the medicine, the issue is familiar (i.e., willful noncompliance). If he did take it, then the issue is biological resistance and suggests considering different neuroleptics, including atypical antipsychotics (such as Zyprexa [olanzapine], Risperdal [risperidone], Seroquel [quetiapine], Geodon [ziprasidone], and Abilify [aripiprazole]) and clozapine. The second area requiring clarification is Mr. Simpson's legal status. Is he remanded by court to the long-stay institution? Who does he have to answer to, if anyone? Of pivotal importance is whether the treating psychiatrist has any leverage in this matrix. Unless the patient is required by the court to be a patient, Mr. Simpson will exercise his civil right to deny intervention. For patients like Mr. Simpson, treatment often depends on a loss of civil rights.

The treating psychiatrist's first meeting with Mr. Simpson will be crucial if the effort is to have any chance of success. The doctor should be ready to face someone who is lined up against any encounter. A conservative and supportive approach, especially in the early phases of treatment, is necessary if there is to be some chance of developing a working alliance. Because such patients often enter treatment feeling coerced and exhibiting great mistrust and hostility, they are best greeted by the therapist with a removed but matter-of-fact attitude. A high degree of professionalism and reliability, and no evident desire to be liked by the patient, will enhance the possibility of success in establishing some trust. The reality of the patient's delusions should neither be accepted nor argued, and observations should be offered as hypotheses. Attempts to modify or diminish paranoid defenses should be made only after a reasonable working alliance has been established and should be undertaken without ambitious expectations on the part of the therapist.

The doctor should explicitly address his or her understanding that Mr. Simpson is being seen under coercion—that he is here because of the police. The doctor should also make explicit his or her role in this situation and inform the patient who it was that recruited him or her to intervene, for what purpose, to what end, and with what contingencies (i.e., what Mr. Simpson has to do in order to resecure his freedom and autonomy). The doctor should be nonjudgmental with respect to the patient's guilt or innocence, or whether Mr. Simpson's behavior was justifiable or not, given his delusional conviction about his neighbor's persecution. The doctor should state that he or she is willing to explore all these issues with Mr. Simpson, with the goal being how Mr. Simpson can react so as to not have any further trouble with the police.

The doctor should be truthful and unambiguously state who he or she is, what he or she believes is going on with Mr. Simpson at this time, and what he or she can and cannot do with or for Mr. Simpson. He or she should acknowledge up front being a psychiatrist brought in by the court because Mr. Simpson assaulted his neighbor and add that Mr. Simpson's act was judged by the court to have occurred because Mr. Simpson was psychotic and delusional. The doctor may share the diagnosis given by the court (i.e., Schizophrenia) and offer to elaborate on what that means at some future time if Mr. Simpson is at all interested.

The doctor should also say that he or she assumes mental illness is involved because he or she was called into the case as a psychiatrist but that he or she is willing to listen to Mr. Simpson's side of the story, again with the aim not of assigning blame or determining whether the events were real but to help Mr. Simpson avoid trouble with the police and to secure greater personal freedom. The doctor then outlines what the process involves—regular meetings to get to know each other and to explore the events that led to Mr. Simpson's trouble.

The doctor should also be clear in the first encounter about the "rules" of this "process" (the word *treatment* should be avoided). The rules include a clear delineation of the limits of confidentiality in the doctor-client relationship such as limits relating to responsibilities the doctor has for reporting back to court and especially limits relating to dangerousness. Regarding the latter, the doctor should be explicit with Mr. Simpson that he or she will warn any potential victims of the patient's wrath and that he or she will inform the courts and police of any plans Mr. Simpson has to hurt himself or anyone else. If it seems appropriate, the doctor may predict that Mr. Simpson may become suspicious of him or her (or more suspicious than he already is), much like he is suspicious of just about everyone else, but that this in no way suggests they cannot work together, especially if Mr. Simpson can talk about his misgivings.

At this point, the doctor says something such as, "That's who I am and what I see myself doing here. What did you expect? I think I can be useful to you. What do you think?" Hopefully, Mr. Simpson will engage and elaborate. If he does, the doctor can elaborate further on what to expect in the sessions and, over time, include more active treatment modalities such as medication and cognitive-behavioral techniques. Before these are introduced, however, time and effort must first be invested in establishing a relationship.

Because of suspiciousness, disorganization, indifference, or ambivalence about human attachments, establishing a relationship with a patient with Schizophrenia can be challenging. Analytic strategies of passive neutrality and anonymity can easily be misinterpreted as disinterest or dislike and are generally discouraged. Consistency, straightforwardness, and an active effort to establish rapport are advocated. Within bounds, a reasonable degree of self-disclosure on the therapist's part can help to counter distortions by allowing the patient to become comfortable with the therapist as a person. A relationship should be sought on the patient's terms. If the patient initially wants the therapist only to meet some immediate need (e.g., to secure discharge from a hospital or intervene with the patient's family), this is taken as the starting point and viewed positively as a sign that the therapist is seen as potentially useful. At times, engaging in activity (walking or playing a game), finding a neutral topic of common interest (sports, music), or placidly accepting periods of silence will further promote establishing a relationship. Creativity and patience are the only rules.

The process of engagement is often hard, unrewarding, and sometimes scary. The latter, especially, should never be ignored. The aggressive patient requires great care and some experience for one-to-one interactions to be safe. The maintenance of mutual respect, firmness, and an undistorted awareness of one's own anxiety are all strongly recommended. Limit setting, ranging from verbal remonstrance to meeting in the presence of readily available help, to the use of restraints, to timely termination of a volatile session, can be instituted as the situation dictates. Very frequently, the open and candid admission by the therapist to a highly threatening patient that he or she is frightened will defuse the patient's need to be defensively attacking. In all of these situations, it is important that the therapist acknowledge his or her own difficulties in becoming comfortable with the patient. Should these difficulties prove insurmountable, the therapist should seek supervision or consider a change of therapist. It is highly unrealistic to expect oneself to be both comfortable and effective with all patients.

What could be talked about? The events surrounding Mr. Simpson's assault on his neighbor will need to be elaborated eventually, but initially, the doctor might fruitfully focus on what Mr. Simpson has done right over the last 5 years rather than focus on what he did wrong. The doctor should observe out loud that Mr. Simpson avoided hospitalization and trouble with the law (with one exception) for the past 5 years and that it might be useful to explore how he has managed to do that.

If Mr. Simpson takes up the offer, an opening into his life and experiences may be created. The doctor remains nonjudgmental and focuses on how the patient successfully coped with his delusional and hallucinatory "experiences" in his everyday life for the last 5 years. These experiences are not labeled as psychotic but are dealt with as real enough to Mr. Simpson that he probably struggled many times to keep from doing what he ultimately did to his neighbor. The doctor focuses on the times Mr. Simpson was successful in that struggle (i.e., when he remained in behavioral control) and what he did to achieve that control. The process highlights the patient's rational capacities and strengths; it provides models for successful coping in the future, and it does so without getting into contentious debates about the "reality" of the patient's experiences.

Only after a certain degree of familiarity and comfort has been established can the patient's psychotic symptoms be approached in any systematic and technical fashion. Cognitive-behavioral strategies become relevant at this point. The patient's rational cognitive capacity is called on to challenge and scrutinize his delusional realities. As outlined by Dickerson (2000), cognitive-behavioral therapy (CBT) approaches include belief modification, focusing/reattribution, and normalizing the psychotic experience, among other strategies.

In belief modification, evidence for delusional belief is challenged in reverse order to the importance of the delusion to the patient and the strength with which it is held. In Mr. Simpson's case, this might be applied to the sequence about his shoes being altered. He reported being quite surprised by this turn of events, suggesting that he might be willing to entertain alternative hypotheses about what was happening. Focusing/reattribution targets auditory hallucinations such as the voices that Mr. Simpson hears at times. The phenomenology of the voices is explored in detail: who is talking, how frequently, how loud, etc. The patient is asked to keep a daily diary of the voices' frequency and content. The patient and therapist examine the beliefs the patient has elaborated around the voices, their source, and their aim. By elaborating and embedding the patient's hallucinations in the matrix of everyday life, including the patient's concomitant thoughts and feelings, the therapist attempts to help the patient reattribute the voices to him- or herself. Asking Mr. Simpson to elaborate the details surrounding the moments when the "joker" talks, for example, may link the experience to other aspects of the patient's mental state and thereby suggest an internal rather than an external origin of the voice.

In normalizing the patient's psychotic experience, the therapist tries to put the patient's thinking in the frame of antecedent stressful events to "explain" the patient's symptoms in a stress-diathesis context. This helps to make the psychotic experience appear less bizarre and "crazy" to the patient. With Mr. Simpson, it might be useful to focus on the event bringing him into treatment—his assault of the elderly neighbor who operated one of the "voice machines." Despite countless days and nights filled with harassing voices and plots, he lost control only this once. Something different was probably happening around this event, and careful detailing of the experience might reconstruct the link between symptoms, assault, stress, and personal history. Highlighting the emergence of stress and personal history in the elaborated story can possibly help Mr. Simpson "normalize" the experience and take some personal responsibility for it.

CBT strategies, such as that described above, could be tried with Mr. Simpson's extensive paranoid delusions and auditory hallucinations should he ever be sufficiently motivated and develop a relationship with the doctor that is strong and trusting enough to manage the effort. If he proved he was able to negotiate such a sequence of exercises, sufficient rationality and alliance may be present to introduce other treatment modalities for consideration, particularly medication. It is highly unlikely that Mr. Simpson would ever reach this level. Nevertheless, should he reach the level of CBT exercises, his treatment could be regarded as highly successful, even if he remained delusional, unemployed, and socially isolated. He would have a realistic chance of achieving what is most precious to him—his freedom to resume a paranoid lifestyle to which he has become accustomed and adapted but to resume it with a greater capacity for containing it safely.

Reference

Dickerson FB: Cognitive behavioral psychotherapy for schizophrenia: a review of recent empirical studies. Schizophr Res 43:71–90, 2000

Suggested Reading

Dingman CW, McGlashan TH: Psychotherapy, in A Clinical Guide for the Treatment of Schizophrenia. Edited by Bellack AS. New York, Plenum, 1989, pp 263–282

Fenton WS, McGlashan TH: Individual psychotherapy, in Kaplan and Sadock's Comprehensive Textbook of Psychiatry, 7th ed. Edited by Sadock BJ, Sadock VA. Philadelphia, PA, Lippincott Williams & Wilkins, 2000, pp 1217–1231

McGlashan TH: Intensive individual psychotherapy of schizophrenia: a review of techniques. Arch Gen Psychiatry 40:909–920, 1983

Emilio

Emilio is a 40-year-old man who looks 10 years younger. He is brought to the hospital, his twentieth hospitalization, by his mother because she is afraid of him. He is dressed in a ragged overcoat, bedroom slippers, and a baseball cap and wears several medals around his neck. His affect ranges from anger at his mother ("She feeds me shit...what comes out of other people's rectums") to a giggling, obsequious seductiveness toward the interviewer. His speech and manner have a child-like quality, and he walks with a mincing step and exaggerated hip movements. His mother reports that he stopped taking his medication about a month ago and has since begun to hear voices and to look and act more bizarrely. When asked what he has been doing, he says "eating wires and lighting fires." His spontaneous speech is often incoherent and marked by frequent rhyming and clang associations.

Emilio was first hospitalized when he was 15. His development was apparently normal until the family moved from Puerto Rico when he was 9. He made no friends in his new neighborhood, dropped out of school in ninth grade because he felt victimized by the older boys, and began to hang out with homosexual male prostitutes. He has apparently never held a job for more than a few weeks. Living with his mother and sister, he became increasingly disorganized, wandering the apartment all night, talking and laughing to himself, refusing to bathe, eating very little, throwing things out of the window, and lighting fires in the apartment. He sometimes said a monster was after him or a white bird was flying over him trying to grab his hair. During each hospitalization he was quickly stabilized on antipsychotic medication, but after discharge he refused to continue taking medication, and within a few months he was either again psychotic, leading to readmission to a hospital, or else he disappeared for months at a time before turning up at his mother's house incoherent and unwashed. There is no evidence that he ever abused drugs or alcohol. His sister suspects that when he is relatively well, he finds older men to take care of him, and in this manner has made his way back and forth across the country without ever having a steady job.

DSM-IV-TR Casebook Diagnosis of "Emilio"

The combination of a chronic illness with marked incoherence, inappropriate affect, auditory hallucinations, and grossly disorganized behavior leaves little doubt that the diagnosis is chronic Schizophrenia (DSM-IV-TR, p. 312). The course would be noted as Continuous because he apparently never has prolonged remissions of his psychosis. The prominence of his disorganized speech and behavior, grossly inappropriate affect, and the absence of prominent catatonic symptoms indicate the Disorganized Type.

Follow-Up

Emilio has been hospitalized five more times in the 10 years after this admission to the hospital. During each of his hospitalizations, he was treated with high doses of antipsychotic drugs and within a few weeks began to behave appropriately and to be able to ignore the voices of his auditory hallucinations. During the first hospitalization, he was able to establish a relationship with a therapist and talk thoughtfully and with a full range of appropriate affect about his unhappy life, his inability to do any work because "nobody wants me," and his desire to be taken care of. However, soon after leaving the hospital, Emilio stopped taking his medication, failed to keep clinic appointments, and within a few months was again grossly disorganized and psychotic.

Emilio's last hospitalization was 2 years ago when he was 48. His mother was now too feeble to care for him, and arrangements were made for him to live in an adult home after he left the hospital—supported by welfare and with medication managed by the staff of the institution. In that setting he does fairly well.

Discussion of "Emilio"
by E. Fuller Torrey, M.D.*

The challenge with a patient like Emilio is treating a dysfunctional patient in a dysfunctional psychiatric care system. On any given day, it is a toss-up as to which of the two is in worse shape.

Diagnostically, Emilio's case is straightforward: He has classic, bread-and-butter, chronic Schizophrenia, and everyone working in public sector psychiatry has seen hundreds of cases like his. The most important piece of diagnostic data missing from the history is his human immunodeficiency virus (HIV) status. Given his apparent homosexual lifestyle and episodes of psychosis, he is likely to have been exposed to the virus. If he is HIV-positive, I would make sure that he received antiretroviral medications and that he was assessed for active tuberculosis. If and when he progressed to active acquired immunodeficiency syndrome, he would then be susceptible to secondary infections of the brain, such as toxoplasmosis, which might also cause symptoms of psychosis or dementia and thus further complicate his clinical picture.

The most striking thing about Emilio's clinical course is his 30-plus hospitalizations and its revolving-door aspect. Unfortunately, for the last three decades of American psychiatry, for patients like Emilio, this has been the rule rather than the exception. Emilio's downward clinical spiral could, and should, have been interrupted early in its course. Two essential elements—assisted treatment and rehabilitation—appear to have been completely neglected.

Assisted treatment is important because Emilio appears to have a substantial degree of anosognosia, or lack of awareness of his illness. This is not merely denial but rather a biologically based deficit in understanding one's condition and need for treatment (Amador and David 1998). Current studies suggest that anosognosia is caused by schizophrenia-related

*Dr. Torrey is Professor of Psychiatry at the Uniformed Services University of the Health Sciences; Associate Director for Laboratory Research of the Stanley Medical Research Institute (SMRI) in Bethesda, Maryland; and President of the Treatment Advocacy Center (TAC) in Arlington, Virginia. With an annual budget of approximately $40 million, SMRI conducts and supports research on schizophrenia and bipolar disorder (http:// www.stanleyresearch.org). TAC advocates for improved state laws to encourage the treatment of individuals with severe psychiatric disorders before they become homeless or incarcerated due to their illness (http://www.psychlaws.org). Dr. Torrey worked for 8 years at St. Elizabeths Hospital in Washington, D.C., and volunteered for 16 years at a community clinic for homeless individuals with severe psychiatric disorders.

damage to the frontal and parietal lobes. Because Emilio has limited awareness of his illness, he is unlikely to ever comprehend the importance of taking his medication on a regular basis to remain well. Sending him home with his bottle of pills as he exited the hospital from each of his multiple admissions was an act of predictable and repeated futility.

Instead, early in the course of his illness, Emilio should have been put on some form of assisted treatment that would have required him to take his medication (Torrey and Zdanowicz 2001). This could have been done by a legal mechanism, such as conditional release (as used in New Hampshire), outpatient commitment (as used in New York under "Kendra's Law"), or guardianship. Experience with various forms of assisted treatment has shown that it markedly reduces readmissions (Swartz et al. 1999). Emilio would probably have met criteria for assisted treatment on the grounds of being a danger to himself (repeated exposure to HIV during periods of psychosis) or to others (his mother was afraid of him).

The choice of antipsychotic medication for treating Emilio depends on several factors. His clinical history and improvement of symptoms while hospitalized suggest that he is a relatively good responder to medication. The choice of antipsychotics should be discussed with both Emilio and his mother and should include consideration of his experience with side effects and his clinical response to the medications that he has tried. If physical appearance and a slim figure are very important to Emilio, I would avoid those second-generation antipsychotics that have a propensity for causing weight gain (e.g., Zyprexa [olanzapine] or Risperdal [risperidone]) until I exhausted possibilities with the first-generation agents (e.g., Haldol [haloperidol] or Trilafon [perphenazine]). If, on the other hand, medication compliance continued to be a problem despite implementation of assisted treatment, then I would have Emilio try long-acting, injectable haloperidol or fluphenazine.

Rehabilitation is the second major piece missing from Emilio's treatment plan. If he is living in New York City, he would be a good candidate for Fountain House, the original of more than 200 clubhouses in existence in the United States (Flannery and Glickman 1996). Fountain House would provide him with a place to go during the day, a social network, an opportunity to go into a job-training program, and a network of apartments and living facilities. His ability to survive in the community living off of older men when he was relatively well suggests that Emilio had good social skills that might have been developed for a job, such as a receptionist position.

In implementing the treatment plan involving assisted treatment and rehabilitation, it would be important to also educate Emilio, his mother, and other family members about Schizophrenia. That should be done in a straightforward way, exactly as if one were educating a person about Parkinson's disease or diabetes. I would recommend that they purchase one of the many useful books about Schizophrenia written for families. If pushed for a specific recommendation, I would (immodestly) suggest *Surviving Schizophrenia* (Torrey 2001), which has been translated into Spanish and might be more accessible for Emilio's mother, who was born in Puerto Rico.

So why hasn't Emilio been offered assisted treatment and rehabilitation? Why has he been allowed to continue cycling through repeated hospitalizations, ultimately ending up in an adult home where he will likely live out his days sitting in a poorly lit room with a television perpetually on in the corner? If he is very lucky, the home in which he lives is run by caring people who make sure he gets his medication and organize some activities for him. More likely, the major activities in the home are the movement of cockroaches, and the drug dealers living next door may steal Emilio's discretionary Social Security income funds on a regular basis. This is the fate of large numbers of individuals in today's public psychiatric non-care system.

Emilio might not have been offered assisted treatment for one of many reasons. He may live in one of the nine states (e.g., Massachusetts, New Jersey) that do not yet have an adequate legal provision for assisted treatment. Or, his psychiatrist and treatment team may not be fully aware of recent research on the importance of anosognosia. Or, they may be intimidated by well-meaning but misguided civil libertarians who believe that nobody should ever be required to take medication. And, finally, there is the laziness factor: It is much easier for the treating psychiatrist to simply discharge Emilio from the hospital than to initiate an assisted treatment plan that is likely to require an appearance in court.

Emilio has not been offered rehabilitation because the economics of public psychiatric care are organized in such a way that there is no incentive to do so (Torrey 1997). When Emilio is hospitalized in a state psychiatric hospital, the state pays for virtually all the cost. When he is living in the community, the federal government pays for the majority of his support through Social Security income, Medicaid, HUD-202 housing support, etc. Both the state and the federal government gain financially by providing as little care as possible for Emilio, and each segment of government tries to shift existing costs to the other. Nobody except Emilio and his family stand to benefit from investing in a good, but relatively expensive, rehabilitation program such as Fountain House. One can argue that, in the long run, the state and federal governments would benefit from his rehabilitation by reducing Emilio's rehospitalizations and getting him into a paying job and eventually off Social Security income. But state and federal officials rarely take the long-term perspective into account.

In recent years, this situation has been further exacerbated in many states by the implementation of for-profit managed care systems for public sector psychiatry. For-profit managed care would lose money if it provided patients like Emilio with rehabilitation. Instead, most managed care companies exert great efforts to provide Emilio with no rehabilitation and as little treatment as possible. They require approval for rehospitalization, restrict the medications available to him, and discourage any use of rehabilitation programs. That is how for-profit managed care companies become profitable and why their executives are paid very handsomely. Managed care has almost nothing to do with managing care; it is simply a mechanism for managing costs.

So Emilio, and many patients like him, end up living in an adult home or similar institution, and Emilio is among the lucky ones. Many patients like Emilio end up living on the street in a homeless shelter or rotating through jail, charged with various misdemeanors. It is a sad situation for Emilio, for the psychiatric profession, and for our claims of being a civilized society.

References

Amador XF, David AS (eds): Insight and Psychosis. New York, Oxford University Press, 1998

Flannery M, Glickman M: Fountain House: Portraits of Lives Reclaimed From Mental Illness. Center City, MN, Hazelden, 1996

Swartz MS, Swanson JW, Wagner HR, et al: Can involuntary outpatient commitment reduce hospital recidivism? findings from a randomized trial with severely mentally ill individuals. Am J Psychiatry 156:1968–1975, 1999

Torrey EF: Out of the Shadows: Confronting America's Mental Illness Crisis. New York, Wiley, 1997

Torrey EF: Surviving Schizophrenia: A Manual for Families, Consumers and Providers, 4th ed. New York, HarperCollins, 2001

Torrey EF, Zdanowicz M: Outpatient commitment: what, why, and for whom. Psychiatr Serv 52:337–341, 2001

Late Bloomer

A single, unemployed, college-educated 35-year-old woman, Ms. Fielding, was escorted to the emergency room by the mobile crisis team. The team had been contacted by the patient's sister after she failed to persuade Ms. Fielding to visit an outpatient psychiatrist. Her sister was concerned about the patient's increasingly erratic work patterns and, more recently, her bizarre behavior. The patient's only prior psychiatric contact had been brief psychotherapy in college.

Ms. Fielding had not worked since losing her job 3 months ago. According to her boyfriend and roommate (both of whom live with her), she had become intensely preoccupied with the upstairs neighbors. A few days earlier, she had banged on their front door with an iron for no apparent reason. She told the mobile crisis team that the family upstairs was harassing her by "accessing" her thoughts and then repeating them to her. The crisis team brought her to the emergency room for evaluation of "thought broadcasting." Though she denied having any trouble with her thinking, she conceded that she had been feeling "stressed" since losing her job and might benefit from psychotherapy.

After reading the admission note, which described the patient's bizarre symptoms, the emergency room psychiatrists were surprised to encounter a poised, relaxed, and attractive young woman, stylishly dressed and appearing perfectly normal. She greeted them with a courteous, if somewhat superficial, smile. She related to the doctors with nonchalant respectfulness. When asked why she was there, she ventured a timid shrug, and replied, "I was hoping to find out from you!"

Ms. Fielding had been working as a secretary and attributed her job loss to the sluggish economy. She denied having any recent mood disturbance and answered no to questions about psychotic symptoms, punctuating each query with a polite but incredulous laugh. Wondering if perhaps the crisis team's assessment was of a different patient, the interviewer asked, somewhat apologetically, if the patient ever wondered whether people could read her mind. She replied, "Oh yes, it happens all the time," and described how, on one occasion, she was standing in her kitchen planning dinner in silence, only to hear, moments later, voices of people on the street below reciting the entire menu. She was convinced of the reality of the experience, having verified it by looking out of the window and observing them speaking her thoughts aloud.

The patient was distressed not so much by people "accessing" her thoughts as by her inability to exercise control over the process. She believed that most people developed telepathic powers in childhood and that she was a "late bloomer" who had just become aware of her abilities and was currently overwhelmed by them. Although she had begun having occasional telepathic experiences around 5 months ago, they had become almost constant in the 3 months since losing her job. She was troubled most by her upstairs neighbors, who not only would repeat her thoughts but would bombard her with their own devaluing and critical comments, such as "You're no good!" and "You have to leave." They had begun to intrude upon her mercilessly, at all hours of the night and day.

She was convinced that the only solution was for the family to move away. When asked if she had contemplated other possibilities, she reluctantly admitted that she had spoken to her boyfriend about hiring a hit man to "threaten" or, if need be, "eliminate" the couple. She hoped she would be able to spare their two children, who she felt were not involved in this invasion of her "mental boundaries." This concern for the children was the only insight she demonstrated into the gravity of her symptoms. She did agree, however, to admit herself voluntarily to the hospital.

DSM-IV-TR Casebook Diagnosis of "Late Bloomer"

It is extremely unusual for patients with bizarre delusions, such as Ms. Fielding's delusion that her thoughts were "accessed" by others, to appear otherwise perfectly normal. Nevertheless, the presence of 3 months of frank bizarre delusions and hallucinations, causing marked social and occupational impairment in the absence of a mood disorder, substance use, or general medical condition that could account for the disturbance, justifies a diagnosis of Schizophreniform Disorder (DSM-IV-TR, p. 319). Her good premorbid functioning and the absence of blunted or flat affect indicate the further specification of With Good Prognostic Features.

When the diagnosis is made without waiting for recovery, as in this case, it is further qualified as Provisional, because if continuous signs of the disturbance persist for at least 6 months, the diagnosis would change to Schizophrenia.

Follow-Up

Once admitted to the hospital, Ms. Fielding immediately began pressing for discharge and disavowed her previous symptoms. Her behavior, thinking, and affect seemed otherwise normal. After 2 weeks of observation, she was discharged to her treating physician's clinic. Within a month, however, she again admitted having frightening experiences of hearing voices and of reading other people's thoughts, as well as a general inability to plan for finding work. She agreed to try medication.

She was treated with an antipsychotic drug, and her frightening hallucinations, as well as the belief that she was clairvoyant, remitted. Within 3 months after discharge, she had obtained work with a temporary employment agency. Soon afterward, feeling completely well, she stopped attending the clinic and was lost to follow-up.

Note: This case is discussed first by Drs. Graham and Lieberman and then by Dr. Kane.

Discussion of "Late Bloomer"
by Karen A. Graham, M.Sc., M.D.,*
and Jeffrey A. Lieberman, M.D.**

Ms. Fielding clearly has a psychotic disorder. She has thought broadcasting—the bizarre delusion that others can hear her thoughts—delusions of reference, paranoid delusions that her neighbors are harassing her, auditory hallucinations that the neighbors are repeating her own thoughts to her and making derogatory comments, and bizarre behavior—banging on the neighbor's front door with an iron. She reports that telepathic experiences began approximately 5 months ago and have become almost constant in the last 3 months. It is likely that the job loss 3 months earlier was due to a decline in her performance, which often accompanies the development of frank psychosis. Whether one counts the initial onset of sporadic "telepathic experiences" 5 months ago or the development of frank psychosis 3 months ago as the beginning of the disturbance, the total duration falls within the 1- to 6-month range that is part of the diagnostic criteria for Schizophreniform Disorder. If the duration extended beyond 6 months, the diagnosis would be Schizophrenia.

When trying to differentiate between Schizophreniform Disorder and Schizophrenia, it is important to consider the period of time before the development of frank psychosis. These early symptoms, called *prodromal symptoms*, include nonspecific changes in mood or sleep schedule; attenuated positive symptoms, such as sensory illusions (e.g., seeing faces among the leaves of the trees, hearing music when it is actually just noise of a fan) or brief intermittent hallucinations (e.g., hearing one's name called or "hey you" when no one is around); ideas of

---

*Dr. Graham is Assistant Professor of Psychiatry at the University of North Carolina at Chapel Hill School of Medicine. She works extensively with first-episode psychotic patients. Her research interests focus on the prodrome to Schizophrenia, treatment of first-episode psychosis, and the mechanism of antipsychotic-induced weight gain.

**Dr. Lieberman is the Thad and Alice Eure Distinguished Professor of Psychiatry, Pharmacology, and Radiology and Director of the Mental Health and Neuroscience Clinical Research Center at the University of North Carolina at Chapel Hill School of Medicine. He also serves as Adjunct Professor of Psychiatry and Radiology at Duke University School of Medicine. Dr. Lieberman's research has focused on the neurobiology, pharmacology, and treatment of Schizophrenia and related psychotic disorders. In this context, his work has advanced our understanding of the natural history and phenomenology of Schizophrenia and its pathophysiological basis and the mechanism of action and clinical effectiveness of antipsychotic drugs.

reference that are not delusional (e.g., "it feels as if everyone is looking at me and laughing, but I know that isn't true"); mild to moderate negative symptoms such as social withdrawal; and decline in functioning in school, work, or relationships. Sometimes these symptoms will bring the person to the attention of a psychiatrist or other mental health professional, but, more often, the symptoms will progress to psychotic intensity before this contact occurs. The prodrome of Schizophrenia is a retrospective concept, diagnosed only after the development of the full syndrome. A prodromal period of 2–5 years is not uncommon in the early development of Schizophrenia.

Patients experiencing a first episode of psychosis, such as Ms. Fielding, are often brought to the emergency room by friends or family members who have noticed bizarre thinking or dangerous behavior. In these cases, the safety of the patient, family, and staff is a primary concern. Often, urgent admission to a psychiatric unit is warranted, but some patients can begin treatment as outpatients if the symptoms are not dangerous, there is good family support, and there is adequate access to a mental health professional. Unfortunately, people with psychotic symptoms often remain untreated for lengthy periods, on average between 1 and 2 years, and not infrequently up to 5 years (McGlashan 1999). It is not known whether psychosis is "toxic" to the brain and, therefore, whether a long duration of untreated symptoms is damaging, but ongoing research is addressing this question. What is known is that a long delay in attaining treatment results in prolonged suffering, disability, and loss of opportunity for the individual.

Treatment of the person with psychosis who is presenting to the mental health system for the first time should be comprehensive and flexible. Comprehensive treatment recognizes that although antipsychotic medication is the foundation of the treatment of psychosis, alone this treatment is not sufficient. Individual and family education and therapy are essential to success. Flexible treatment tailors the amount and type of medication, education, and counseling to the needs of the patient and his or her family.

The initial choice of antipsychotic medication is important, because rapid response and minimal side effects will help current, and possibly future, treatment adherence. The atypical antipsychotics (Zyprexa [olanzapine], Risperdal [risperidone], Seroquel [quetiapine], Geodon [ziprasidone], and Abilify [aripiprazole]) are considered first-line treatment for Schizophrenia in most clinical situations (McEvoy et al. 1999) owing to comparable efficacy with conventional drugs for positive symptoms and superior efficacy for negative and cognitive symptoms. In general, the dose of antipsychotic medication for treatment of a first psychotic episode should begin low and increase slowly, with a final dose often lower than typically used for chronic psychosis. This is partly because of the greater efficacy that these medications often have for treating this population and because these patients are more prone to developing side effects. Daily doses as low as 2.5–5.0 mg of Zyprexa, 1–2 mg of Risperdal, and 200–300 mg of Seroquel are common early in treatment. Helpful at times are the antipsychotic formulations that enhance adherence, with olanzapine available in a dissolving tablet (Zydis) and risperidone available as a liquid.

The atypical agents generally have a more favorable side-effect profile; particularly, they have fewer extrapyramidal symptoms, such as acute dystonic reactions and symptoms that resemble Parkinson's disease. However, side effects of the atypical agents may still be significant, distressing, and potentially dangerous and should not be minimized. Weight gain is a significant side effect of a number of the atypical (and typical) antipsychotics. A meta-analysis by Allison and colleagues (1999) estimated that weight gain at 10 weeks on Zyprexa would be approximately 4.17 kg, and on Seroquel and Risperdal it would be approximately 2.47 kg and 1.67 kg, respectively. The reasons for weight gain are multifactorial, with antipsychotic medications potentially causing changes in food intake, metabolism, and energy expenditure (McIntyre et al. 2001). Unfortunately, preventing and treating the weight gain has been very challenging and largely unsuccessful. Another potentially serious side effect is diabetes, often, although not always, associated with obesity. Geodon and Abilfy are the two newest atypical antipsychotics, and early data support their claim of weight neutrality. Ziprasidone is associated with a rare but theoretically possible side effect of QT_c prolongation. Prolongation of the QT_c interval refers to a finding on an electrocardiogram (which measures the conduction of electricity through the heart) indicating that conduction of electricity is slowed down. If it becomes too slowed down, "heart block" can develop, which can lead to potentially serious arrhythmias. Although it is not clear how much more likely Geodon is to cause this side effect as compared to the other antipsychotic medications, it is prudent to obtain a baseline electrocardiogram before starting a patient on Geodon.

Returning to Ms. Fielding's case in particular, we would begin treating Ms. Fielding with both psychoeducation and medication, with visits optimally every 1–2 weeks in the early stages of treatment. Psychoeducation would focus on improving her understanding of psychotic illness and its treatments and provide practical ways to decrease risk of relapse (i.e., reduce stress, avoid recreational drugs, take antipsychotic medications) and improve overall functioning. A good initial choice of antipsychotic would be Zyprexa, 2.5 mg po qhs, but any other atypical antipsychotic would be a good choice as well. Pretreatment weight, body mass index (weight [kg] divided by height^2 [m^2]), fasting glucose and triglycerides, and liver function tests will be helpful baseline measures. Weight and body mass index should be measured at least monthly initially, and lab tests can be rechecked in 6 months to monitor for side effects of the medication.

The duration of treatment with an antipsychotic medication after a first psychotic episode is often foremost in the mind of the individual taking the drug and should be carefully considered by the psychiatrist as well. At the outset of treatment, a plan must be formulated to take into account the risks and benefits of taking, and not taking, medication. Treatment guidelines suggest that patients who have had resolution of psychotic symptoms after a first psychotic episode should continue taking antipsychotic medication for 1–2 years (McEvoy et al. 1999). The decision to have the patient continue taking medication is based on evidence that shows that the risk of relapse is very high, with 78% of those with Schizophrenia relapsing within 1 year and 96% within 2 years of discontinuing medication (Gitlin et al. 2001). If the patient is also using recreational drugs, the chances of relapse are even greater. With each successive relapse, time to remission is longer and extent of remission is poorer (Lieberman et al. 1998). With each psychotic episode comes major disruption to educational, career, and social domains that will have long-lasting effects. Psychotic relapse can also lead to aggressive acts toward people or property. Shortly after a psychotic episode, suicide attempts are common, occurring in 5%–25% of those with early Schizophrenia. Death by suicide occurs in up to 10% of those with Schizophrenia (Wiersma et al. 1998). It is ultimately the patient's decision whether to take medication, so it is vital that patients are educated early and often about the risk of relapse and the possible long-term consequences.

Antipsychotic medications are an essential part of the treatment, but, as in Ms. Fielding's case, the patient may believe differently. Insight into the presence of psychotic symptoms and need for treatment are often poor or even lacking altogether. This is not denial but part of the illness itself. The patient will often see no need for medication: How will taking a medication stop the harassing behavior of neighbors? Where is the logic in that? This is where compassion for the patient's distress is important. Often, patients will agree with you that "things are not going well" even if they don't agree that their senses are playing tricks on them or that their thinking has changed. Focusing on the benefit of the medication to help the person "put things in perspective," improve distractibility, or "get a good night's sleep" so that he or she can cope better can often be early goals. Once individuals have been taking medication for several months, they often develop some awareness that before starting antipsychotic medication, they were unable to distinguish real from unreal experiences. At this point, take the opportunity to educate the patient about psychotic illness and the risk of relapse when one is not taking medication, as well as the long-term side effects of the medication, so that together, you and the patient can plan for the future. The first months to years of treatment for psychosis can be rocky, but taking the time and effort to educate the patient about the illness and its treatment can make a lasting impression.

Patients recovering from their first psychotic episode are in the process of forming beliefs about their diagnosis and attitudes toward treatment. They are ideal candidates for interventions emphasizing attitudes and beliefs that enhance adaptation and coping with the illness (D. Penn, D. Perkins, J.M. Nieri, unpublished data, 2000). Cognitive and behaviorally oriented psychotherapeutic interventions can be very useful and include the techniques of motivational interviewing, normalizing rationales, inductive questioning, reflective listening, reframing, and summarizing. Motivational interviewing explores the options that a subject is considering and his or her views of the positive and negative aspects, as well as suggesting benefits and drawbacks that may be overlooked. An example of a normalizing rationale is to inform the subject that people without mental illness can have psychotic experiences under circumstances such as extreme stress or sleep or sensory deprivation, thus helping the patient to feel more normal. Inductive questioning uses open-ended questions to flesh out the subject's ideas about an issue. Reflective listening, reframing, and summarizing involve reflecting back to the patient what he or she has said in a way that pulls together a number of his or her own thoughts or comments to improve insight. These techniques can improve insight into illness, treatment adherence, and adaptive coping strategies. In addition, first-episode patients require help to regain and maintain premorbid social and occupational functioning. They can greatly benefit from support and education to better navigate the process of grief over losses in school, jobs, independence, and friendships and to accept their vulnerability to future psychotic episodes.

The first psychotic episode is a very traumatic experience for patients and their families. As clinicians, we have an important role to play in resolving the psychosis and enabling the patient to return to a productive and independent life. Treatment of the person with a first psychotic episode is both challenging and rewarding.

References

Allison DB, Mentore JL, Heo M: Antipsychotic-induced weight gain: a comprehensive research synthesis. Am J Psychiatry 156:1685–1696, 1999

Gitlin M, Nuechterlein K, Subotnik KL, et al: Clinical outcome following neuroleptic discontinuation in patients with remitted recent-onset schizophrenia. Am J Psychiatry 158(11):1835–1842, 2001

Lieberman JA, Sheitman B, Chakos M, et al: The development of treatment resistance in patients with schizophrenia: a clinical and pathophysiologic perspective. J Clin Psychopharmacol 18 (2 suppl 1):20S–24S, 1998

McEvoy JP, Scheifler PL, Frances A (eds): Expert Consensus Guideline Series. The Expert Consensus Guideline Series treatment of schizophrenia. J Clin Psychiatry 60 (suppl 11):1–80, 1999

McGlashan TH: Duration of untreated psychosis in first-episode schizophrenia: marker or determinant of course? Biol Psychiatry 46(7):899–907, 1999

McIntyre RS, Mancini DA, Basile VS: Mechanisms of antipsychotic-induced weight gain. J Clin Psychiatry 62 (suppl 23):23–29, 2001

Wiersma D, Nienhuis FJ, Slooff CJ, et al: Natural course of schizophrenic disorders: a 15-year followup of a Dutch incidence cohort. Schizophr Bull 24(1):75–85, 1998

Discussion of "Late Bloomer"
by John Kane, M.D.*

Despite enormous advances in the diagnosis and treatment of Schizophrenia, the challenge of treating patients at the initial presentation of the illness poses one of the most difficult tests of our skills as clinicians.

I first began studying patients during their initial episode of Schizophrenia in 1975. With the assistance of my mentors Donald Klein, Arthur Rifkin, and Frederic Quitkin, I took responsibility for the completion of data analysis and publication of one of the first and few double-blind, placebo-controlled trials of maintenance medication in first-episode patients who had achieved a stable remission (Kane et al. 1982). At that time (and continuing to a less extent even today), many clinicians were reluctant to continue medication for more than a few months after recovery. This study helped to establish a database supporting the importance of relapse prevention even after the very first episode.

The National Institute of Mental Health Clinical Research Center for Schizophrenia, which I have directed for the past 17 years, subsequently undertook an extensive series of studies in first-episode patients, which continues to this day.

Ms. Fielding's case illustrates a number of important and potentially difficult treatment issues. The first is the presentation of an apparent first episode at the age of 35, which is not rare, but not the norm. The potential advantages from a treatment standpoint are the apparent good premorbid adjustment and lack of negative or deficit signs and symptoms. This would bode well for treatment response but, at the same time, would contribute to uncertainty or hesitation on the part of the clinical team in prescribing long-term treatment (and in all likelihood resistance on the part of the patient in accepting such treatment).

A common mistake that clinicians commit with these patients is hesitancy to make and to share a diagnosis that is so frightening and so widely misunderstood. The availability of better-tolerated medications, the increasing presence of support groups for patients and fami-

---

*Dr. Kane is Executive Director of the Zucker Hillside Hospital and Vice President for Behavioral Health Services for the North Shore–Long Island Jewish Health System. He also holds the Dr. E. Richard Feinberg Chair in Schizophrenia Research at the Albert Einstein College of Medicine, where he is also Professor of Psychiatry, Neurology, and Neuroscience.

lies, and more evidence-based treatment guidelines have helped to make this process somewhat easier but still very difficult.

Ms. Fielding also illustrates an important point in conducting diagnostic interviews. There are patients who present in a manner such that clinicians might feel apologetic about asking certain questions and in some cases might be tempted to skip them because it seems so unlikely that certain symptoms or signs might be present. Clearly, for a patient such as Ms. Fielding, this would have been a serious mistake.

Although from a technical, diagnostic standpoint Ms. Fielding does not meet criteria for Schizophrenia, the duration is almost sufficient, and such a presentation would certainly not argue against the short-term use of antipsychotic medications.

I would choose to use a second-generation antipsychotic with recognition of the likelihood that Ms. Fielding would probably respond to lower doses than patients with multiepisode or chronic diagnosis. The possible occurrence of extrapyramidal symptoms is a particularly important concern in first-episode patients because early experiences with medication can have a strong influence on subsequent attitudes toward and compliance with pharmacotherapy. In fact, in a sample of first-episode patients, early-occurring parkinsonian side effects were the single most powerful predictor of subsequently stopping medication (Robinson et al. 2002). (Other significant predictors were lower socioeconomic status or educational level, depression, and poorer executive functioning on cognitive testing.)

Response to antipsychotic medication is often quite good in first-episode patients (in terms of positive symptoms such as delusions and hallucinations), although full response is often not as rapid as some clinicians expect. In the Hillside first-episode study, median time to response was 9 weeks (Robinson et al. 1999).

Unfortunately, in terms of social and vocational functioning, the results of treatment can be discouraging. In the same first-episode study, applying criteria for functional recovery (requiring relatively good, although not necessarily normal, functioning for 2 consecutive years), fewer than 20% of patients achieved this outcome after 5 years of follow-up (Robinson et al., in press).

The greatest challenge in treating first-episode patients is really a psychotherapeutic and psychosocial one. As with the onset of any devastating illness, the psychological consequences for the patient and family can be very serious. Personality and environmental factors can influence response to such circumstances, and the therapeutic team needs to work closely with the patient (and significant others when available) to manage the psychological and social sequelae. A psycho-educational approach is also critical in attempting to provide important knowledge about the disease and its treatment. Among the most difficult aspects is balancing the realities of the situation with some sense of optimism and possibility. To do so, it is important to focus on premorbid strengths that can be built on and to help the patient set reasonable and achievable goals to promote a sense of self-esteem and satisfaction. Because there are no consistent and highly powerful predictors of functional outcome, it is often difficult, however, to provide guidance as to realistic expectations.

Ideally, the clinical team should have considerable experience working with first-episode patients. It is often difficult for clinicians accustomed to treating chronic, multiepisode patients to be optimally sensitive to the special needs of first-episode patients and their families.

As alluded to previously, a critical decision with Ms. Fielding, once an acute response is obtained, is how long to continue antipsychotic medication. I am not aware of any data specifically focusing on Schizophreniform patients, but for individuals who meet the DSM-IV diagnosis for Schizophrenia, the data are compelling in suggesting high rates of relapse—82% after 5 years (Robinson et al. 1999). The single most powerful predictor of relapse was stopping antipsychotic medication (a fivefold greater risk among those who stopped compared to those who continued).

Treatment guidelines have not necessarily recommended maintaining pharmacotherapy for more than 1 year after recovery from a first episode, but these data would suggest that longer-term medication administration would be appropriate. Some past hesitation is probably due to the risk of tardive dyskinesia with conventional antipsychotics (Chakos et al. 1996), even within 1–2 years of the initiation of treatment. However, this risk appears to be substantially lower with the second-generation antipsychotics (Correll et al., in press).

One critical question in the management of such patients is what, if anything, can be done to protect against, diminish, or delay the "deterioration" in functioning that is often associated with Schizophrenia; are there strategies that, if applied early, can help in this regard? This is an area of research that remains promising but very difficult in terms of design, implementation, and interpretation.

If, for example, each subsequent relapse or exacerbation is associated with some biological and/or psychological sequelae leading to a poorer long-term outcome, then relapse prevention becomes an even more critical goal. As yet, the data in this regard are far from clear, and other aspects of whatever process(es) lead(s) to deterioration are far more hypothetical.

Clinicians can have some immediate impact on reducing rates of relapse, as discontinuing care and inadequate attention to medication adherence are obvious contributors. With regard to the latter, as previously mentioned, Robinson et al. (1999) in the Hillside first-episode program showed that those patients who discontinue medication after recovering from their first episode are five times more likely to relapse than those who continue. In some cases, such discontinuation may be due to physician uncertainty, but in many cases, it is due to nonadherence.

Clinicians are generally quite poor at identifying when and to what extent patients are nonadherent, and better methods to identify and manage this eventuality are sorely needed. Specific approaches to compliance, such as focused group sessions (Kemp et al. 1998), can be helpful, and, for some patients, the use of long-acting injectable medications should be considered (Kane et al. 2003). It can be particularly helpful for patients and families to talk to others who have been through similar experiences (e.g., the patient who stopped medication and subsequently relapsed). Such individuals can be powerful allies to the clinical team in explaining the importance of medication adherence.

As always, the ultimate treatment decisions should be consensual ones between the patient, significant others, and the clinical team based on an appropriate review of relevant benefits and risks of specific treatments or discontinuation of treatments.

References

Chakos MH, Alvir JM, Woerner MG: Incidence and correlates of tardive dyskinesia in first-episode schizophrenia. Arch Gen Psychiatry 53:313 319, 1996

Correll C, Leucht S, Kane JM: Reduced risk for tardive dyskinesia associated with second generation antipsychotics: a systematic review of one-year studies. Am J Psychiatry (in press)

Kane JM, Quitkin F, Rifkin A, et al: Fluphenazine versus placebo in patients with remitted acute first episode schizophrenia. Arch Gen Psychiatry 39:70–73, 1982

Kane JM, Eerdekens M, Lindenmayer JP, et al: Long-acting injectable risperidone: efficacy and safety of the first long-acting atypical antipsychotic. Am J Psychiatry 160:1–8, 2003

Kemp R, Kirov G, Everitt B, et al: Randomised controlled trial of compliance therapy: 18-month follow-up. Br J Psychiatry 172:413–419, 1998

Robinson DG, Woerner MG, Alvir JM, et al: Predictors of treatment response from a first episode of schizophrenia or schizoaffective disorder. Am J Psychiatry 156:544–549, 1999

Robinson DG, Woerner MG, Alvir JM, et al: Predictors of medication discontinuation by patients with first episode schizophrenia and schizoaffective disorder. Schizophr Res 57:209–219, 2002

Robinson DG, Woerner MG, McMeniman M, et al: Symptomatic and functional recovery from a first episode of schizophrenia or schizoaffective disorder. Am J Psychiatry (in press)

Sitting by the Fire

Paddy O'Brien is a 26-year-old bachelor, living with his mother and two older brothers on the family farm in the west of Ireland. He is interviewed as part of a family study of mental disorders in Ireland.

Paddy is described by his mother as having been a "normal" youngster up until 14. He was average to slightly below average in his schoolwork. He had friends he played with after school, and he helped his brothers and father with the chores around the farm. When he was 14, he began to "lose interest" in his schoolwork. His teacher noted that he was "staring into space" while in class and rarely followed the work. Soon thereafter, his mother noticed that he no longer played with his friends after school but would just come home and sit in front of the turf fire. It also became harder and harder to get him to do the farm chores. Sometimes he would come in and say the work was finished. Only hours later would they notice that only some of the cows had been milked or only some of the eggs collected.

When he was 16, because his condition had become progressively worse, Paddy was withdrawn from school and was admitted to the county psychiatric hospital. The hospital records indicate that he was socially withdrawn and had a flat affect. It was not possible to interest him in ward activities. No psychotic symptoms could be elicited.

Paddy has been in psychiatric care intermittently ever since that time. For the last year and a half, he has been attending a day care center 2 days a week.

When interviewed by the research team, Paddy is observed to be an obese, rather disheveled young man. He replies to most questions with a yes, no, or "could be." He denies any psychotic symptoms, feelings of depression or elation, or difficulty with appetite or energy. He does, however, admit to unspecified problems with his "nerves" and problems in sleeping. On probing, he admits to feeling uncomfortable around "people," except his family. Eye contact is poor; he looks at the floor during most of the interview. His affect is flat. Despite all attempts, the interviewer is unable to establish rapport with him.

252

he would be given a diagnosis of Schizoptypal Personality Disorder. In my experience clinically as well as in a research program that has entered hundreds of people with Schizotypal Personality Disorder, a history like that of Paddy almost invariably suggests a diagnosis of Schizophrenia when the patient is closely examined and followed. We have received referrals from numerous schizophrenia clinical research programs, as well as from outpatient clinics, of people who initially are presumed to have Schizophrenia but, because psychotic symptoms could not be elicited in the initial evaluation, were considered to be "schizotypal." In almost all of these cases, a thorough evaluation in our program did indeed establish a diagnosis of Schizophrenia.

There are two relatively common scenarios that occur that permit us to establish the diagnosis of Schizophrenia. Our evaluations with patients can take up to 7 or 8 hours over two sessions. We also conduct an evaluation with a close family member or friend who serves as an informant. Our interviews establish a rapport with these patients, who, over the course of the scheduled interviews, may reveal more of themselves than they do in their ordinary circumstances, in which they may be quite guarded. Often, even when family and psychiatric staff had not elicited any psychotic symptoms, patients will reveal delusions and hallucinations to our clinical raters in the context of an extended discussion of their history and problems. In other cases, we have sought and received permission to gather prior clinical records that do suggest some symptoms of psychosis despite reports from the mental health professionals currently treating the patient indicating that there are no and never have been such symptoms. On the basis of this experience, I am not persuaded that Paddy is indeed free of these symptoms based on the lack of psychotic symptoms reported to psychiatric staff or family.

However, it certainly is conceivable, and I have been convinced after extensive and longitudinal evaluation in other cases, that there are patients such as Paddy who indeed do not exhibit psychotic symptoms even after we have worked with them for a long time and know them quite well. I would agree with the discussion that such patients conform more to the traditional Bleulerian concept of simple schizophrenia and that the primary symptoms of autism, loose associations or other "thought disorder," and affective blunting are present in the absence of any secondary psychotic symptoms. I do not necessarily agree, however, that such patients have to be diagnosed with Schizotypal Personality Disorder, as the patients I have seen who would meet criteria for the older concept of simple schizophrenia also meet current DSM-IV-TR criteria for Schizophrenia. Because of their "thought disorder" and attendant disorganization, such patients generally meet criteria not only for negative symptoms, which Paddy clearly meets, but also for disorganized speech and/or behavior. It is noted in the discussion that Paddy's speech is "odd," but the extent of the disorganization, which is implied by the statement that he had "thought disorder," is not clear. My suspicion is that a closer examination of his thinking and speech pattern would suggest more than an unusual or odd speech style, such as more serious disorganization of thinking patterns. Furthermore, I would wonder, in light of the fact that Paddy was finding it increasingly difficult to do his chores at home, including milking the cows and collecting the eggs, and that he worked only for brief periods at simple tasks and occupational therapy, whether indeed he had serious praxis difficulties in organizing his behaviors to accomplish more complex tasks that he may have been able to complete before. Paddy's inability to bathe or change his clothes unless prompted also suggests rather gross disorganization of behavior. Thus, even without confirmation of underlying psychotic symptoms, which were not elicited in this case, I believe it is likely that Paddy's illness would still be diagnosed as schizophrenic. Another possibility is that his current clinical state is the prodrome of Schizophrenia, and the full-blown psychosis has yet to emerge.

The distinction between Schizophrenia and Schizotypal Personality Disorder is an important one, because Paddy's picture, as acknowledged, is typical of residual symptoms of chronic Schizophrenia and clearly reflects deterioration from a previous level of functioning. This is not what is ordinarily thought of as a "personality disorder" as stated in the discussion, whereas my experience with people meeting criteria for Schizotypal Personality Disorder is that rather than showing the pronounced deterioration from previous functioning described in Paddy's case, they indeed are people with maladaptive patterns of behavior and experiences that are relatively inflexible and lead to impairment that is relatively stable over time. Rather than being incapacitated as Paddy was, they are often, although certainly not always, employed in solitary occupations, including jobs such as a mail sorter, security guard, surveyor, technician, or computer analyst, which do not challenge their more limited interpersonal resources but do require a minimal degree of organization that is usually missing in Schizophrenia even in the face of relational detachment, cognitive/perceptional distortions, and eccentricity. They do exhibit fairly recognizable affective flattening or blunting, anhedonia, and profound interpersonal discomfort.

Rather than being misdiagnosed as having Schizophrenia, in most instances, people who truly meet criteria for Schizotypal Personality Disorder are more often misdiagnosed as dysthymic, chronically depressed, or socially phobic. Although they may have at some point in the past or may sometimes concurrently meet criteria for Mood or Anxiety Disorders, their interpersonal and occupational limitations extend clearly beyond any episodes of mood- or anxiety-related overt symptomatology. Their anhedonic flattening is mistaken for depression, and their detachment from others may be mistaken for social anxiety. However, their blunted affect persists even in the absence of any documented depressive mood or symptoms and is not generally responsive to standard antidepressant medication. Their social anxiety is not easily treated with pharmacologic intervention with selective serotonin reuptake inhibitors or cognitive-behavioral therapy used effectively for classic social anxiety, as this kind of anxiety does not lessen even with familiarity with the people whom they encounter. They are often left inadequately treated with doses of multiple antidepressants and mood stabilizers. It is only on close questioning that a pervasive suspiciousness, perhaps unusual perceptual symptoms, and relatively invariant social anxiety are established. Especially if psychotic-like symptoms are present, atypical antipsychotic medications can be helpful, not only for the more "positive" symptoms but also to a lesser degree for the underlying affective flattening and other negative symptoms, at least as suggested by available evidence from controlled clinical trials in schizotypal volunteers and patients. People who are relatives of individuals with chronic Schizophrenia may, in some instances, exhibit Schizotypal Personality Disorder or symptoms, but, again, it would be unusual if they showed the degree of impairment that Paddy displays. Indeed, the stereotype of Schizotypal Personality Disorder as an attenuated psychotic disorder (as in Paddy's case history)—close to Schizophrenia—does not reflect the negative symptoms commonly present in patients with the disorder. This misconception often interferes with the clinical recognition of schizotypal pathology. It is also worth noting that, in clinical treatment settings, the less dramatic schizotypal symptomatology may not be recognized because the clinician focuses on the more dramatic symptoms, such as prominent dysphoria, interpersonal difficulties, and social anxiety, that lead the patient to seek treatment.

There has been little systematic study of psychosocial treatments of people with Schizotypal Personality Disorder, and those studies that have been undertaken suggest only very modestly successful outcomes. There have been reports of using social skills training and supportive and behavioral interventions with people with this disorder. Cognitive remediation, which is beginning to be explored in the treatment of Schizophrenia, has not been tested in this population. In working with these patients, longer-term, supportive psychotherapies with some attempts at remediation and skills training may be helpful, but this is an area that requires empirical study.

Schizotypal Personality Disorder remains underdiagnosed and underrecognized in clinical and community settings and, as a result, has been understudied in terms of treatment options. It has served as a valuable resource in terms of understanding the underlying pathophysiology of the schizophrenia spectrum, and, indeed, people with Schizotypal Personality Disorder have been found to share cognitive, structural brain, and functional brain abnormalities with patients who have Schizophrenia.

Suggested Reading

Kirrane RM, Siever LJ: New perspectives on schizotypal personality disorder. Curr Psychiatry Rep 2:62–66, 2000

Siever LJ, Bernstein DP, Silverman JM: Schizotypal personality disorder, in DSM-IV Sourcebook, Vol 2. Edited by Widiger TA, Frances AJ, Pincus HA, et al. Washington, DC, American Psychiatric Association, 1996, pp 685–702

Siever LJ, Koenigsberg HW, Harvey P, et al: Cognitive and brain function in schizotypal personality disorder. Schizophr Res 54:157–167, 2002

Discussion of "Sitting by the Fire" by Ming Tsuang, M.D., Ph.D.*

Paddy's case highlights a variety of ideas about the schizophrenia spectrum, both past and present. The severity of his negative symptoms, their apparent onset at age 14 (with the resultant reduced level of function), and the absence of obvious positive psychotic symptoms are reminiscent of Schizophrenic Reaction, Simple Type, in DSM-I (called Schizophrenia, Simple Type, in DSM-II). The absence of psychosis is perhaps even more characteristic of Schizophrenic Reaction, Chronic Undifferentiated Type in DSM-I, which was called Schizophrenia, Latent Type, in DSM-II. Although psychosis has been a core diagnostic feature of Schizophrenia for much of the last century, recent DSMs make the requirement of psychosis more explicit for the diagnosis of Schizophrenia than did DSM-I or -II (Tsuang et al. 2000). A nonpsychotic disorder in the schizophrenia spectrum, such as Paddy's appears to be, is more likely to be classified currently as a Personality Disorder. In this case, DSM-IV-TR diagnostic criteria for Schizotypal Personality Disorder are met.

Three additional diagnostic issues should also be addressed. First, is this a typical case of Schizotypal Personality Disorder? Personality Disorders are usually considered to be lifelong problems, and, according

Dr. Tsuang is University Professor and Director of the Institute of Behavioral Genomics in the Department of Psychiatry at the University of California at San Diego; Director of the Harvard Institute of Psychiatric Epidemiology and Genetics in the Department of Epidemiology at the Harvard School of Public Health and Harvard Medical School Departments of Psychiatry at Massachusetts Mental Health Center and Massachusetts General Hospital in Boston, Massachusetts. Dr. Tsuang studied genetic epidemiology at the Institute of Psychiatry and Galton Laboratory at the University of London. He participated in the World Health Organization International Pilot Study of Schizophrenia in the 1960s to identify common characteristics of schizophrenia among nine different countries. He undertook a long-term field follow-up and family studies of Schizophrenia and Affective Disorders (Iowa 500) and atypical Schizophrenia (Iowa non-500) from 1972 to 1982 while he was running an inpatient service at the University of Iowa Psychiatric Hospital. He then moved to Brown University in 1982 and Harvard in 1985, where he continued his genetic epidemiological work on Schizophrenia and Mood Disorders, extending his research using molecular genetics, neuropsychology, and neuroimaging. His current interest is in the identification of people at risk for severe mental disorders. The ultimate goal is to use all of the research results on genetics and pre- and postnatal environmental factors to discover whether early identification of these severe mental disorders could lead to prevention of their onset in the future.

to his family, Paddy did not demonstrate symptoms until the age of 14. Actually, the extent to which this is true is unclear. We would want to know more about Paddy's interpersonal relationships before age 14, both at home and at school. For example, did he show evidence of social anxiety or acting-out behaviors that, especially compared to his later symptoms, seemed emotionally healthy? Also, we know that he may have been a below-average student, which raises the question of whether Paddy experienced any of the neuropsychological difficulties (e.g., in attention) that often occur in Schizotypal Personality Disorder (Voglmaier et al. 1997). Such "preschizotypal" symptoms often occur in children before the appearance of the more stable adult syndrome (Olin et al. 1997). Even in the absence of childhood precursors, however, Paddy's symptoms, once they occurred, remained stable for the 12-year period covered by the vignette. This in itself is consistent with his diagnosis. Although no mention is made of similar symptoms in other members of Paddy's family, confidence in his diagnosis might also increase if we knew whether other members of his family demonstrated evidence of any related psychiatric conditions.

The second diagnostic issue involves the severity of the symptoms. Can Paddy's inability to function since the age of 14 result from Schizotypal Personality Disorder? The answer appears to be yes. The absence of psychotic symptoms and the stability of the negative symptoms, however severe, are certainly consistent with the conception of a severe Personality Disorder that prevents normal functioning in daily life. Moreover, Paddy's difficulties emphasize a dimensional component to the disorder, whereby symptoms exist on a continuum of severity. The third diagnostic issue is related to the second one. Can Schizotypal Personality Disorder present primarily as a cluster of negative symptoms? In fact, we have argued elsewhere that Schizotypal Personality Disorder with mainly negative symptoms ("negative schizotypal personality disorder") may be considered as a subtype of Schizotypal Personality Disorder (Tsuang et al. 2002a). This conception may be a particularly useful construct, both as a meaningful clinical syndrome and as a marker of the liability to Schizophrenia. Thus, while Paddy's clinical presentation may not be modal, it is consistent with the DSM-IV-TR diagnosis of Schizotypal Personality Disorder.

Nevertheless, a first treatment recommendation would be to obtain a neurological evaluation to rule out other kinds of problems (e.g., a metabolic disorder or a cerebrovascular problem). He would also benefit from a clinical neuropsychological evaluation to determine whether cognitive deficits contribute to his clinical picture. Assuming that no other disorders can account for Paddy's symptoms, how would we approach treatment? Several modalities would be appropriate, but medication is a reasonable place to start. Based on evidence that Schizotypal Personality Disorder is actually in the schizophrenia spectrum (Tsuang et al. 1999), the spectrum disorder is likely to share at least some common psychopathological and pathophysiological elements with Schizophrenia. The same reasoning leads to the view that treatments that alleviate symptoms in Schizophrenia will also do so in schizophrenia spectrum disorders. Antipsychotic medications are thus a good starting point. Typical neuroleptics are not likely to be useful in treating negative symptoms and may cause significant side effects. They are better for treating positive symptoms, but Paddy showed few positive and no obvious psychotic symptoms. One of the newer antipsychotic medications, however, might be helpful.

We used this logic in a pilot study to treat nonpsychotic, adult relatives of patients with Schizophrenia (Tsuang et al. 2002b). These individuals were all first-degree relatives of a patient with Schizophrenia, who themselves had not met DSM-IV diagnostic criteria for any Schizophrenia-related psychiatric diagnosis. They all had negative symptoms and neuropsychological deficits, which means that their symptoms were similar to Paddy's, at least in part, although milder. The subjects received low doses of risperidone for 6 weeks. Side effects were temporary and mainly mild. Out of six subjects (who were approved for this treatment by our Human Subject's Committee), five showed reductions of negative symptoms and improvements in attention. The one subject who did not show improvement had an IQ score in the borderline range of cognitive ability and may not have been able to benefit from treatment. Although larger, well-controlled studies are needed before antipsychotic medications can be recommended for nonpsychotic patients on a routine basis, Paddy is a good candidate for such treatment. As for the subjects described above, a low dose of risperidone or another of the newer antipsychotic medications is recommended for Paddy. The treatment should be explained to Paddy as an attempt to treat his attention and memory difficulties so that he may enjoy more of the world around him. The dose will need to be titrated to minimize side effects.

Other types of treatments should also be considered. If, as is likely, Paddy has neuropsychological deficits, a number of compensations are possible to improve his attention, organize his thoughts, and help him remember new information. For example, he could be taught to centralize important information in a "memory notebook," which is a strategy that is useful for people with Attention-Deficit/Hyperactivity Disorder and related conditions. He could also learn to make an outline before attempting a new task to obtain the "big picture." Strategies such as these will not help, however, until his negative symptoms are reduced and he attains higher levels of energy and motivation. Similarly, focused cognitive-behavioral psychotherapeutic approaches will help Paddy function better inside and outside his home, but only after a successful course of psychopharmacological treatment.

The real question here, then, is whether medication will work well enough to allow the use of other forms of treatment. Unfortunately, we are only just learning how to use medication effectively in nonpsychotic conditions and especially in ones as severe as Paddy's. Therefore, a trial and error approach will be needed. My experience with both mild and severe conditions in the schizophrenia spectrum, however, tells me that this looks like the right general direction in which to go at this point.

References

Olin SS, Raine A, Cannon TD, et al: Childhood behavior precursors of schizotypal personality disorder. Schizophr Bull 23:93–103, 1997

Tsuang MT, Stone WS, Faraone SV: Schizophrenia: a review of genetic studies. Harv Rev Psychiatry 7:185–207, 1999

Tsuang MT, Stone WS, Faraone SV: Towards reformulating the diagnosis of schizophrenia. Am J Psychiatry 147:1041–1050, 2000

Tsuang MT, Stone WS, Tarbox SI, et al: An integration of schizophrenia with schizotypy: identification of schizotaxia and implications for research on treatment and prevention. Schizophr Res 54(1–2):169–175, 2002a

Tsuang MT, Stone WS, Tarbox SI, et al: Treatment of nonpsychotic relatives of patients with schizophrenia: a pilot study. Neuropsychiatric Genetics 114(8):943–948, 2002b

Voglmaier MM, Seidman LJ, Salisbury D, et al: Neuropsychological dysfunction in schizotypal personality disorder: a profile analysis. Biol Psychiatry 41:530–540, 1997

Goody Two Shoes

Maryann West is an attractive, single, 35-year-old woman, originally from San Diego, now working as a magazine editor and living by herself in a deteriorating Boston neighborhood. She was referred for psychotherapy by her female family doctor, who suggested she needed to work on problems in her relationships with men. Maryann resisted following through on the referral for a year, saying, "I don't like getting help. I like giving it."

When interviewed, Maryann appeared to be highly intelligent; she was affable and articulate and spoke in a breathy, girlish voice. She had metal-black hair, was dressed all in black—leather skirt and jacket and black top—and wore "punkish" glasses. She said, at the beginning of the interview, that she didn't want a male therapist because she was mistrustful of men, who, in her experience, wanted only to exploit women. However, with the exception of her family doctor, she had no close women friends.

Her story was that she had just extricated herself from a "destructive" relationship with a man, "my outlaw love," who was a heroin addict, and she was fighting her wish to return to him. Once, 4 years earlier, he had hit her and made her cry, but she told him that if he did that again, she would leave, and it never recurred. She claimed she was not frightened of him and actually blamed herself for his attacking her. "I often tell him things he should know about himself, and he gets furious. I only do it to motivate him. I hit his soft spot."

Her lover's addiction persisted, and Maryann continued to support him financially whenever he needed help. She said she received many indications that this relationship could not make her happy. The man had gone out with other women while dating Maryann, served a brief jail sentence for selling drugs, and never wanted to engage in mutually entertaining activities, except sex, which was enjoyable. Maryann had gone to a university, but her lover had never completed high school. She felt that he was like a little child who needed mothering. He would tell her to get lost when she insisted he stop using drugs, but she continued to call him regularly in spite of his ungrateful behavior. She felt resentful and embittered because of all she had done for him, but she always helped him when he, typically, came back to her, late at night, asking for money or assistance. As a result, she said she felt "more like a Mother Teresa than a girlfriend."

Maryann is now seeing another "exciting" man, also a substance abuser. Although she considers herself "left-wing," her new friend is a collector of Nazi memorabilia. She knew that he treated his previous girlfriend cruelly by being unfaithful and abusive but didn't think about whether this might happen to her. She has seen this man on and off for a year. He insisted he wanted a close relationship but did not tell her he was seeing one of her acquaintances on the side. When she found out about this, she was very upset but continues to have an intense interest in him. A number of nicer men who had monogamous intentions have tried to date her, but she has avoided them because they were all "boring."

In her other relationships, Maryann always gives help, but never asks for it, even when she is in real need. Most of her friends and ex-boyfriends have been drug addicts or ex-addicts. She herself has never abused drugs. She often visits these people in jail and offers to help them, but when they are released, they hardly ever visit her.

At her job, Maryann is hardworking and good at solving disputes, but she has sometimes gotten into trouble with her boss for arranging to use the magazine's resources to raise money for needy groups. She feels that her female colleagues "gang up on her" because of envy of her abilities and capacity for hard work, in spite of all the benefits that she has helped them obtain.

Maryann is the oldest of four children and often had to grudgingly care for her younger siblings. She became a "goody two shoes," whereas her younger brothers were permitted to "act up." In church and school she did well and won many awards, until she was in her teens, when she rebelled and left home. Her parents predicted she would "go to hell." She went through a period of "sexual liberation" during which she had about 50 lovers, often in one-night stands, which she rarely enjoyed "because I didn't love those guys." As a young adult she was always involved in some worthy cause for the underprivileged, the poor, or the politically disadvantaged.

DSM-IV-TR Casebook Diagnosis of "Goody Two Shoes"

Maryann seems to have gone through life playing the role of martyr. She has repeatedly been attracted to and chosen boyfriends who were inappropriate and mistreated her. She does not like to take help from others, and this has delayed her seeking treatment, even though she has realized for a long time that her relationships with people are harmful to her. She incites angry responses from others and then feels hurt when she is rejected (telling her boyfriend his failings). She is not interested in boyfriends who treat her well because they are "boring," and she engages in excessive self-sacrifice that is unsolicited by the recipients (visiting people in jail).

Behavior that appears to an outside observer as "self-defeating" may be observed when a person is in a situation in which he or she is afraid of being psychologically or physically abused, or when a person is depressed. In Maryann's case, however, it seems to be a pervasive personality pattern that expresses itself in many situations and relationships of her own choosing. This personality pattern has been called masochistic personality or self-defeating personality disorder. Many clinicians, particularly those who do psychodynamically oriented treatment of Personality Disorders, believe that this is a common and important diagnosis, which is nearly as common in males as in females. On the other hand, many clinicians, particularly those concerned with the potential for misuse of psychiatric diagnoses, have argued that the underlying construct of the disorder has no validity and that the diagnosis perpetuates blaming victims (primarily females) who have been abused. The category was included in an appendix of DSM-III-R after much controversy but was eliminated entirely from DSM-IV. Such a case can still be diagnosed according to DSM-IV-TR as Personality Disorder Not Otherwise Specified (DSM-IV-TR, p. 729).

Discussion of "Goody Two Shoes" by Arnold M. Cooper, M.D.*

One of the great puzzles of human psychology is the irresistible attraction of some people to situations and persons that are damaging to themselves. This behavior, known for many years as *self-defeating* or *masochistic* behavior, constitutes a prominent—often the most prominent—aspect of some individuals' personalities. Unfortunately, although the term *masochism* was coined by Kraft-Ebbing with reference to Sacher-Masoch's description of a man in an utterly self-destructive enslaving love for a woman, historically the term came to be confused with attitudes of passivity and self-abasement that, during much of the nineteenth and early twentieth centuries, were associated with femininity. At the time of the construction of DSM-III, a time of heightened feminist activism, the concept of masochism was opposed because of the fear that it would be a diagnosis used to pathologize victimized women. Women, it was held, would be labeled masochistic and held responsible for their abuse and exploitation by men. There are no studies that clarify the issue of gender ratios in self-defeating personality disorder. It is, however, the opinion of many clinicians that as many males as females present with prominent self-defeating character traits. Unfortunately, the absence of the diagnosis in DSM-IV has inhibited a focused research attempt to understand better this very complex disorder.

Psychoanalytic literature has used the word *masochism* in two quite different ways. *Perversion masochism* refers to attraction to sexual practices that involve experiencing pain and/or fear. *Masochistic personality disorder* refers to a character type in which self-defeating or self-damaging behaviors are prominent.

Dr. Cooper is the Stephen P. Tobin and Dr. Arnold M. Cooper Professor Emeritus in Consultation Liaison Psychiatry at Cornell Weill Medical College. He is a Supervising and Training Analyst at the Columbia University Psychoanalytic Center for Training and Research. He is a past President of the American Psychoanalytic Association. He has served as North American Editor of the International Journal of Psychoanalysis. *From 1993 to 2003, he was Deputy Editor of the* American Journal of Psychiatry. *He has been an Adjunct Professor of Comparative Literature at Columbia University. He is a widely published author and has been especially interested in psychoanalytic theory and technique and the psychotherapy of narcissistic and masochistic personality disorders.*

Maryann demonstrates several typical features of self-defeating personality disorder:

1. Relationships that are predictably disappointing, dangerous, or damaging are repetitively sought.
2. What for another individual would be a warning sign of trouble and lead to avoidance is an attraction leading to engagement.
3. The prospect of repeated damage is overtly or secretly "exciting," or "gratifying."
4. The individual creates a pseudomoral justification for self-damaging behavior. (Maryann claims to be helping people, although in her intimate relationships the more prominent feature is the damage to herself.)
5. There is a spectacular inability to learn from experience.

The brief case description omits another typical aspect of this behavior—a period of angry depression and feelings of innocent victimization that follows the perceived mistreatment, self-damage, and disappointment. Usually relationships end with angry and bitter feelings of hurt ("I have been taken advantage of again") and the feeling of being unappreciated.

Edmund Bergler (1961) some years ago described what he called the "oral triad" or the mechanism of injustice collecting, a three-step process that rather well describes the behavior of a large group of patients with self-defeating personality disorder. These individuals 1) either by the misuse of an existing situation or by provocation and the creation of a new damaging situation experience actual or fantasized injury to themselves, quite unaware of their role in making themselves the victim; 2) in an effort to ward off the guilt of inner accusations of responsibility for their self-defeat, respond with "pseudo-aggression," a display of aggressive-seeming activity that, because it is poorly timed or poorly dosed, results, in fact, in an increase of the original damage; and 3) then subside into a self-pitying depressive state of feeling personally singled out for unfair treatment, unlucky, and not responsible.

I have written of these patients as "narcissistic-masochistic characters" (Cooper 1988) referring to the struggle of these individuals to maintain a sense of narcissistic well-being and control in childhood situations in which they felt the passive victims of powerful adults denying them gratification. In effect, they maintain a sense of power by taking over the task of hurting themselves before anyone else can do it.

They attempt, unconsciously, to perceive their victimizers as doing their bidding rather than their being the passive recipients of abuse. They salvage remnants of self-esteem by putting themselves in charge of their deprivation. This psychic situation is further complicated by their inner guilt over secretly deriving some satisfaction from their manipulation of their own self-damage.

These patients may also attempt, defensively, to perceive themselves or have others label them as the active aggressor (e.g., Maryann in black leather and "punkish" glasses). Close examination reveals that they are, in most areas of their lives, conspicuously passive and unable to assert themselves appropriately. Maryann is not advancing in her job, despite her intelligence. Provocative aggressive behaviors, which are often inappropriately dosed and timed (i.e., striking out at a lover who will hit her back harder)—starting fights that cannot be won—substitute for genuine self-assertion.

Except that Maryann was the coerced caretaker of her younger brothers, we lack any detailed developmental history, family or interpersonal history, or exploration of her inner life, her fantasies, or her dreams. One might guess that further investigation would reveal that beneath Maryann's facade of helping people is a bitter burning anger and that the show of helping is designed as unconscious demonstration of how every time she helps she is exploited, which is perhaps how she regarded her childhood setting. She probably has unconscious fantasies, or even conscious memories, of being the unloved, abused child and believes that even her self-sacrifice was not appreciated. Maryann goes through life making this point over and over again.

To the extent that Maryann flirts with violence and is overtly attracted to potentially violent situations, she departs from the more usual characterological self-defeating disorder. She is atypical in her flirtation with psychopathy, drugs, breaking the law, and violence. The battered-woman syndrome, which is something that Maryann may be heading toward, is not the prototypical case of self-defeating personality disorder. The absence of close or lasting friendships is important and may indicate more borderline features that are not necessarily typical of the self-defeating personality. If we make an assumption that her repetitive behaviors represent some combination of wishes and defenses, then her "helping" behavior conceals her identification with those who need help, and she is enacting what she wishes would be done for her but never is. By choosing people on the fringes of society as "friends" to receive her charitable ministration—people who are unstable and unsuccessful—she wards off any possibility of intimacy, which she feels incapable of, and supports a fragile self-esteem by being superior to her dependents and avoiding relationships that would reveal the emptiness and inadequacy that she feels about herself. This may be an indicator of the depth of her self-loathing—the sense that no one could be her friend—as well as a somewhat paranoid conviction that everyone else is untrustworthy, exploitive, and undeserving of her friendship. One would guess that there is a significant history of physical, sexual, or emotional abuse in her family history and an unconscious personality structure in which she perceives herself as an undesired, unlovable child dependent on unloving parents whom she sees as the only people in the world who could tolerate her. She carries on a pseudo-rebellious stance, whereas she is in actuality enslaving herself.

Maryann is averse to treatment and is likely to break off a number of psychotherapies before she ups the ante of her self-damage and becomes even more provocative at work than she has been, thereby getting into serious trouble. I would predict she would then be overtly depressed, and then therapy would have some leverage.

She is a candidate for a trial of psychodynamic psychotherapy at a minimum of twice or, preferably, three times a week. Any treatment less intensive than this has almost no chance of breaking through the armor of her moralistic, self-pitying defenses and her unconscious attraction to harm under the guise of excitement. A course of cognitive-behavioral therapy might also be helpful and less frightening initially. Treatment will be difficult, and one can predict endless provocation, both angry and sexual, of the therapist. It will be important early in treatment to try to assess her capacity for introspection.

Her pose of "tough guy," her remoteness from any warm interpersonal engagement, and her gratification from her pose as "rebel" are indications of a fragile self-structure to which she clings rather desperately with the accompanying inner fear that she is otherwise empty and powerless. It will be important for the therapist to establish early on a rather paradoxical stance of sympathetic understanding of the need for her behaviors and the impossibility of her immediately relinquishing them, while simultaneously being able to give her a clear sense of the therapist's capacity to "see through" her facade and understand both her fragility and the ferocity of her self-damaging campaign. She will make every effort to sabotage the treatment, just as she has sabotaged every human relationship in which she has ever participated. It would probably be useful to predict these efforts to her and to inform her in advance that they are behaviors to be understood and not simply enacted. Psychotherapy with these patients is complex and, in my experience, rarely brief. The same self-defeating patterns of their lives are carried out in their therapy, and the patient is likely to find multiple causes for grievance against the therapist, proving his or her ineptitude and helplessness and finding many subtle ways of attempting to provoke the therapist into anger or neglect. One can hope, through the therapy, to help the patient to begin to see the self-defeating pattern of his or her behavior and to develop an awareness of the unconscious sense of injury that is maintained to help shift the balance of inner guilt from self-punitive behaviors to self-restraining ones.

There is no evidence that pharmacologic interventions are helpful for treating patients with self-defeating personality disorder. These individuals are prone to depression at one time or another, and medication may then be useful, although most of these depressions are transient. It is my clinical perception that, for a subgroup of these patients who also have dysthymia, antidepressant medication seems to help ameliorate the chronic resentment that they experience. Treatment efforts for Maryann should include gathering a far more complete history of her early and current relationships, a careful description from her of why she thinks her relationships and her life always go wrong, and the available evidence from her of the degree to which she is conflicted about her performance in the important areas of her life. Is Maryann disappointed by her personal and vocational failures? What are or were her ambitions? Does she have positive feelings for anyone? The prognosis is better if there is a history of her having had some emotionally meaningful and supportive relationships at some point in her life.

The odds are high that several attempts will be required before she is able to participate constructively in treatment. It is possible that, because of her quasi-antisocial attitudes, a group therapy with other chronic "losers" might help Maryann shed her protective fantasy that she is a rebel against bourgeois society, when in fact she is only injuring herself.

It is unfortunate that self-defeating personality disorder is not a part of DSM. I will not attempt to go through all the arguments, pro or con, but will suggest that the two major reasons for excluding it—1) that it was directed against women and 2) that it was merely a side effect of all neurotic behaviors—are, I believe, invalid. The disorder is at least equally prominent among males, and one has little difficulty separating out those for whom the pursuit of self-damage is preeminent, therefore distinguishing them from individuals with other neurotic patterns that are also damaging. Further research on self-defeating personality disorder—unlikely with its exclusion from DSM-IV—would be a blessing.

References

Bergler E: Curable and Incurable Neurotics. New York, Liveright, 1961

Cooper A: The narcissistic masochistic character, in Masochism: Current Psychological Perspectives. Edited by Glick RA, Myers DI. Hillsdale, NJ, The Analytic Press, 1988

A Perfect Checklist

Billy, a 7-year-old child, was brought to a mental health clinic by his mother because "he is unhappy and always complaining about feeling sick." He lives with his parents, his younger brother, and his grandmother. His mother describes Billy as a child who has never been very happy and never wanted to play with other children. From the time he started nursery school, he has complained about stomachaches, headaches, and various other physical problems. They are most intense in the morning when he is getting ready to go to school. In the last few months, his somatic complaints have escalated, prompting a complete medical examination, including a neurologic examination and electro-encephalogram, all of which were normal.

Billy did well in first grade, but in second grade he is now having difficulty completing his work. He takes a lot of time to do his assignments and frequently feels he has to do them over again so that they will be "perfect." Because of Billy's frequent somatic complaints, it is hard to get him off to school in the morning. If he is allowed to stay home, he worries that he is falling behind in his schoolwork. When he does go to school, he often is unable to do the work, which makes him feel hopeless about his situation. In order to get through the day, he carries a note that he has instructed his mother to write for him: "You are not getting out of school early today. If you feel that you have to do your papers over and over again, please just do the best you can. Do not think about the time of day and it will go quickly."

His worries have expanded beyond school, and frequently he is clinging and demanding of his parents. He is fearful that if his parents come home late or leave and go somewhere without him, something may happen to them. For the past 2 weeks, he has insisted that his little brother sleep with him because he is afraid to go to sleep at night alone.

Although Billy's mother acknowledges that he has never been really happy, in the last 6 months, she feels, he has become much more depressed. He frequently lies around the house, saying that he is too tired to do anything. He has no interest or enjoyment in playing. His appetite has diminished. He has trouble falling asleep at night and often wakes up in the middle of the night or early in the morning. Three weeks ago, he talked, for the first time, about wanting to die and said that maybe he would shoot himself.

Billy's mother became pregnant 2 months after she was married. She did not feel ready for a child. She was hypertensive during the pregnancy and was emotionally upset. Delivery was complicated because of increasing hypertension. At the time of delivery, Billy reportedly went into cardiac arrest. During the first week of his life, he developed projectile vomiting, which persisted for 2 weeks. He had nocturnal enuresis until a year ago.

During the assessment, Billy allowed his mother to go to another room to be interviewed, but after 20 minutes, he became very upset, began crying, and insisted on being taken to her. He then was willing to sit outside the room where his mother was, as long as the door was open and he could see her.

Billy was unable to finish a symptom checklist (designed for children his age) given at the time of the evaluation. He felt that he had to have a perfect checklist and requested that he be allowed to take the papers home so that he could finish them. He became very worried about not being able to complete the list, and although he was told that it was not necessary for him to take the papers home, he insisted on doing so.

DSM-IV-TR Casebook Diagnosis of "A Perfect Checklist"

This case was submitted as an example of Dysthymic Disorder in a child with a recent superimposed Major Depressive Episode. There is little doubt about the latter, because Billy is clearly depressed; has lost interest and enjoyment in playing; and has trouble sleeping, poor appetite, low energy, and suicidal thoughts. In cases such as this, in which there has been a long history of depressed mood before the onset of a full depressive syndrome, the question is whether to regard the chronically depressed mood as a prodrome of the Major Depressive Disorder or to make another diagnosis of Dysthymic Disorder. The DSM-IV-TR rule is that, in a child, a 1-year period of sustained depressed mood or irritable mood accompanied by at least three symptoms of the dysthymic syndrome justifies an additional diagnosis of Dysthymic Disorder. In Billy's case, however, we do not have enough information about specific symptoms before the recent episode of Major Depressive Disorder to justify the diagnosis of Dysthymic Disorder. Because this is the first episode and the symptoms cause marked impairment in functioning, the diagnosis would be Major Depressive Disorder, Single Episode, Severe Without Psychotic Features (DSM-IV-TR, p. 375).

Billy has many other symptoms, including perfectionism, worrying about his performance in school, somatic complaints, and anxiety about being separated from his mother. The perfectionism raises the question of Obsessive-Compulsive Personality Disorder or Obsessive-Compulsive Disorder. He is too young to be considered for a Personality Disorder diagnosis, and there is no evidence of frank obsessions or compulsions. His worrying about his work and school performance, accompanied by somatic complaints, suggests the additional diagnosis of Generalized Anxiety Disorder. However, because these symptoms apparently occur only during the presence of a Mood Disorder, the DSM-IV-TR rule is to regard these symptoms as associated features of the Mood Disorder, rather than as an independent Anxiety Disorder.

The diagnosis of Separation Anxiety Disorder (DSM-IV-TR, p. 125) requires at least three of eight symptoms of excessive anxiety concerning separation from those to whom the child is attached. We count at least four: unrealistic worry about possible harm befalling major attachment figures, reluctance to go to school, avoidance of being alone (including clinging), and complaints of physical symptoms on school days.

The many somatic complaints suggest Undifferentiated Somatoform Disorder, but a more parsimonious approach is to regard these symptoms as a manifestation of either the Separation Anxiety Disorder or the Major Depressive Disorder.

Discussion of "A Perfect Checklist" by Rachel Klein, Ph.D.*

Billy has an unusual presentation for a child of 7 years. The picture of separation anxiety is typical enough in that Billy worries that something bad will happen to his parents and thinks it has happened when they are delayed or out without him. However, the comorbid perfectionistic and depressive symptoms are not common in early childhood.

Billy cannot sleep alone and requires the presence of his younger brother. It is almost always the case that sleep is affected in children with Separation Anxiety Disorder. Nighttime is a relatively stressful time for young children in general. They are left alone in the dark without immediate access to their parents. Evolution probably did not program us to sleep in our own rooms away from caretakers at an early age. If so, it is understandable that nighttime is especially provocative for children with separation anxiety.

In addition, Billy has stomachaches and other physical complaints. The form and timing of Billy's somatic symptoms are very common in children with separation anxiety. Note that the symptoms emerged when Billy started nursery school—a major separation experience for a young child. Also, children typically present with gastrointestinal distress (stomachaches, nausea, and even vomiting) rather than cardiovascular symptoms, commonly reported by anxious adults. At the time we meet Billy, his physical complaints are worse in anticipation of separation—while preparing to leave for school.

It is important to emphasize that children with Separation Anxiety Disorder are anxious not only during separation events but also while they anticipate them. Anticipatory anxiety is manifested, in part, through physical symptoms. Thus, in my opinion, Billy's clinical picture is not somatic complaints associated with a depressive or Generalized Anxiety Disorder. If they were, they would not have a relationship to imminent separation experiences, as is the case with Billy.

---

*Dr. Klein is Professor of Psychiatry and Director of the Institute for Anxiety and Mood Disorders at the Child Study Center of the New York University School of Medicine. Dr. Klein began her research with children with Anxiety Disorders in the 1970s and has continued her studies ever since. She has contributed to the field through controlled treatment and longitudinal studies of children and adolescents with Anxiety Disorders. In addition, Dr. Klein was a major contributor to the formulation of childhood Anxiety Disorders from DSM-III on. Under the aegis of a grant from the National Institute of Mental Health, with colleagues, she is studying children who are at high risk for Anxiety Disorders.

Billy's perfectionistic and depressive symptoms are unusual for a young child. Perfectionism is not common in young children. The fact that the perfectionistic concerns are reported to revolve only around Billy's performance in school is also unusual (I view the request to fill out a self-rating scale as analogous to a school assignment). He is not reported to have unrealistic standards about any other expectation or situation. For diagnostic and therapeutic purposes, it would be helpful to know whether Billy is nervous about doing school-related tasks even if no one is going to see what he has done. If someone is perfectionistic, the self-imposed tyranny of doing things "just so" occurs whether someone else will view the work or not. If unreasonable concerns about performance arise in situations in which the work will be judged or graded, they indicate performance anxiety, which is a form of Social Anxiety Disorder.

The information about Billy that is provided to us is insufficient to select a differential diagnosis between perfectionism and performance anxiety. This issue has treatment implications. For example, if we were dealing with social anxiety, we would provide Billy with corrective experiences through analogue performance situations in which he would be assisted to make mistakes and experience others' benign reactions. If we were dealing with perfectionism, a similar approach to making the child produce imperfect work would be applied without the added social intervention. In the latter instance, it would be important to involve the parents in performing certain homework assignments with Billy to help him risk performing less than perfectly. These approaches require considerable cooperation from the parents and the child. From the clinical summary, Billy seems highly motivated to control his difficulties, because he values carrying a note from his mother reassuring him. This augurs well for his progress.

Billy's depressive symptoms are classic. However, it would be informative to know whether his sleep and appetite problems are present during school holidays. Often, children with severe separation anxiety have unusual sleep patterns and become poor eaters during the school year. These normalize when the child is out of school. The same does not occur in depression. In sum, knowledge about Billy's functioning during school vacations would clarify whether the sleep and appetite changes are more related to depression or anxiety.

Because Billy is so distressed and appears anhedonic, it is legitimate to consider medication as a first-line treatment. There is now evidence of efficacy for selective serotonin reuptake inhibitors (SSRIs) to treat childhood depression and anxiety. Billy seems to be an excellent candidate for such treatment. In addition, one would attempt to treat Billy with behavior modification. To address the separation anxiety, together with Billy, the therapist would identify separation events that Billy was willing to attempt. Such events would include being taken to his room at night by his mother, staying with her in his room for a few minutes, and then remaining alone in the room for a specified short interval until mother returns. Essentially, a plan of graduated exposure would be implemented. It is critical to involve the child in the process, because a hallmark of anxiety is dread of uncertainty. The child must know exactly what he or she has agreed to try. Moreover, no changes can be made (through requests by parents or teachers). This is done to reassure the child that there will be no surprises. The treatment progresses with gradual increases in separation experiences. In most children, this treatment is very effective in altering their resistance to separation. However, many patients remain uncomfortable, and there is still an undercurrent of anxiety, even though it is not manifest in overt behavior. In such cases, it is helpful to add medication to remove all, or at least most, traces of anxiety.

There are several SSRIs available, and there is no evidence of them having distinct efficacy. However, it is, in general, wise to use a short-acting medication, such as sertraline or fluvoxamine, in children because disinhibition is not an uncommon side effect. If disinhibition occurs during treatment with a long-acting SSRI, it will not disappear quickly on discontinuation of the medication. For this reason, a short-acting compound is preferable. Although, in general, it is good practice to hold off medication in depressed and anxious children until behavioral treatment has been attempted for a few weeks, Billy's condition is so severe and chronic that the immediate use of medication seems to be indicated.

I would suggest delaying treatment of Billy's perfectionistic symptoms until his depression and separation anxiety symptoms are alleviated. It is entirely possible that they will disappear when he no longer experiences separation anxiety and his mood has normalized. If not, then behavioral exposure interventions will be appropriate. To institute these interventions from the start might pose too much of a burden to the child and the family. It is often best to be patient and tackle one set of problems at a time when applying exposure treatment.

Billy's treatment requires the involvement of his family. Parents often fail to appreciate the nature of their child's difficulties, and having the child explain what he or she feels often decompresses the tension between the parent and child and the parents' exasperation at their child's inability to perform ordinary behaviors comfortably, such as going to school or sleeping in his or her bed. Also, it is important for Billy's parents to learn skills that will facilitate his ability to push himself to overcome his fears and anxieties. Often, and understandably, parents accommodate the child's difficulties—for example, in Billy's case, insisting that his brother sleep in his room. Billy's parents need assistance and support designed to promote his comfort and well-being to establish appropriate expectations of the child. In addition, because Billy is so anxious in school, it is appropriate to involve his teachers in efforts to help him cope better. To develop an appropriate plan, we would need more information about exactly what happens to Billy in school—what his worries and concerns are. Are his concerns only about his performance, or are they also about his mother's welfare? If the latter is true, it may be helpful to allow Billy to call home at specified times (but at no other times). This is just an example, and other strategies might be indicated. These decisions require the understanding of school personnel and cannot be made without their cooperation.

Thus, Billy's treatment should not be focused on him alone. It should involve his parents—at least his mother—and possibly the school as well.

Suggested Reading

Gittelman R, Klein DF: Childhood separation anxiety and adult agoraphobia, in Anxiety and the Anxiety Disorders. Edited by Tuma AH, Maser JD. Hillsdale, NJ, Laurence Erlbaum, 1985, pp 389–402

Gittelman-Klein R, Klein DF: Controlled imipramine treatment of school phobia. Arch Gen Psychiatry 25:204–207, 1971

Gittelman-Klein R, Klein DF: Separation anxiety in school refusal and its treatment with drugs, in Out of School. Edited by Hersov L, Berg I. London, Wiley, 1980, pp 321–341

Klein RG: Is panic disorder associated with childhood separation anxiety disorder? Clin Neuropharmacol 18 (suppl 2):7–14, 1995

Klein RG, Pine DS: Anxiety disorders, in Child and Adolescent Psychiatry: Modern Approaches. Edited by Rutter M, Taylor E. London, Blackwell Science, 2002, pp 486–509

Klein RG, Koplewicz HS, Kanner A: Imipramine treatment of children with separation anxiety disorder. J Am Acad Child Adolesc Psychiatry 31:21–28, 1992

Pine DS, Coplan JD, Papp LA, et al: Ventilatory physiology of children and adolescents with anxiety disorders. Arch Gen Psychiatry 55:123–129, 1998

The RUPP Anxiety Study Group: Fluvoxamine treatment of anxiety disorders in children and adolescents. N Engl J Med 344:1279–1285, 2001

The RUPP Anxiety Study Group: Treatment of pediatric anxiety disorders: an open-label extension of the research units on pediatric psychopharmacology anxiety study. J Child Adolesc Psychopharmacol 12:175–188, 2002

Frustrated Librarian

Mr. Jones, a 47-year-old married librarian with a strong family history of depression, presented for treatment when he became so fatigued and anxious that he was unable to work. He slept excessively, felt anxious, was unable to concentrate, and sometimes thought life was not worth living. Mr. Jones had previously had several bouts of depression with marked anergia that remitted after 6–8 months without treatment. His only medical problem was mild hypertension, which was well controlled on atenolol, 50 mg/day. He drank alcohol infrequently and had no history of mania or hypomania. He was once treated for depression with imipramine, but he stopped using it because of intolerable dry mouth, constipation, and worsened anxiety. Mr. Jones had entered psychotherapy once before but stopped the therapy because he was embarrassed to talk about his problems. Treatment with fluoxetine, 20 mg/day, was chosen for Mr. Jones and yielded significant improvement in all depressive symptoms after 3 months.

During a follow-up visit 6 months after starting treatment, Mr. Jones reported that he felt back to his normal self. At the end of the session, however, the patient asked whether the medication could affect his sex life. The patient reported that although he never had a high sex drive, his sexual desire was now even lower than when he was depressed. He was also having difficulty reaching orgasm and maintaining an erection until orgasm. These problems appeared within the first 2 weeks of starting use of fluoxetine but had become more bothersome in the last few months when his depression improved.

A more detailed sexual history was obtained. The patient noted that he was a "late bloomer" because of his painful shyness as an adolescent and young adult. He felt very uncomfortable meeting new people and meeting women in particular. He had very few dates before he was 25. He eventually met and married a woman who was also shy through a work colleague. Although he was interested in sex, he felt uncomfortable initiating sex and worried about sexual performance. Sometimes he would go for long stretches without initiating sex with his wife for fear of rejection or inadequate performance. He had inter-mittent difficulties with premature ejaculation and inability to attain erections, although these difficulties were tolerable. He was able to enjoy sex more after drinking one or two beers, although alcohol some-times affected his ability to develop an erection. He felt that his libido had declined after fluoxetine use, and sex became more of an issue for him after he was feeling better. He and his wife had sex approximately three times per month. He masturbated approximately once a week. Delay in orgasm was present during sexual intercourse and during masturbation after the start of the use of fluoxetine. He had no other medical problems that could affect his sexual functioning. He did not smoke. There was no peripheral vascular disease and no history of en-docrine disease, peripheral neuropathy, or genital trauma. He used no illicit drugs.

DSM-IV-TR Diagnosis of "Frustrated Librarian"

The patient's current depressive symptoms and past history are consistent with the diagnosis of Major Depressive Disorder, Re-current. After treatment, the diagnosis would be Major Depres-sive Disorder, In Full Remission. He also appears to have Social Phobia, although this was not the reason for clinical presentation. Social Phobia, however, is a common comorbid condition with de-pressive disorders. Even though Mr. Jones had mild sexual prob-lems before treatment, he developed a clinically significant sexual disorder after fluoxetine treatment. Because fluoxetine and other antidepressants are thought to be the direct cause of sexual dysfunction, he would meet DSM-IV-TR criteria for Substance-Induced (fluoxetine) Sexual Dysfunction with impaired desire, arousal, and orgasm (DSM-IV-TR, p. 565). Substances may affect any of the three phases (desire, arousal, or orgasm) of the sexual cycle. The other potential specifier for Substance-Induced Sexu-al Dysfunction is sexual dysfunction with sexual pain. This diag-nosis of Substance-Induced Sexual Dysfunction requires that the sexual dysfunction begin within 1 month of starting the culpable drug.

Discussion of "Frustrated Librarian" by Lawrence A. Labbate, M.D.*

This case illustrates the common clinical problem of sexual dysfunction developing after successfully treating a depressive illness with a serotonin reuptake inhibitor (SRI) antidepressant. Although the SRIs may be helpful in treating depressive illness, side effects may be troublesome and generate another focus for treatment. Mr. Jones's case brings up the vexing conundrum of how to evaluate and treat SRI-associated sexual dysfunction. The case also illustrates how patients may delay bringing the problem to clinical attention until after they are feeling better and how psychological or other medical problems may complicate the assessment and treatment of SRI-associated sexual problems.

Mr. Jones's problems are typical in that he developed sexual problems after treatment with an SRI, but he also has a few additional factors that contribute to his current sexual dysfunction. His hypertension (via vascular effects) or antihypertensive medication may make him more prone to sexual dysfunction. In addition, his social anxiety may lead to cognitive distortions or catastrophic interpretations of his current sexual problem that may amplify the sexual dysfunction. Mr. Jones's problems are relatively uncomplicated, but, often, patients have many more medical and interpersonal contributors to their sexual problem.

In clinical samples, between one-third and one-half of patients develop sexual dysfunction while taking SRIs (Montejo-González et al. 1997). In addition, many patients have risk factors for sexual dysfunction, including depression, peripheral vascular disease, tobacco smoking, alcohol or drug dependence, endocrine disorders, hypertension, and diabetes, and may be taking other medications that affect sexual functioning (e.g., antihypertensives, antipsychotics). Because sexual dysfunction is common in the general population (Laumann et al. 1999) and in psychiatric clinical populations (Labbate and Lare 2001),

---

*Dr. Labbate is Professor of Psychiatry at the Medical University of South Carolina and Associate Director of Mental Health at the Veterans Administration Medical Center in Charleston, South Carolina. Dr. Labbate was a fellow in clinical psychopharmacology with Jerrold F. Rosenbaum, M.D., and Mark Pollack, M.D., at the Massachusetts General Hospital and is the coauthor of an e-book, Psychiatric Drug Therapy (available on PDA and CD-ROM; Lippincott Williams & Wilkins, 2002), with Dr. Rosenbaum and George W. Arana, M.D.

investigation of sexual function before treatment with SRIs is critical to help establish baseline sexual functioning. The clinician or patient may be uncomfortable talking about this life facet early in the evaluation process, but only through careful inquiry can the problems be examined or treated.

The SRIs appear to primarily affect orgasm, although loss of interest or ability to become aroused is not uncommon (Labbate 1999). Of interest, in women, libido may increase during SRI treatment as the depression remits (Piazza et al. 1997). Sometimes, because of the delay in attaining orgasm, patients may lose the aroused state and only complain of lubrication or erectile dysfunction. It is important to discover all the problems the patient is having. Moreover, when patients have sexual difficulty, they may lose confidence in initiating sex, and then libido may decline as well. Hence, the obvious pharmacologic effects may lead to psychological or behavioral effects. Moreover, the phases of sexual cycle are intimately connected, and difficulty in one phase often affects another phase. All of the SRIs (fluoxetine, sertraline, citalopram, paroxetine, fluvoxamine), as well as venlafaxine, appear to have a similar propensity for causing sexual dysfunction, although paroxetine may be somewhat more problematic than the others.

Mr. Jones's case illustrates that patients frequently do not reveal sexual information early in treatment, and it is imperative to ask directly about problems rather than depend on spontaneous disclosures from the patient. Patients are more likely to respond to direct questioning than to spontaneously report sexual side effects (Montejo-González et al. 1997). Establishing baseline sexual functioning helps ease this line of questioning when starting SRI treatment. A history of the patient's sexual life and current relationship helps put the current problem into perspective. Many patients have some sexual problems before the start of SRI treatment, and the long-standing problems may be addressed earlier this way.

The simplest questions about sexual function include queries about satisfaction in three areas: libido, arousal, and orgasm. Asking about satisfaction is preferable to asking purely physiologic questions about the ability to become aroused or attain orgasm. Is the patient's interest in sex satisfactory compared to normal? What is the current status of the romantic relationship? Is the person able to achieve pleasure during masturbation and with the partner? Is the patient able to become satisfactorily aroused (lubricated for women, erection for men) during sex? Is orgasm uncomfortably delayed? (Sometimes delayed orgasm can be helpful, especially for men with premature ejaculation.) Can the patient attain a satisfactory orgasm? All of these questions ideally lead the patient to put his or her sexual experience in perspective with his or her current emotional life.

If the temporal course of sexual function suggests that the SRI is the proximate cause of the acquired sexual dysfunction, then the clinician is left with several pharmacological options: 1) reduce the SRI dose or wait for tolerance, 2) switch to an agent with fewer sexual side effects, or 3) add an "antidote" treatment. In addition, some patients may choose to switch from pharmacological therapy to psychotherapy.

Reducing the SRI dose is a rational way to reduce toxicity. This method is not well studied, although some anecdotal reports suggest that dose reduction is beneficial. Reducing the dose may also lead to loss of antidepressant effect. Patients may also interrupt treatment and wait for the adverse sexual side effect to resolve, although less than half of patients find this method helpful, and this method is not useful for fluoxetine because of its long half-life. This treatment-interruption method has not been tested under controlled conditions to confirm its use. If this method is used, the SRI must be stopped for several days before the patient has improvement in sexual side effects. After stopping SRIs for a few days, however, some patients will experience the return of depressive or anxiety symptoms or experience an SRI withdrawal syndrome (primarily dizziness and gastrointestinal symptoms) (Rosenbaum et al. 1998).

Switching antidepressant agents—from an SRI to an agent with lower propensity for sexual dysfunction—has intuitive appeal. This option also has very limited empirical data. Because the SRIs appear to have a very similar propensity for inducing sexual dysfunction (although sometimes an individual may have fewer problems with one or another), a switch to a non-SRI antidepressant is a logical choice, but it is not free of problems. Three antidepressants with limited propensity for inducing sexual dysfunction appear reasonable switch choices: bupropion (Wellbutrin), mirtazapine (Remeron), and nefazodone (Serzone).

A potential problem with switching to any of these substitute agents is that some patients fare less well with the new agent than with the SRI that was working. In addition, as in the case of Mr. Jones, the patient may have an undiagnosed anxiety disorder, such as Social Phobia, that responds to an SRI but not to another agent, such as bupropion. The other two agents, mirtazapine or nefazodone, although sometimes useful for anxiety disorders, may not be as well tolerated because of their side effects: sedation for nefazodone and weight gain and sedation for mirtazapine. Making a change is probably best done with a gradual introduction of the new agent and a gradual tapering of the SRI performed over 4–6 weeks.

Adding an antidote treatment is a popular method for treating SRI-associated sexual dysfunction. Many pharmacologic options that are theoretically plausible are available, although very few agents have controlled-study data supporting their use. Psychotropic agents potentially benefiting sexual dysfunction theoretically serve to enhance dopamine or norepinephrine transmission (methylphenidate, dexamphetamine, amantadine, pramipexole, bupropion, yohimbine), reduce serotonin transmission (cyproheptadine or buspirone), or increase genital blood flow (sildenafil [Viagra]). For all of these agents, anecdotal reports suggest sexual function benefits, but, with the exception of sildenafil, the few available placebo-controlled trials suggest marginal, if any, benefits.

Some patients have partially responsive depressive illness and sexual dysfunction that may improve once the depression remits. This pattern may be particularly true for women (Piazza et al. 1997). For patients in whom there is partial improvement of depression with SRI treatment and new or lingering sexual dysfunction, it may be useful to add methylphenidate (5–20 mg bid), dexamphetamine (5–10 mg bid), or bupropion (150–300 mg/day) to improve the depression and sexual dysfunction (Bartlick et al. 1995; Labbate et al. 1997). Bupropion has been studied more than methylphenidate or dexamphetamine as an adjunctive agent for SRI-associated sexual dysfunction. Although open-label studies suggest benefits of bupropion use for libido, arousal, or orgasm, the limited controlled data suggest that bupropion benefits for depressed patients with sexual dysfunction may be modest and limited to sexual desire (Clayton et al. 2001). Otherwise, placebo benefits in the studies may be affecting the findings on bupropion.

A number of drugs are anecdotally useful on an as-needed basis. The psychostimulants (methylphenidate, 20–40 mg, or dexamphetamine, 10–20 mg), as well as bupropion, amantadine (100–200 mg) (Balon 1996), or pramipexole (Mirapex, 0.125–0.50 mg), may also improve erection or delayed orgasm when used 1–2 hours before sex, although data are very limited, and the benefits may be placebo mediated (Michelson et al. 2000). Unfortunately, the addition of psychostimulants, amantadine, or pramipexole to SRIs may induce anxiety or, rarely, hallucinations. Yohimbine (5.4 mg, 1–2 hours before sex) (Segraves 1994) may potentially improve erectile dysfunction or delayed orgasm in men, although reports are anecdotal. Yohimbine may not be well tolerated because it sometimes induces anxiety.

The additional use of buspirone (BuSpar) may potentially improve sexual dysfunction but perhaps only at fairly high doses (40–60 mg/day) (Norden 1994), and this is not yet confirmed by placebo-controlled trials. There is no evidence for as-needed use of buspirone for sexual dysfunction. Cyproheptadine, an older antihistamine with anti-serotonin properties, given in 4- to 8-mg doses 1 hour before sex, may improve delayed orgasm in men (Aizenberg et al. 1995), but the drug's propensity to induce sleep before intercourse makes cyproheptadine difficult to use.

The only antidote agent for which there is convincing placebo-controlled data is sildenafil. Sildenafil is an effective treatment for all aspects of sexual function in men with improved depressive syndromes who experience a decrease in erectile functioning, orgasm, or libido. Although sildenafil's mechanism of action is peripheral (inhibition of phosphodiesterase-type 5, which allows increased blood flow into the penis), patients report improvement in symptoms that would ordinarily be considered psychological (libido and orgasm). The prolonged erection may allow orgasm to happen, which then further enhances men's confidence and boosts libido. A study found that among 90 men successfully treated for depression who developed sexual dysfunction with an SRI antidepressant, sildenafil was far superior to placebo (Nurnberg et al. 2003). Libido, arousal, and orgasm were all clinically improved with sildenafil.

When using sildenafil to treat sexual side effects associated with antidepressants, the usual starting dose is 25–50 mg, 1–2 hours before sex. Most men can be treated with 50–100 mg. Patients need to be instructed that the drug requires usual sexual stimulation and does not immediately induce erections the way prostaglandin or papaverine injections do. Patients taking nitroglycerin or any nitrate (usually for angina) should not take sildenafil because of the drug's propensity to enhance nitrate-related hypotension. This combination may be lethal and should not be attempted. In general, the drug is well tolerated. Less serious and time-limited side effects include prolonged erections, flushing, headache, or blue-colored haze in the visual field. Sildenafil also appears generally to be safe for use in men with cardiac disease, although patients with recent myocardial infarction should not use sildenafil.

Interestingly, there is some recent evidence that sildenafil may be used to treat sexual dysfunction in women using SRIs (Nurnberg et al. 1999). This is not surprising because of the homology of anatomy and physiology between the clitoris and the penis. The clitoris, like the penis, responds to sildenafil's inhibition of the enzyme phosphodiesterase-type 5 by becoming engorged with blood. The benefits of sildenafil in women, however, may require the presence of estrogen to allow for adequate genital blood flow. An underway placebo-controlled study (Nurnberg et al. 2002) found that women with SRI-associated sexual dysfunction responded to sildenafil during the open-label portion of the study with an overall rate of 80%, far higher than the generally low placebo response rate in this condition. The final results of this study will help define the benefits of sildenafil for women.

In Mr. Jones's case, the simplest treatment for his sexual side effects would be the addition of sildenafil, 50 mg, to his current regimen of fluoxetine and supportive psychotherapy. A starting dose of 25 mg would be worthwhile, although, likely, he will need at least 50 mg, and he may require 100 mg. I would instruct him that the drug takes at least 30 minutes before significant effects occur but that he should generally take it at least 1 hour before attempting intercourse. Less time may be needed if he takes sildenafil on an empty stomach or chews the tablet. Sildenafil may be effective for up to 6 hours, thus allowing for a window of spontaneity. There is no rush to have sex. Because his antidepressant treatment is working, I would not risk switching to another medication. If his treatment were partially effective, then, most likely, I would maximize the depression treatment, perhaps with an addition of bupropion or mirtazapine. A switch to bupropion would be another option, but bupropion would likely not be as effective for treating his social anxiety. Ideally, knowledge of his pretreatment sexual problems would guide antidepressant selection. The problem remains that even though Mr. Jones may have had pretreatment sexual dysfunction, the SRIs continue to be the best treatment option for his constellation of symptoms. Another option for treating Mr. Jones's sexual dysfunction would be use of a vacuum pump device, and although this treatment is effective and is reasonably well tolerated by men with long-standing relationships, most men prefer an oral agent and the natural physiological effects of drugs such as sildenafil.

References

Aizenberg D, Zemishlany Z, Weizman A: Cyproheptadine treatment of sexual dysfunction induced by serotonin reuptake inhibitors. Clin Neuropharmacol 18:320–324, 1995

Balon R: Intermittent amantadine for fluoxetine-induced anorgasmia. J Sex Marital Ther 22:290–292, 1996

Bartlick BD, Kaplan P, Kaplan HS: Psychostimulants apparently reverse sexual dysfunction secondary to selective serotonin reuptake inhibitors. J Sex Marital Ther 21:264–271, 1995

Clayton A, Warnock J, McGarvey EL, et al: Placebo controlled trial of bupropion SR as an antidote for SSRI-induced sexual dysfunction (NR 421). Paper presented at the annual meeting of the American Psychiatric Association, New Orleans, LA, May 2001

Labbate LA: Sex and serotonin reuptake inhibitor antidepressants. Psychiatric Ann 571–579, 1999

Labbate LA, Lare SB: Sexual dysfunction in male psychiatric outpatients: validity of the Massachusetts General Hospital Sexual Functioning Questionnaire. Psychother Psychosom 70:221–225, 2001

Labbate LA, Grimes JB, Hines AH, et al: Bupropion in the treatment of SRI induced sexual dysfunction. Ann Clin Psychiatry 9:241–245, 1997

Laumann EO, Paik A, Rosen RC: Sexual dysfunction in the United States, prevalence and predictors. JAMA 281:537–544, 1999

Michelson D, Bancroft J, Targum SD: Female sexual dysfunction associated with antidepressant administration: a randomized placebo controlled study of pharmacological intervention. Am J Psychiatry 157:239–243, 2000

Montejo-González AL, Llorca G, Izquierdo JA, et al: SSRI-induced sexual dysfunction: fluoxetine, paroxetine, sertraline, and fluvoxamine in a prospective, multicenter, and descriptive clinical study of 344 patients. J Sex Marital Ther 23:176–194, 1997

Norden MJ: Buspirone treatment of sexual dysfunction associated with selective serotonin reuptake inhibitors. Depress Anxiety 2:109–112, 1994

Nurnberg HG, Lauriello J, Hensley PL, et al: Sildenafil for sexual dysfunction in women taking antidepressants. Am J Psychiatry 156:1664, 1999

Nurnberg HG, Gelenberg AJ, Fava M, et al: Sildenafil citrate for serotonergic reuptake inhibitor-antidepressant associated female sexual dysfunction. Presented at the annual meeting of the American Psychiatric Association, Philadelphia, PA, May 2002

Nurnberg HG, Hensley PL, Gelenberg AJ, et al: Treatment of antidepressant-associated sexual dysfunction with sildenafil: a randomized controlled trial. JAMA 289(1):56–64, 2003

Piazza LA, Markowitz JC, Kocsis JH, et al: Sexual functioning in chronically depressed patients treated with SSRI antidepressants: a pilot study. Am J Psychiatry 154(12):1757–1759, 1997

Rosenbaum JF, Fava M, Hoog SL, et al: Selective serotonin reuptake inhibitor discontinuation syndrome: a randomized clinical trial. Biol Psychiatry 44:77–87, 1998

Segraves RT: Treatment of drug-induced anorgasmia. Br J Psychiatry 165:55, 1994

Mike DeBardeleben

James Mitchell "Mike" DeBardeleben was born in 1940 as the elder son of an upper-middle-class Texan family. His father was a lieutenant colonel in the Army, known within the family for his punitiveness toward his sons. When Mike was 5 years old, for example, his father would hold him underwater as a punishment for various childhood peccadilloes. His father also beat him on many occasions.

Mike was the middle child and also happened to be the most disobedient of the three children, so he drew the most thrashings and switchings from his father. His mother was a chronic alcoholic, whose behavior oscillated between the violent and the promiscuous. Both of his parents had numerous sexual affairs with other partners, but this was especially true of his mother. The eldest of the three children was a daughter who took on the mother role for her brothers because their mother spent much time in bars drinking and picking up men, even more so when her husband was stationed away from home.

Mike was an excellent student with a high IQ (approximately 127) who received mostly As until his behavior began to deteriorate in high school. At age 16, he was booked for the first time for assaults on his mother. He threatened her at times with a hatchet or with a letter opener. He also threatened his father with a razor. Both parents viewed Mike as capable of murdering them. His next arrest was for reckless driving, after having rammed a police car with his car.

At that point, he was expelled from high school and sent to military school in an effort to cure his delinquent tendencies. At age 18, while in basic training in the Air Force, he was court-martialed for disorderly behavior and various breaches of conduct and then given a less-than-honorable discharge. Diagnostically, he was labeled a "sociopath."

Mike, living at home for a while, terrorized the family. He set fires in his room and knocked down doors. He embarked on the first of what was to be five marriages. He intimidated and tortured his wives, one after the other; each wife fled when she had the chance. Three daughters were born from these unions, one by the first wife (the marriage ended after 3 months) and two by the second wife. He subjected the third wife to bondage and took nude photos of her to blackmail her into assisting him in bank robberies and in bilking elderly women out of money. When in his mid-20s, Mike kidnapped several women, including a banker's wife, from whose husband he demanded ransom. As an outgrowth of his hatred toward his mother, he considered all women "whores and sluts."

Having contracted gonorrhea and hepatitis in his 20s, he had a sallow complexion and was unhealthy looking. This led to his having obsessive concerns about his appearance.

At age 30, Mike was married for a fourth time to a high school girl, whom he subjected to the same degradations he had visited on his earlier mates. He became abusive and scatological under the influence of either alcohol or marijuana (his drug of choice).

By this time, he exhibited multiple paraphilias, including transvestism and a penchant for anal rape and homosexual pornography, as well as a pronounced (and predominantly heterosexual) hypersexuality. His ambition was to build a torture house, akin to the ones fashioned by other sexual sadists such as Herman Mudgett and Gary Taylor. As he himself wrote of it, "I would need secret hidden compartments built into the house…as well as a fun area—a secret fun area—which would include a cage so that I could have a female victim locked up!" (Michaud 1994, p. 21).

Altogether, Mike's crime spree spanned 19 years, from 1964 to 1983. He was arrested in 1983 for counterfeiting, an art that he had for some time practiced with exceptional skill. Many of his violent felonies—rape, kidnap, murder, and robbery—had remained undiscovered until that arrest. Ultimately, he was convicted and sentenced to 400 years in prison.

What was remarkable about Mike was the extensive documentation he had left behind: "trophies" of bloody underwear of victims, audiotapes of torture sessions (some devoted to the torture of his fourth wife), and voluminous notes—including a kind of manifesto about the rationale for sadism. It is believed that Mike kidnapped and murdered more than 20 young women whom he disposed of in swamps. When Mike cross-dressed, as he did with some of his victims, he would pretend that he was the "victim," begging the kidnapped woman to "bite my titties." At other times, he would force his victims to acknowledge that they "loved the pain." Of importance, inflicting pain in these various ways—through torture, bondage, and rape—and then *witnessing the suffering of his victims* was the key element that was sexually arousing for him.

In personality, Mike showed marked schizoid and narcissistic traits, along with the traits of psychopathy. His shifts from his agreeable facade to cruelty earned him the appellation of a Jekyll-and-Hyde personality. Furthermore, he exemplified all eight of the traits described in the Appendix of DSM-III-R (American Psychiatric Association 1987) under the heading of Sadistic Personality Disorder.

The following is the essence of Mike's manifesto of sadism:

> Sadism: The wish to inflict pain on others is not the essence of sadism. The central impulse is to have complete mastery over another person, to make him/her a helpless object of our will, to become the absolute ruler over her, to become her god, to do with her as one pleases—are means to this end. And the most radical aim is to make her suffer. Since there is no greater power over another person than that of inflicting pain upon her. To force her to undergo suffering without her being able to defend herself. The pleasure in the complete domination over another person is the very essence of the sadistic drive. (Hazelwood and Michaud 2001, p. 88)

James Mitchell "Mike" DeBardeleben, the serial killer and sexual sadist, committed murders in many states. He was tried in a Virginia court in 1987 and found guilty. He will not be eligible for parole there until 2059 (at age 119!), at which point he would face an additional 31 years for crimes committed in New Jersey.

DSM-IV-TR Diagnosis of "Mike DeBardeleben"

Mike's terrible behavior has been punished by the criminal justice system, and many readers may wonder about the appropriateness of trying to assess his behavior from the perspective of a psychiatric diagnosis. This case provides vivid examples of extremely antisocial behavior that is symptomatic of several mental disorders.

Perhaps the most frightening aspect of Mike's behavior is that the link between sexual arousal and sadistic behavior is so extreme that it involves torturing and killing his victims. Such behavior is a symptom of Sexual Sadism (DSM-IV-TR, p. 574), which is a Paraphilia in which the person is sexually excited by the psychological or physical suffering of a victim.

Mike's sadism is not only in the service of sexual excitement, as in Sexual Sadism. He also demonstrates a lifelong pattern of cruel, demeaning, and aggressive behavior. Mike has been physically cruel to others to establish dominance in relationships, he humiliates and demeans other people, and he gets other people to do what he wants by intimidating them. This personality pattern indicates Sadistic Personality Disorder, which was a category added to the appendix of DSM-III-R and ultimately deleted from the manual in DSM-IV. Even though it has not received official status in DSM, the clinician can indicate this diagnosis by using the category Personality Disorder Not Otherwise Specified.

Finally, Mike demonstrates a lifelong pattern of irresponsible and antisocial behavior, beginning with threatening his family with violence as an adolescent and progressing to robbery, kidnapping, assault, and murder as an adult. This pattern indicates Antisocial Personality Disorder.

Discussion of "Mike DeBardeleben" by Michael Stone, M.D.*

The case of Mike is typical of Sexual Sadism as the term is understood and used by experts in the forensic field, such as by Roy Hazelwood of the Federal Bureau of Investigation; Park Elliot Dietz, M.D.; and Janet Warren, D.S.W. In their study of 30 sexual sadists, Dietz et al. (1990) emphasized that all of them intentionally tortured their victims to arouse themselves. Citing the above-mentioned writings of Mike and of another sexual sadist, Hazelwood et al. (1992) also stress the same point: It is the suffering of the victim that is sexually arousing to someone who is sadistic.

*Dr. Stone is Professor of Clinical Psychiatry at Columbia College of Physicians and Surgeons. He has worked in the area of severe Personality Disorders, specializing in Borderline Personality Disorder and the various forms of antisocial psychopathology. Among his books are The Fate of Borderline Patients: Successful Outcome and Psychiatric Practice (Guilford Publications, 1990)—an outgrowth of his large-scale long-term follow-up of Borderline and Other Personality Disorders—and also Abnormalities of Personality (WW Norton, 1992), which deals with all of the Personality Disorders in DSM and also psychopathy. He conducts outcome studies at a forensic hospital, where he has followed psychiatric patients who have committed murder (including infanticide) but have been judged not guilty by reason of mental defect.

Others, like Hucker (1997), use a broader definition of Sexual Sadism to encompass a variety of behaviors, not all of which involve experiencing the suffering of a conscious victim. Relying on the earlier classification of Krafft-Ebing (1886/1965), Hucker enumerates several categories: 1) lust-murder (in which there is a connection between sexual arousal and killing, although not necessarily the previous suffering of a victim); 2) mutilation of corpses, or necrophilia; 3) injury to the victim via stabbing or flagellation, etc.; 4) defilement; 5) symbolic sadism, in which a nonharmful act such as cutting the hair of the victim is substituted for a harmful act; 6) "ideal" sadism or sadistic fantasies without acts; 7) sadism with "other objects," such as whipping boys; and 8) sadistic acts with animals. All of the categories include actual behaviors, except for number 6, in which the sadism is restricted to the realm of one's "ideas" (i.e., fantasies).

A number of background factors figure commonly among those who exhibit the Paraphilia of Sexual Sadism, even in cases in which this is more broadly defined (as in Hucker's taxonomy). In Dietz's study of 30 males, for example, 43% had a history of homosexual experience, 20% showed the Paraphilia of Transvestism, approximately half had been raised in families in which there was infidelity or divorce, and approximately one-fourth had been physically or sexually abused (or both) as children. Careful planning of their offenses was nearly universal in this group; 40% kept "trophies" taken from their victims (clothing, jewelry, or other objects). Drug abuse and alcoholism were noted in half of the offenders.

The definition of Sexual Sadism in DSM-IV-TR (p. 574) consists of two features: "A) over a period of at least 6 months, recurrent, intense sexually arousing fantasies, sexual urges, or behaviors involving acts…in which the psychological or physical suffering…of the victim is sexually exciting to the person; and B) the person has acted on these sexual urges with a nonconsenting person, or the sexual urges or fantasies cause marked distress or interpersonal difficulty."

The problem with the DSM definition is the use of the word "or" in criterion A. To allow for persons who either experience sadistically tinged sexual urges (but who never carry them out) *or* who depend on the suffering of victims whom they sexually attack for their sexual arousal is to conflate an ostensibly harmless group of sexually "mis-programmed" persons (i.e., those who fantasize about sadistic acts but never act on these fantasies), with the admittedly smaller but extremely dangerous group of offenders for whom Sexual

Sadism (as defined by Hazelwood or Dietz) is their primary para-philic perversion.

There are inadequacies even with the B descriptor in DSM. There may be some persons who experience the kind of "distress or impair-ment" mentioned in DSM, but these people would be the exception. In 40 years of practice (7 spent at a forensic hospital), I have encountered only one such individual. He was a man of 20 referred to the New York State Hospital some years ago because he had spoken to his internist about his lurid sexual fantasies, which involved skewering women with swords or spikes after he raped them. To that point, he was a vir-gin, schizoid, and painfully shy, who had never assaulted anyone or committed a crime of any sort. He spent 3 years at the hospital, where at first he frightened the female patients when he began to verbalize his fantasy life. His mother had been cold and rejecting; his father used to taunt him about his sexual inadequacies—for example, by promis-ing to bring home a pretty young girl for him to have sex with, only to have sex with the girl himself, while his son listened to the love mak-ing from the next room. There was much less sadistic tinge to his sex-ual fantasies by the time he left the hospital, and he has never committed any antisocial acts in the postdischarge years.

This is in contrast to the typical sexual sadist, who enjoys his sadis-tic fantasies and enjoys even more carrying them out, with no twinge of remorse and no sense of doing wrong. As Mike put it: "All women are tramps: they asked for what they got" (Michaud 1994, p. 171).

Although DSM and the authors cited above use gender-neutral words like "person" in their descriptions of sexual sadists, they are, for all intents and purposes, males. The only female sexual sadist (i.e., de-fined via *actions*) who I am aware of was the Hungarian countess, Erzsébet Báthory (1560–1614), who had her servants capture young virgins from the countryside to be strung up in her castle. There, she would proceed to slit their bellies, experiencing orgasm as she pressed her body against the dying bodies of the girls (Penrose 1996).

From the standpoint of a differential diagnosis, Hazelwood, Dietz, and their colleagues identify several varieties of sadistic behaviors that need to be distinguished from Sexual Sadism as defined here (sexual arousal dependent on the suffering of a hetero- or homosexually attacked victim). Seven such varieties are identified: 1) nonsexual sadism (e.g., humiliation of subordinates in the workplace), 2) cruelty during a crime, 3) pathologi-cal group behavior (e.g., gang-rape), 4) state-sanctioned cruelty (e.g., rape of Bosnian women by Serbian soldiers), 5) revenge-motivated cruelty (e.g., a criminal gang's torture of a rival gang-member), 6) interrogative cruelty (e.g., torture of political opponents by Saddam Hussein's henchmen, torture by the Communists in Moscow's Lyubyanka prison), and 7) postmortem mutilation.

Hazelwood and Warren (2000) underline certain differences in sexually violent offenders, in that some show little advanced planning and commit their crimes without a specific sexual "script." These offenders are the *impulsive* types. Most rapists fall into this category and commit their crimes in an opportunistic manner—when an enticing situation presents itself. In contrast, the *ritualistic* offender is prompted by various paraphilic fantasies and has nourished a specific sadistic "script" in his fantasy over a long period, thence to be acted out in a sexually sadistic crime. The ritualistic type of offender, of whom Mike is a paradigmatic example, is often clever at eluding arrest (19 years, in Mike's case) and is compelled to repeat the crime, often in a highly specific fashion and at fairly predictable intervals. Serial killers of the sexually sadistic type will often, besides carrying out the assault in a carefully scripted way (using bondage, gagging, or duct tape taken from a "rape kit" or forcing the victim to speak or act in certain ways, etc.), "stage" the corpse in a humiliating posture as a final demonstration of the sexual sadist's fury and god-like superiority over the victim.

Apropos of the "sadist" part of Sexual Sadism, there is an important distinction to be made: Not all persons with sadistic personality (see DSM-III-R) exercise their sadism through the sexual channel. The tyrannical boss, for example, may reduce his subordinates to tears, yet be gentle and considerate with his spouse. However, almost all sexual sadists also demonstrate the attributes of sadistic personality (Stone 2001). Curiously, Sadistic Personality Disorder, which was relegated to the Appendix of DSM-III-R, was dropped altogether from DSM-IV. The disappearance of this personality type from DSM was not, however, accompanied by its elimination from the human community. A glance at yesterday's newspaper confirms this.

Spitzer et al. (1991) have drawn attention to some of the politics that underlie the removal of Sadistic Personality Disorder from our official nomenclature. For example, certain feminist groups were concerned that inclusion of the disorder would serve the interests of defense attorneys representing sadistic offenders: They could claim that their clients "suffered" from Sadistic Personality Disorder, which could then be exculpatory of their wife-bashing, rape, or other sadistic crimes. Or, if not exculpatory of their crimes, the diagnosis could at least argue for "diminished responsibility" ("my Sadistic Personality Disorder made me do it!"). This argument fails, in my estimation, for two main reasons. First, DSM is not a guidebook for judges to help determine whether or for how long a defendant should serve time. DSM is an exercise in taxonomy, and its mission is only to identify and describe with some accuracy what is actually "out there." Second, it strains credulity to imagine that the men and women who serve on juries are in such thrall to the arcana of a psychiatric manual or to the casuistical arguments of a defense attorney as to believe that they would grant freedom to a sexual sadist whom they are convinced "did it" (whatever his crimes were) simply because he manifests a psychiatric condition enshrined in our DSM. The public may be naive about psychiatric diagnosis, but it is not naive about human nature.

In my study of serial sexual homicide (Stone 1998, 2001), I note that of 119 serial killers (here, limited to men committing sexual sadism and murder on three or more victims), only 4 received sentences less than "life without parole" or "death." The other sentences were for 25 years to life, 31 years, 40 years, and 120 years. The ages of the defendants were such that none would ever be released back into society. The fears of the feminists are without foundation.

There are, as yet, no definitive, or generally effective, treatments for sexual sadists. Hollin (1997) has written a comprehensive chapter on the evaluation and treatment of "sexual sadism," but, in his discussion, he broadens the topic to include sexual offenders in general, not limited to those who exhibit the type of Sexual Sadism outlined earlier. In his concluding remarks, Hollin asserts that "there are grounds for optimism…for at least some sexual sadists. However, given the current state of knowledge, my overall position is one of extreme caution" (Hollin 1997, p. 220). Much of the research in this area comes from Canada. A more optimistic note was sounded by Marshall and colleagues (1991), who believed that cognitive-behavioral programs yielded encouraging results, but their focus was on child molesters and exhibitionists. They acknowledged that no such effectiveness could be demonstrated for rapists. Quinsey et al. (1993), based at a forensic hospital in northern Ontario, sounded a more pessimistic note, mentioning that the effectiveness in reducing *recidivism* (i.e., the acid test of success in this realm) remained moot. Better success has accompanied the use of libido-lowering medications, such as cyproterone acetate or triptorelin (Rösler and Witzum 1998), than has been achieved with cognitive therapies alone. Traditional dynamic psychotherapy has not proved to be of value for sex offenders; one could expect still fewer benefits when treating sexual sadists, who, as a group, reject therapy of any type—out of their grandiosity and general contempt for psychiatry.

As for the management of sexual sadists who conform to the criteria outlined here (sexual arousal at the suffering of a sexually assaulted victim), approximately three-fourths of whom have already committed a murder when they first draw the attention of the authorities, the very notion of treatment *in the sense of restoring the offender's ability to live peacefully in the community* is illusory. Management for the sexual sadist who has killed can only mean containment within a secure institution. This is the only management for two reasons:

1. In such cases, the public's safety takes precedence over the sexual sadist's desire to be released into the community.
2. In addition, sexual sadists usually score in the clear-cut "psychopathy" range (i.e., 30 or higher) on the Psychopathy Checklist—Revised (PCL-R) of Robert Hare (1991).

But the recidivism rate for men scoring this high on the PCL-R is so great that it justifies extreme caution in the presence of an individual with Sexual Sadism history. This leaves open the question of how best to manage a sexual sadist who has not killed his victim(s) or whose arrest came shortly after his victim escaped. Here, again, the PCL-R score and factors such as the presence or absence of remorse weigh heavily in the balance. Prolonged incarceration is probably in order, in any case. Once within the institution, a lengthy course of behavioral-cognitive therapy, along with a libido-lowering medication, would be the wisest treatment program. Release into the community would be safest if the offender showed sufficient remorse, a low PCL-R score, and the self-discipline to take the libido-lowering drug faithfully and willingness to continue in treatment with appropriate monitoring.

As for men manifesting only sadistic sexual *fantasies*, which I have recommended here to *not* be designated as "sexual sadism," the management and prognosis are difficult to determine. We can never know, for example, whether the young man who spent 3 years in the hospital, in the case cited earlier, would ever have gone on to commit sadistic *acts* absent the extensive treatment he received. The literature on such men is too scanty and sporadic to permit a convincing opinion as to whether the dynamic therapy he received was truly beneficial or a behavioral or other treatment approach would have been more effective in quashing the impulse to move from fantasy to criminal action.

References

American Psychiatric Association: Diagnostic and Statistical Manual of Mental Disorders, 3rd Edition, Revised. Washington, DC, American Psychiatric Association, 1987

Dietz PE, Hazelwood RR, Warren JI: The sexually sadistic criminal and his offenses. Bull Am Acad Psychiatry Law 18:1–16, 1990

Hare RD: Manual for the Revised Psychopathy Checklist. Toronto, Multi-Health Systems, 1991

Hazelwood RR, Michaud SG: Dark Dreams: Sexual Violence, Homicide, and the Criminal Mind. New York, St. Martin's Press, 2001

Hazelwood RR, Warren JI: The sexually violent offender: impulsive or ritualistic? Aggression and Violent Behavior 5:267–279, 2000

Hazelwood RR, Dietz PE, Warren JI: The criminal sexual sadist. FBI Law Enforcement Bulletin 7.1–7.7, 1992

Hollin CR: Sexual sadism: assessment and treatment, in Sexual Deviance: Theory, Assessment and Treatment. Edited by Laws DR, O'Donohue W. New York, Guilford Press, 1997, pp 210–224

Hucker SJ: Sexual sadism: psychopathology & theory, in Sexual Deviance: Theory, Assessment and Treatment. Edited by Laws DR, O'Donohue W. New York, Guilford Press, 1997, pp 194–209

Marshall WL, Jones R, Ward T, et al: Treatment outcome with sex offenders. Clin Psychol Rev 11:465–485, 1991

Michaud SG: Lethal Shadow: The True-Crime Story of a Sadistic Sex Slayer. New York, Onyx/Penguin Books, 1994

Penrose V: The Bloody Countess: The Crimes of Erzsébet Báthory. London, Creation Books, 1996

Quinsey VL, Harris GT, Rice ME, et al: Assessing treatment efficacy in outcome studies of sex offenders. J Interpers Violence 8:512–523, 1993

Rösler A, Witzum E: Treatment of men with paraphilia with a long-acting analogue of gonadotrophin-releasing hormone. N Engl J Med 338:416–422, 1998

Spitzer RL, Fiester SJ, Gay M, et al: Is sadistic personality disorder a valid diagnosis? Am J Psychiatry 148:875–879, 1991

Stone MH: The personalities of murderers: the importance of psychopathy and sadism, in Psychopathology and Violent Crime. Edited by Skodol A. Washington, DC, American Psychiatric Press, 1998, pp 29–52

Stone MH: Serial sexual homicide: biological, psychological and sociological aspects. J Personality Dis 15:1–18, 2001

von Krafft-Ebing R: Psychopathia Sexualis. New York, Stein & Day, 1886/1965

"The Jerk"

Leon is a 45-year-old postal employee who is evaluated at a clinic specializing in the treatment of depression. He claims to have felt constantly depressed since the first grade of school, without a period of "normal" mood for more than a few days at a time. His depression has been accompanied by lethargy; little or no interest or pleasure in anything; trouble concentrating, and feelings of inadequacy, pessimism, and resentfulness. His only periods of normal mood occur when he is home alone, listening to music or watching television.

On further questioning, Leon reveals that he cannot ever remember feeling comfortable socially. Even before kindergarten, if he was asked to speak in front of a group of his parents' friends, his mind would "go blank." He felt overwhelming anxiety at children's social functions, such as birthday parties, which he either avoided or, if he went, attended in total silence. He could answer questions in class only if he wrote down the answers in advance; even then, he frequently mumbled and could not get the answer out. He met new children with his eyes lowered, fearing their scrutiny, expecting to feel humiliated and embarrassed. He was convinced that everyone around him thought he was "dumb" or a "jerk."

As he grew up, Leon had a couple of neighborhood playmates, but he never had a "best friend." His school grades were good but suffered when oral classroom participation was expected. As a teenager, he was terrified of girls, and to this day he has never gone on a date or even asked a girl for a date. This bothers him, although he is so often depressed that he feels he has little energy or interest in dating.

Leon attended college and did well for a while, then dropped out as his grades slipped. He remained very self-conscious and "terrified" of meeting strangers. He had trouble finding a job because he was unable to answer questions in interviews. He worked at a few jobs for which only a written test was required. He passed a civil service examination at age 24 and was offered a job in the post office on the evening shift. He enjoyed this job, as it involved little contact with others. He was offered several promotions but refused them because he feared the social pressures. Although by now he supervises a number of employees, he still finds it difficult to give instructions, even to people he has known for years. He has no friends and avoids all invitations to socialize with co-workers. During the past several years, he has tried several courses of psychotherapy to help him overcome his "shyness" and depression.

Leon has never experienced sudden anxiety or a panic attack in social situations or at other times. Rather, his anxiety gradually builds to a constant high level in anticipation of social situations. He has never experienced any psychotic symptoms.

DSM-IV-TR Casebook Diagnosis of "The Jerk"

Leon presents to the clinic complaining of lifelong depression. Indeed, he has been depressed and has experienced only limited interest and enjoyment ever since he was a child. Although his depressed mood has been associated with pessimism, low energy, and difficulty concentrating, other symptoms of a Major Depressive Episode, such as appetite and sleep disturbance, have not been present. This chronic mild depression is diagnosed as Dysthymic Disorder (DSM-IV-TR, p. 380), which is further qualified as Early Onset (before age 21).

In addition, Leon has lifelong social anxiety that makes it difficult for him to maintain even the most minimal social contact. His fear is that he will have nothing to say and will be thought of as a "jerk." This fear seems to be independent of his Dysthymic Disorder and therefore justifies the additional diagnosis of Social Phobia, Generalized Type (including most social situations) (DSM-IV-TR, p. 456). It should also be noted that Leon's presentation also meets criteria for Avoidant Personality Disorder (i.e., avoids occupational activities that involve significant interpersonal contact, is unwilling to get involved with people unless certain of being liked, is preoccupied with being criticized or rejected in social situations, views self as socially inept). However, including an additional diagnosis of Avoidant Personality Disorder in individuals with early-onset generalized Social Phobia may not be useful, because this "diagnostic comorbidity" more likely reflects conceptual problems regarding whether these two disorders are truly distinct diagnostic entities.

Discussion of "The Jerk"
by Franklin R. Schneier, M.D.*

The assessment of Leon demonstrates the value of an investigation that goes beyond the focus of a patient's chief complaint. Social Phobia (also known as Social Anxiety Disorder) often presents with comorbid Mood Disorders, Anxiety Disorders, Eating Disorders, or substance abuse (Kessler et al. 1994; Schneier et al. 1992). Because Social Phobia remains relatively underrecognized by patients as a disorder, clinicians should specifically inquire about its symptoms when patients present with symptoms of better-known conditions such as depression. Although the mean age at onset of Social Phobia is in the mid-teens, preschool-age onsets are common, and many patients can recall prodromal shyness that intensified and became impairing during adolescence. In more than two-thirds of comorbid cases, Social Phobia precedes the other disorder (Schneier et al. 1992), as is the case for Leon's comorbid Dysthymic Disorder. Social Phobia that occurs first and seems independent of comorbid depressive symptoms is more likely to require specific intervention beyond the treatment of depression. In contrast, social withdrawal and anxiety limited to periods of depressive illness are typically associated with anhedonia and may respond to treatment of the underlying Depressive Disorder.

Leon appears to demonstrate profound social anxiety that likely contributes to his dysphoria and depressive symptoms of low energy and decreased interest that contribute to social avoidance. Asking Leon to describe his perception of the relationship between his social anxiety and depressive symptoms might help prioritize targets for therapeutic interventions to address his vicious cycle of anxiety and depression.

---

*Dr. Schneier is Associate Professor at Columbia University College of Physicians and Surgeons and Research Psychiatrist at the Anxiety Disorders Clinic of New York State Psychiatric Institute in New York City. Dr. Schneier has researched medication and cognitive-behavioral treatments for Social Phobia, has authored more than 60 scholarly publications on the disorder, and served on the Anxiety Disorders Text Revision Work Group for DSM-IV-TR. He is the coauthor of Social Phobia: Diagnosis, Assessment and Treatment (Guilford Press, 1996), and The Hidden Face of Shyness (Avon Press, 1996). His recent work has included positron emission tomography and single photon emission computed tomography imaging of the dopamine system in Social Phobia and related conditions, and he holds an Independent Scientist Career Award from the National Institute of Mental Health.

Even among nondepressed persons with Social Phobia, self-blame, self-criticism, and dysphoria commonly follow perceived social failures.

The broad array of social situations feared and avoided by Leon is characteristic of the Generalized Type of Social Phobia. This subtype is more familial, more severe and impairing, and more likely to be comorbid with other disorders (Mannuzza et al. 1995). As discussed earlier, a comorbid diagnosis of Avoidant Personality Disorder in a patient with Generalized Social Phobia conveys little additional information. Numerous studies investigating the relationship between Generalized Social Phobia and Avoidant Personality Disorder have generally found quantitative rather than qualitative differences (Turner et al. 1992), suggesting that they may not be separate disorders. Furthermore, the relatively sparse literature on the treatment of Avoidant Personality Disorder yields little additional guidance for treatment selection in this case.

After establishing the scope of Leon's social anxiety and dysfunction, I would like to ask him in which situations he *is* comfortable. Even many of the patients with the most severe social phobia report some level of comfort with close family members and friends. Defining a current scope of comfortable activities will remind both Leon and me that Leon is not a "jerk" but has some social capabilities on which he can build during his therapy. I would also want to obtain a sense of his goals for treatment. His social priorities will help me direct him toward those behavioral exposure activities for which he is most motivated and evaluate the personal significance of the gains he achieves in treatment.

The best-established treatments for Generalized Social Phobia are cognitive-behavioral therapies (Heimberg 2002) and the use of medications from one of several classes, including selective serotonin reuptake inhibitors (SSRIs) (Stein et al. 1998), monoamine oxidase inhibitors (MAOIs) (Liebowitz et al. 1992), and benzodiazepines (Davidson et al. 1993). Cognitive-behavioral therapy offers the advantage of better long-term maintenance of gains after discontinuation of treatment, which is an important consideration for people with such a chronic disorder. Medications offer the likelihood of more rapid improvement and possibly a greater magnitude of improvement, although relapse rates of 30%–60% on discontinuation of successful pharmacotherapy have been reported. Combined treatments (medication plus psychotherapy) may offer some advantage, especially for severe or refractory cases, although they have not been well studied.

Cognitive-behavioral therapy for Social Phobia is based on the observations that dysfunction is maintained by avoidance behavior and by a pattern of negative, distorted thoughts about social activities and abilities ("I'm a jerk," "I can never think of anything to say," "Even though she seems friendly, she'll laugh at me if I ask her for a date"). Avoidance of social situations limits opportunities to disprove these negative assumptions and limits social experience, intensifying social fears, which, in turn, lead to more avoidance. Exposure to social situations, when it does naturally occur, may fail to reduce anxiety because of associated cognitive misinterpretations ("My good conversation this time was due to pure luck. Next time I'm sure to fail.") or because of the persistence of more subtle avoidance behaviors (e.g., participating in a conversation but not making any eye contact or initiating any topics of discussion).

In cognitive-behavioral therapy, the clinician and patient first collaborate to identify a hierarchy of feared situations. The cognitive component of therapy involves identifying maladaptive thoughts, teaching a structured approach to questioning these thoughts and developing alternative, more adaptive perspectives, and practicing these techniques during and after exposures conducted in the office and through specified homework assignments. For example, examining his fear of supervising workers, Leon might identify the thought, "He'll think I'm a jerk for acting superior," as commonly associated with his anxiety. The therapist would help Leon examine evidence for and against this belief and develop an alternative coping thought ("I'm just doing my job") that he could use when approaching his next supervision meeting.

The behavioral component involves exposure to feared situations, either in a graded fashion (starting with the easiest first and progressively moving up to harder situations) or more aggressively using flooding (e.g., having Leon attend a party in which he knows hardly anyone). Selection of the situation and specific goals (e.g., not leaving the situation until anxiety has decreased) are developed collaboratively, and the exposures may be conducted in the office through role-playing or in real-life situations. Patients are encouraged to accept that they may experience anxiety but can still achieve their behavioral goals.

Cognitive-behavioral therapy can be conducted in individual or group settings. The latter affords richer opportunities for exposures within office sessions, as group members can be used in role-playing situations. Variations on this approach may place greater emphasis on the behavioral-exposure component or may include social skills training (e.g., therapist modeling of appropriate eye contact or effective ways to initiate a conversation). Psychodynamic and interpersonal therapies have been little studied in Social Phobia.

SSRIs have emerged as the first-line pharmacotherapy for Generalized Social Phobia on the basis of well-established safety and tolerability, efficacy for comorbid depressive symptoms, and several controlled trials in recent years that have proven their efficacy for Social Phobia. Paxil (paroxetine), Zoloft (sertraline), and Effexor-XR (venlafaxine) have been approved by the U.S. Food and Drug Administration for the indication of Social Phobia, and Luvox (fluvoxamine) has also appeared to be effective in controlled trials. Response rates in 12-week trials have averaged approximately 40%–70%, with some evidence for further improvement during longer-term treatment. Dosages are similar to those used in the treatment of depression. Long-term maintenance treatment may be required to prevent relapse.

One alternative to SSRIs is MAOIs, such as Parnate (phenelzine). These older medications have been demonstrated to be effective for treating Social Phobia in several controlled trials, and they are also highly effective for depression. MAOIs are commonly reserved as a third- or fourth-line agent because of the need for dietary restrictions on consumption of cheese and other aged foods and the risk of an acute hypertensive reaction if dietary restrictions are breached.

Another alternative is the benzodiazepine clonazepam, which has appeared highly effective at doses of 2–4 mg/day in a placebo-controlled trial and has rapid onset of action. Its use is limited by the lack of anti-depressant efficacy, need for two- to three-times-per-day dosing, potential for abuse in vulnerable patients, and need to gradually taper off medication at the time of discontinuation. The anticonvulsant gabapentin has also appeared promising in a single controlled trial.

The presence of both Social Phobia and Dysthymic Disorder in Leon's case would influence the approach to his treatment. Significant depression might limit his ability to actively participate and benefit fully from cognitive-behavioral therapy directed at Social Phobia. Although cognitive-behavioral therapy might be adapted to target both dysthymic and social phobic symptomatology, its efficacy in such patients has not been well studied. Unless Leon were highly motivated to undertake cognitive-behavioral therapy, which seems unlikely, given his reported failure of several previous courses of unspecified therapies, I would recommend medication treatment with an SSRI as a first step.

I would encourage Leon to view the medication treatment as likely to improve his mood and anxiety, but, ultimately, his participation in entering challenging social situations is crucial to maximize the benefit of the medication. Even if we were not engaged in formal cognitive-behavioral therapy, I would monitor and encourage his efforts at self-exposure. I would caution him that it takes approximately 8–12 weeks to establish whether a trial of the medication is effective. In addition, owing to the characteristic reticence of patients with Social Phobia, I would place special emphasis on encouraging him to communicate any problems with treatment, so that we could troubleshoot them and pursue a solution.

If Leon showed partial improvement while taking an SSRI, I would reconsider adjunctive cognitive-behavioral therapy or changing his medication regimen. Mood symptoms may improve sooner than social anxiety and avoidance. If depression improved but social anxiety was unresponsive after 12 weeks of SSRI treatment, medication alternatives would include adjunctive clonazepam or gabapentin, switching to another type of SSRI, or switching (after a 2- to 6-week washout period) to an MAOI. With appropriate treatment, most social phobia patients can achieve substantial symptomatic relief and improved quality of life.

References

Davidson JRT, Potts N, Richichi E, et al: Treatment of social phobia with clonazepam and placebo. J Clin Psychopharmacol 13:423–428, 1993

Heimberg RG: Cognitive-behavioral therapy for SAD: current status and future directions. Biol Psychiatry 51:101–108, 2002

Kessler RC, McGonagle KA, Zhao S, et al: Lifetime and 12 month prevalence of DSM III-R psychiatric disorders in the United States. Arch Gen Psychiatry 51:8–19, 1994

Liebowitz MR, Schneier FR, Campeas R, et al: Phenelzine vs atenolol in social phobia: a placebo-controlled comparison. Arch Gen Psychiatry 49:290–300, 1992

Mannuzza S, Schneier FR, Chapman TF, et al: Generalized social phobia: reliability and validity. Arch Gen Psychiatry 52:230–237, 1995

Schneier FR, Johnson J, Hornig CD, et al: Social phobia: comorbidity and morbidity in an epidemiologic sample. Arch Gen Psychiatry 49:282–288, 1992

Stein MB, Liebowitz MR, Lydiard RB, et al: Paroxetine treatment of generalized social phobia (social anxiety disorder): a randomized, double-blind, placebo-controlled study. JAMA 280:708–713, 1998

Turner S, Beidel DC, Townsley RM: Social phobia: a comparison of specific and generalized subtypes and avoidant personality disorder. J Abnorm Psychol 101:326–331, 1992

Sickly

Marion, a 38-year-old married woman, presented to a mental health clinic with the chief complaint of depression. In the past month, she had been feeling depressed, had experienced insomnia, had frequently wept, and had been aware of poor concentration, fatigue, and diminished interest in activities.

Marion relates that she was sickly as a child and has been depressed since her father deserted the family when she was 10. Apparently, she was taken to a doctor for this, and the doctor recommended that her mother give Marion a little wine before each meal. Her adolescence was unremarkable, although she describes herself as having been shy. She graduated from high school at 17 and began working as a clerk and bookkeeper at a local department store. She married at about the same age.

At 19, she began to drink heavily, with binges and morning shakes, which she would relieve by having a drink as soon as she got up in the morning. She felt guilty that she was not caring adequately for her children because of her drinking. At 21, she was admitted to a mental hospital, where she was diagnosed with alcoholism and depression. She was treated with antidepressants. After discharge, she kept drinking almost continually; when she was 29, she was again hospitalized, this time in the alcohol treatment unit. Since then, she has remained abstinent. She has subsequently been admitted to psychiatric hospitals for a mixture of physical and depressive symptoms and once was treated with a course of electroconvulsive therapy, which produced little relief.

Marion describes nervousness since childhood; she also spontaneously admits to being sickly since her youth, with a succession of physical problems doctors often indicated resulted from her nerves or depression. She believes, however, that she has a physical problem that has not yet been discovered by the doctors. Besides nervousness, she has chest pains and has been told by a variety of medical consultants that she has a "nervous heart." She often goes to doctors for abdominal pain and has been diagnosed as having a "spastic colon." She has seen chiropractors and osteopaths for backaches, for pains in the extremities, and for anesthesia of her fingertips. Three months ago, she experienced vomiting, chest pain, and abdominal pain and was admitted to a hospital for a hysterectomy. Since the hysterectomy, she has had repeated anxiety attacks, fainting spells that she claims are associated with unconsciousness that lasts more than 30 minutes, vomiting, food intolerance, weakness, and fatigue. She has had surgery for an abscess of the throat.

Marion is one of five children. She was reared by her mother after her father left. Her father was said to have been an alcoholic who died at 53 of liver cancer. Despite a difficult childhood financially, the patient graduated from high school and worked 2 years. She was forced to quit because of her sickliness.

Marion married her present husband at age 17 and has remained married, although she describes her marriage as "troubled." They have frequent arguments, in part related to her sexual indifference and pain during intercourse.

Her husband is said to be an alcoholic who has had some periods of work instability. They have five children, ranging in age from 2 to 20 years old.

Marion currently admits to feeling depressed but thinks that it is all because her "hormones were not straightened out." She is still looking for a medical explanation for her physical and psychological problems.

DSM-IV-TR Casebook Diagnosis of "Sickly"

It is first necessary to separate the immediate problem that prompted Marion's current consultation (depression) from her long-standing problems (physical symptoms and excessive use of alcohol). She is apparently now having a recurrence of a Major Depressive Episode (1 month of depressed mood, accompanied by diminished interest, insomnia, poor concentration, and fatigue). The mood disturbance is diagnosed on Axis I as Major Depressive Disorder, Recurrent, Mild (DSM-IV-TR, p. 376).

Nearly all of Marion's many physical symptoms that have plagued her for so many years are apparently not adequately explained by a known general medical condition. She has received "physical" diagnoses from doctors in the past, such as "nervous heart" and "spastic colon," but these do not represent disorders with known pathophysiology. Therefore, the physical symptoms suggest a Somatoform Disorder. In her case, the large number of symptoms involving multiple organ systems suggests the Axis I category Somatization Disorder (DSM-IV-TR, p. 490). The cardinal feature of Somatization Disorder is a history of many physical complaints beginning before age 30 and occurring over a period of several years, which result in treatment seeking or functional impairment. In addition, the diagnosis requires four pain, two gastrointestinal, one sexual, and one pseudoneurological symptom. Marion reports pain during intercourse, chest pain, abdominal pain, backaches, and extremity pain; vomiting, food intolerance, and diarrhea (colitis); sexual indifference; and periods of "unconsciousness" and weakness (pseudoneurological symptoms).

Marion has also had periods of heavy alcohol consumption, with binge drinking, accompanied by morning shakes, which she treated by drinking more alcohol, and difficulty functioning as a mother. These problems all indicate the Axis I diagnosis of Alcohol Dependence (DSM-IV-TR, p. 213).

Discussion of "Sickly"
by C. Robert Cloninger, M.D.*

Attention must be directed to both Marion's acute psychological state of depression and the recent exacerbation of her chronic somatization

*Dr. Cloninger is the Wallace Renard Professor of Psychiatry, Genetics, and Psychology at the Washington University School of Medicine in St. Louis, Missouri. Dr. Cloninger trained with Drs. Eli Robins and Samuel Guze, who initially described and validated criteria for chronic hysteria, later known as Briquet's syndrome and now Somatization Disorder. Dr. Cloninger developed and field-tested the current DSM-IV criteria for Somatization Disorder based on a follow-up study of psychiatric outpatients with Drs. Guze and Paula Clayton. He carried out the family and adoption studies of Somatoform Disorders that demonstrated the interaction of genetic and environmental factors in their development. Later, he developed a model of individual differences in personality to explain the differences between Somatization Disorder, Generalized Anxiety Disorder, and depressive disorders, which developed into the widely used Temperament and Character Inventory. He has carried out controlled trials on the treatment of Major Depressive Disorder and Somatization Disorder and has an active clinical practice in addition to directing the basic and clinical research of the Center for Psychobiology at Washington University.

in establishing a therapeutic alliance and diagnosis that will be accepted and understood by the patient. There are three major reasons for this multifaceted approach. First, patients with Somatization Disorder often change doctors after a short time or may go to several doctors at the same time. They quickly reject the conclusion that there is nothing wrong with them physically and then seek another evaluation and more tests from another physician. Second, they also quickly reject the suggestion that their depressive and somatic symptoms are due to psychological distress or psychiatric disorder if this is equated with the absence of a physical basis to their complaints. Third, Somatization Disorder is nearly always associated with a Personality Disorder, which impairs the quality of the history due to little or no self-awareness.

I find it useful to begin by directly communicating my interest, hope, and compassion for patients' very real suffering and to reinforce my words and manner by taking an exhaustively thorough history of their medical, psychological, and social problems. In addition, I request to see all available medical records from childhood to the present if the patient agrees. I suggest that it is important to bring some order and certainty to the diagnosis and treatment, which for the patient have often been a series of disorganized and narrow reactions to isolated complaints. At the same time, I conduct a thorough psychological assessment, including personality testing with my Temperament and Character Inventory as a guide for pharmacotherapy and psychotherapy (Cloninger et al. 1993; Svrakic et al. 1993). With the patient's permission, I seek collateral information from his or her current treating physicians and family members because this often uncovers information the patient has failed to communicate because of limited self-awareness.

After assuring the patient that thorough assessments are under way, I also quickly initiate pharmacotherapy and educate the patient in relaxation techniques to increase calmness. I explain that treatments can help the patient to feel more relaxed and happy regardless of the particular biopsychosocial causes that are exacerbating her problems. I try to validate a patient's dignity to foster responsibility for him or her to manage his or her own life with a sense of freedom and self-respect.

The plan of therapy depends on the patient's configuration of temperament and character traits (Cloninger and Svrakic 1997). *Temperament traits* refer to individual differences in basic emotional reactions, such as anxiety, anger, and disgust, whereas *character traits* refer to individual differences in higher cognitive processes that influence a person's goals and values. Commonly, such sickly patients have mixtures of cluster B and C personality disorders. In temperament, they have high scores in Novelty Seeking (i.e., the impulsiveness typical of cluster B disorders) and Harm Avoidance (i.e., the anxiety proneness typical of cluster C disorders). In character, patients with somatization often have low scores in Self-Directedness—that is, they have little sense of responsibility, purpose, or resourcefulness, indicating the immaturity of their self-concept and self-object relations. These personality deviations are strongly correlated with individual differences in emotional reactivity and in regional brain activity that are measurable using functional magnetic resonance imaging (Cloninger 2002a; Gusnard et al. 2003). Most such patients are treated best by the combination of a selective serotonin reuptake inhibitor or selective norepinephrine reuptake inhibitor (e.g., venlafaxine) plus a mood stabilizer (e.g., salts of lithium or valproic acid) because of their mixture of anxiety proneness and impulsiveness (Cloninger and Svrakic 2000). I recommend long-term maintenance of the combination of medications that the patient responds to and tolerates acutely until the patient has made substantial and sustained improvements in character development and tolerates gradual discontinuation of the maintenance medications.

From the beginning of treatment, I emphasize to my patients that they should not expect a cure of their problems by any medication. The medications will help to calm and stabilize them so that they can learn how to manage their lives better. Teaching brief relaxation techniques, as I describe elsewhere (Cloninger 2004), helps to facilitate a growing sense of self-awareness and self-directedness and decreased emotional instability. This teaching provides a basis for patients to begin to recognize the psychosocial factors that exacerbate their psychosomatic distress.

Immediately after personality testing, which occurs early in therapy, I review with the patient the description he or she has given me of his or her personality and what that means. This allows us to work together to seek better ways of adapting without making the patient feel defensive or judged, blamed, or rejected. Only later in therapy will I give him or her the diagnosis of Somatization Disorder. The diagnosis of Somatization Disorder should be described after we have thoroughly reviewed all available biomedical and psychosocial information and established a strong therapeutic alliance.

After a few outpatient visits, the accumulated psychosocial information and medical records can be reviewed with the patient carefully, giving him or her an opportunity to correct what he or she sees as errors or to add information for perspective. This helps him or her grow in self-awareness and to recognize my interest and knowledge of his or her whole life. Fundamentally, I regard Somatization Disorder as a form of impairment in self-awareness, which leads to frequent depression, anxiety, conversion, dissociation, substance abuse, and somatization. The impaired self-aware consciousness can be directly observed during mental status examination in the patient's vagueness, circumstantial flow of associations, and difficulty recognizing relationships between biomedical and psychosocial events (Cloninger 1986). Patients with Somatization Disorder have little understanding of themselves, their relationships with other people, or the relationships among their many biopsychosocial problems. For them, life is an unpredictable series of crises in which they are clueless victims.

Once there is a stable working alliance with the patient, I explain that his or her clinical syndrome has been recognized for centuries, that it is partially heritable, and that it has a complex biopsychosocial etiology. I explain that biological, psychological, and social factors are all important interdependent causes of the problem, so it is useful to pay attention to each of these aspects of his or her being. It is essential to communicate to patients that they have a real disorder that leads to their experiencing characteristic symptoms that distinguish their disorder from other disorders that lead to progressive physical deterioration and from other psychiatric disorders that do not have such prominent physical complaints. Many patients are reassured that their disorder has been recognized by physicians as a valid entity, that it has a name, that it is heritable, and that it does not lead to progressive physical deterioration. However, they will not be much reassured by this information alone because they are uncomfortable, disabled, seeking relief of their discomfort, and seeking help to reduce their disability. It is important to communicate about a realistic treatment plan and goals.

The long-term goal of treatment in Somatization Disorder is to increase self-awareness so that the patient can manage his or her own life more effectively. The goal is not for the physician to cure and relieve all symptoms of the patient passively, although patients may ask for that repeatedly and may try to avoid responsibility for growing in self-awareness. If a passive cure is promised or expected, both the patient and the physician will be frustrated and disappointed. Realistic, concrete indicators of improvement in Somatization Disorder include reduced frequency and severity of physical complaints, improved social adjustment, and reduced cost and frequency of medical treatment.

These practical outcomes can usually be achieved by adherence to a few treatment principles. First, it is essential to limit the number of doctors the patient is seeing. Often, a primary care physician alone can effectively manage a patient with Somatization Disorder. However, if there is prominent depression, substance abuse, work disability, or marital problems, as is the case with Marion, then a psychiatrist is needed. Regular consultation between the psychiatrist and other physicians can reduce unnecessary and costly diagnostic evaluations. Generally, diagnostic and treatment procedures should be undertaken only in response to objective evidence of disease and not in response to subjective complaints alone. Of course, patients with Somatization Disorder are not immune to physical disorders. A physician who is responsible for all of the health care needs of a patient over many years has much more knowledge of the patient's usual status and so is in the best position to recognize the emergence of another disorder. Sometimes a patient may be frustrated with the physician for not performing more tests or not prescribing a desired medication and will threaten to change physicians. This threat should be met with an empathic but firm response that such a change would be unfortunate because the physician knows the patient's history well. Extensive knowledge permits the physician to be effective in providing the best possible care of the patient in the long run. A thorough annual physical examination and routine tests can also provide reassurance to the patient.

It is important to recognize that patients with Somatization Disorder often have anxiety and depressive symptoms that are reactive to their personal and social problems and unmet psychological needs. For example, Marion is in an unsatisfying marriage with an alcoholic who has an unstable work history, which all leads to frequent arguments. Why has she stayed in this marriage? What has she done to improve it? She has responsibility for five children ranging from 2 to 20 years of age. What is the quality of her relationships with her children? Marion's alcoholic father deserted her family when she was 10 years old, which led to her financial and personal problems as a child. How does she feel about her parents or about men in general? Has she ever had a sexually satisfying relationship with a man? Does she have any friends? What are her sources of enjoyment? To understand these psychosocial issues, Marion's understanding must be supplemented by collateral information, as mentioned earlier. In the course of following Marion, the relevance of the psychosocial context to fluctuations in her complaints will become clarified by the quality of the doctor-patient relationship and the observed course of illness. The disorganized and crisis-oriented nature of the lives of patients with Somatization Disorder is a consistent feature of their psychopathology. Accordingly, an essential part of therapy for the patient is attention to these issues in psychotherapy.

I have found it crucial to focus on facilitating the development of self-awareness in my patients and not on chronic management of clinical syndromes reified as fixed disease entities. If a doctor indicates that he or she thinks that the patient has a chronic disorder of unknown etiology, this concept becomes a self-fulfilling prophecy for the patient. The patient will then be treated throughout his or her life with medications and/or psychotherapy until he or she learns to manage the disability, but he or she will never recover fully. Instead, it is possible to help patients to recover fully by facilitating growth in self-understanding, which leads to psychobiological integration manifested by both coherence of personality and remission of vulnerability to depression, anxiety, and somatization. This growth in self-understanding requires specific mental exercises to stimulate the integration of mind-brain networks and increasing levels of self-aware consciousness (Cloninger 2004). The general principles of such coherence therapy are fourfold. First, patients are encouraged to let go of all struggles, including all fighting, judging, blaming, and criticizing of oneself and others. Second, patients are encouraged to work in the service of others, rather than being preoccupied with self-gratification. Third, patients are helped to grow in intrapsychic and psychosomatic awareness by specific mental exercises, including meditation and contemplation. Fourth, patients are educated in the interdependent processes of thought that modulate emotional reactivity and well-being (Cloninger 2002b, 2004). The rate and extent of progress depends on the patient, but the psychiatrist must be prepared to advise and assist the patient with his or her knowledge of the stages of development of self-aware consciousness and the obstacles that may occur along the way. Coherence therapy is applicable to the full range of psychopathology. The biopsychosocial disorganization of patients with Somatization Disorder provides a clear example of the need to integrate biomedical and psychosocial approaches to psychiatric disorders to develop well-being.

References

Cloninger CR: A unified biosocial theory of personality and its role in the development of anxiety states. Psychiatr Dev 4:167–226, 1986

Cloninger CR: Functional neuroanatomy and brain imaging of personality and its disorders, in Biological Psychiatry. Edited by D'haenen H, den Boer JA, Willner P. Chichester, England, Wiley, 2002a, pp 1377–1385

Cloninger CR: Implications of comorbidity for the classification of mental disorders: the need for a psychobiology of coherence, in Psychiatric Diagnosis and Classification. Edited by Maj M, Gaebel W, Lopez-Ibor JJ, et al. Chichester, England, Wiley, 2002b, pp 79–106

Cloninger CR: Feeling Good: The Science of Well Being. New York, Oxford University Press, 2004

Cloninger CR, Svrakic DM: Integrative psychobiological approach to psychiatric assessment and treatment. Psychiatry 60:120–141, 1997

Cloninger CR, Svrakic DM: Personality disorders, in Kaplan and Sadock's Comprehensive Textbook of Psychiatry, 7th Edition. Edited by Sadock BJ, Sadock VA. New York, Lippincott Williams & Wilkins, 2000, pp 1723–1764

Cloninger CR, Svrakic DM, Przybeck TR: A psychobiological model of temperament and character. Arch Gen Psychiatry 50:975–990, 1993

Gusnard DA, Ollinger JM, Shulman GL, et al: Persistence and brain circuitry. Proc Natl Acad Sci U S A 100(6):3479–3484, 2003

Svrakic DM, Whitehead C, Przybeck TR, et al: Differential diagnosis of personality disorders by the seven factor model of temperament and character. Arch Gen Psychiatry 50:991–999, 1993

Appendix A

Index by Case Name

Appendix B

Index by Discussant

Appendix C

Index by DSM-IV-TR Diagnosis

Appendix D

Subject Index